Foundations of Biosocial Health

Foundations of Biosocial Health

Stigma and Illness Interactions

Edited by Shir Lerman, Bayla Ostrach,
and Merrill Singer

LEXINGTON BOOKS
Lanham • Boulder • New York • London

Published by Lexington Books
An imprint of The Rowman & Littlefield Publishing Group, Inc.
4501 Forbes Boulevard, Suite 200, Lanham, Maryland 20706
www.rowman.com

Unit A, Whitacre Mews, 26-34 Stannary Street, London SE11 4AB

British Library Cataloguing in Publication Information Available

Library of Congress Cataloging-in-Publication Data

Names: Lerman, Shir, editor. | Ostrach, Bayla, editor. | Singer, Merrill, editor.
Title: Foundations of biosocial health : stigma and illness interactions / edited by Shir Lerman, Bayla Ostrach, and Merrill Singer.
Description: Lanham : Lexington Books, [2017] | Includes bibliographical references and index.
Identifiers: LCCN 2017011602 (print) | LCCN 2017013824 (ebook) | ISBN 9781498552127 (Electronic) | ISBN 9781498552110 (cloth : alk. paper)
Subjects: LCSH: Public health—Social aspects. | Diseases—Social aspects. | Social medicine. | Stigmatization.
Classification: LCC RA418 (ebook) | LCC RA418 .F653 2017 (print) | DDC 362.1—dc23
LC record available at https://lccn.loc.gov/2017011602

™ The paper used in this publication meets the minimum requirements of American National Standard for Information Sciences—Permanence of Paper for Printed Library Materials, ANSI/NISO Z39.48-1992.

Printed in the United States of America

Contents

Introduction

Merrill Singer, Shir Lerman, and Bayla Ostrach

In this book, the authors conceive of health as a product of the enduring interaction of diverse biological and social factors. As skillfully demonstrated by the contributors to this volume, health is socially contextualized and produced, and, in turn, has dramatic impacts on society. Stigma, as a social factor, has particular effects on the biological and structural dimensions of health and as such drives many deleterious health interactions.

Consider the example of Human Immunodeficiency Virus (HIV) disease, a recurring theme in this edited volume. While indisputably a biological condition working at the cellular level through gradual viral destruction of the immune system, HIV became a global pandemic because of social factors (e.g., globalization); it is disproportionately an affliction of the poor and other socially marginalized groups because of the immediate effects of social hierarchy on risk exposure and on risky behavior (Brennan et al. 2012; Jha and Madison 2009; Logie et al. 2012). Except for heuristic purposes—such as focused biological assessment of CD4 (white cell) penetration, reorganization, and cell death—it is not possible to fully understand HIV disease in population health separate from its social contexts, determinants, and consequences. Of special concern in these two volumes is the role of social stigma in this and other mutually exacerbating health interactions.

As a health and social science concept, stigma has a fifty-year history that first gained attention with Erving Goffman's seminal work (1963). Its roles in disease processes, human social suffering, life chances, and social control have been addressed in a broad, multidisciplinary literature (Goffman 1963; Hopper 1981; Kleinman and Hall-Clifford 2009; Jenkins and Carpenter-Song 2008; Puhl and Heuer 2010). Central to the understanding of stigma is the assertion of consequential social difference. In its original connotation in ancient Greek society, stigma referred to brand marks burned into the flesh of slaves to demarcate ownership. Frederick Douglas described precisely the same practice among slave owners in the antebellum South as a means of: "imprinting upon [flesh] the name of the monster who claimed the slave" (quoted in Hoenig 2012:271). Through this act, an individual was both marked as different and as having a significantly inferior social standing—that is, as being an inherently different kind of being than the slave owner—and inflicted by the process of branding and its social implications to profound misery and social disgrace. As Erving Goffman (1963:12) commented in his groundbreaking book *Stigma: Notes on the Management of Spoiled Identity*, "Today the term is widely used in something of the original sense, but is applied more to the disgrace itself than to the bodily evidence of it."

In short, as used in contemporary analysis, physical marks of ignominy (e.g., the skin lesions of karposi sarcoma that came to be a stigmatizing condition among individuals with dual infection of herpesvirus and HIV), are not required to subject a socially linked set of individuals to damaging opprobrium (e.g., as seen in abortion stigma, a topic explored in the second book in this set, *Stigma Syndemics: New Directions in BioSocial Health*). Stigma does not merely develop due to pre-existing differences among human groups (e.g., hair color) or segments of society, most of which are not elevated to the level of determinant social status, but rather commonly "feeds upon, strengthens and reproduces existing inequalities of class, race, gender and sexuality" among other distinctions (Parker and Aggleton 2003:13).

Link and Phelan (2006) assessed stigma as involving a set of five components: 1) identification and labelling of socially charged human differences; 2) stereotypic association of certain differences as undesirable or even threatening; 3) some form of social separation of the stigmatized from others in society through discrimination or other mechanisms; 4) harmful loss of social status among those in a stigmatized social grouping; and 5) the exercise of power and social control with corresponding loss of rights, access, and privacy.

Stigma, including the expectation of prejudice and discrimination and the internalization of stigma (i.e., accepting as true negative stereotypes about one's group), has significant health implications (Lewis et al. 2006). Stress is a key biological mechanism in stigmatization, an intermediate variable, and process, linking stigma to the production of disease (Rüsch et al. 2013). Stress includes two observable types: acute stress, produced by sudden and usually unexpected events that disrupt everyday social life and relationships (e.g., divorce), and chronic social stress, referring to enduring and often emotionally damaging problems (e.g., poverty) that threaten an individual's personal and social identity, and in turn, his/her health.

While the healthy body can readily handle acute stress, chronic stress, like that caused by stigma, does not allow the body to achieve or return to homeostasis. Rather, body parameters (e.g., blood pressure, blood glucose, immune system functioning), change and do not drop to pre-stress levels but may be re-set at a more harmful level. This change is referred to as allostasis and the build-up of such changes is called allostatic load. Over time, the increase of allostatic load in the body can lead to disease onset (Dressler 2007; McEwan 2000). Stigma stress also can promote various coping behaviors that are, in turn, notably risky and lead to additional harm (e.g., smoking, illicit drug use, unprotected sex) (Lick et al. 2013). Moreover, stigma discrimination can push people to inhabit unsafe places (ecologically degraded, toxic, and polluted environments) or deny them access to resources (food, health care) that also are sources of disease promotion. The end result is the potential for a clustering of diseases in a stigmatized population as seen in the chapters in this volume. Increasingly, the study of epigenetics also draws attention to the intergenerational health threats of chronic stress (Gudsnuk and Champagne 2012; Stankiewicz et al. 2013), revealing the long-term toll of this product of social inequality.

In this book, the contributors analyze specific forms, perpetuators, and targets of stigmatization in the biosocial generation of adverse disease interactions known as syndemics. The term syndemic is a portmanteau derived from the Greek word *synergos*, meaning two or more agents working together to create a greater effect than each working alone, and demos or "people," commonly used in the public health concept of epidemic (Singer 2009; Singer and Clair 2003). The syndemics concept focuses attention on multiple detrimental interconnections that occur among co-present or clustered diseases and other health-related conditions in a population and the social and socioenvironmental factors that promote and enhance negative effects produced by disease interaction. A syndemics approach involves the identification of: (1) disease concentrations affecting a social group; (2) the pathways through which disease interaction(s) unfold biologically within individual bodies and within populations causing an intensification of overall disease burden; (3) the ways in which social and structural environments, especially conditions of social inequality and injustice (and stigma), contribute to disease clustering and interaction; and (4) methods to prevent and treat these biosocial threats to health.

The third editor of this book and the related volume introduced the syndemics concept into the social science and epidemiological literature in the mid-1990s in the context of the AIDS pandemic, based on ethnographic research with illicit street drug users (Singer 1996). This population not only reported multiple serious diseases but, notably, had high rates of mortality related to many factors beyond HIV disease in interaction with opportunistic infections (e.g., exposure to violence, injection-site skin infections, endocarditis, drug overdoses) (Singer and Clair 2003). Since then, researchers from a growing array of health-related disciplines adopted the concept and use it to interpret and explain a wide range of disease interactions among diverse populations (Chukwuanukwu et al. 2016; Coulter et al. 2015; González-Guarda et al. 2011; Romanowski et al. 2016), including the other two editors of this two volume set. Most recently, the March 2017 issue of *The Lancet* was dedicated to how syndemics can holistically impact health inequalities.

Like all diffusing concepts, new adopters may interpret the meaning of syndemics in novel ways or use the intended theoretical framework and related conceptual models less than fully. There has thus been some tendency, for example, to emphasize biological disease interaction while paying lesser or no attention to the social forces that can drive biological processes. Wright et al. (2016) even suggest that a shift from a biosocial model to a more traditional biomedical model of syndemics began in 2003. In fact, however, as emphasized by Singer and Clair (2003:428):

> Beyond the notion of disease clustering in a location or population, and processes of biological synergism . . . the term syndemic points to the determinant importance of social conditions in the health of individuals and populations.

This clarifying point has been stressed repeatedly by multiple syndemic researchers (Bulled et al. 2014; Everett 2009; Mendenhall 2012; Ostrach and Singer 2012), and the failure to acknowledge it by more recent would-be syndemics scholars suggests a troubling tendency to overlook recent research in syndemics in favor of citing an early publication rather than thoroughly reading the body of syndemics work. Underscoring the long tradition of closely examining the role of social contexts and structural dynamics in biosocial health and suffering, the particularly important common social driver of syndemics examined in this book is stigmatization.

To take an example, viral respiratory tract infections are an independent risk factor for the frequency, intensity, and expression of asthma episodes. Viral microbial agents appear to interfere with complex immunological pathways, thus contributing to, inducing, and exacerbating asthma. Asthma patients, in turn, are at heightened risk for viral respiratory infection. The interactions between environmentally triggered asthma and rhino, syncytial, or influenza A virus infection, and the particular clustering and interactions among these conditions in a particular population, such as economically marginalized and socially stigmatized ethnic minorities which tend, because of social conditions, to have significantly higher rates of asthma, comprise a syndemic (Singer 2009, 2010, 2013). Moreover, because ethnic minorities, at greater risk for asthma due to structural factors and politically produced disadvantaged living conditions, also receive poorer treatment when seeking health care (Forno and Celedón 2009; Leong 2006). The suffer the doubly stigmatizing experience of first being subjected to disproportionate environmental risk factors for asthma episodes, and then being less likely to have access to adequate prevention and treatment for flare-ups, while being stigmatized and judged for not properly 'managing' their chronic asthma. These processes layer stigma onto other social aspects of this persistent syndemic. Notably, research shows that children in North America limit their use of inhalers in the company of peers and that stigma diminishes treatment adherence among asthma sufferers (Jessop and Rutter 2003; Penza-Clyve et al. 2004). Moreover, a medical anthropology content analysis of 66 movies that featured one or more scenes showing an individual with asthma affirmed that this disease has been systematically stigmatized in the entertainment, including films seen by children (Clark 2012). Stigma and asthma syndemics are fatefully entwine, as are the various syndemics examined on the pages to follow.

The central unifying question addressed in the diverse but thematically connected chapters of this book is: How and through what mechanisms does social stigmatization play a role in increasing the likelihood that specific diseases will cluster in a population and produce or worsen the conditions for harmful disease synergy? Also addressed is the nature of stigma-driven syndemics, including the pathways and health burdens of specific disease interactions. These are critical issues because stigma-driven syndemics are an important dimension in the marked, unjust, and costly health disparities that characterize all societies.

The chapters in this volume present an exploration of the role of stigma as a structural factor that drives biological interactions among diseases by creating the social conditions that promote disease clustering that is the foundation of syndemic production. In addition, structural factors, through the stress they produce for the people living in affected communities, and/or through their exposure to emotional trauma (e.g., discrimination), physical violence (e.g., discriminatory policing), toxins (e.g., environmental racism), and deteriorated environments (e.g., slum conditions) create vulnerabilities that facilitate disease interaction by weakening bodily systems. Finally, adverse structural conditions promote the spread of key syndemogenic diseases like HIV or diabetes that are particularly interactive with co-present diseases because of the types of damage they do to human bodies. With their foci on HIV, violence, and substance abuse, chapters 1 (Singer and Ziegler), 2 (McKinley), 6 (Pfeiffer et al.), 7 (Emard), and 8 (Gideonse) echo, update, and build on the interactions proposed in the original syndemics theory (Singer 2009). Chapter 7 examines interactions among HIV stigma, substance abuse, unprotected sexual intercourse, and reduced medication adherence. The chapter presents the multiple ways in which both enacted and perpetuated stigma—stigma that is internalized and reproduced in others within HIV communities—act on HIV-positive bodies to affect the overall health of community members. He also addresses the ways in which individuals with HIV maintain healthy behaviors, which he terms "biomedical moralities." In Chapter 8, on HIV/AIDS, homelessness, methamphetamine addiction, homosexuality, and mental illness syndemics and the shame attached to HIV/AIDS, addiction, and mental illness, the author illustrates the embeddedness of multiple stigmas in the everyday life of HIV-positive gay men. Chapter 2 explores how social conditions, constructed in racist colonial systems, contribute to the development of a syndemic of substance abuse, violence, and suicide among Aboriginal youth in Northwestern Ontario. The author frames this syndemic within the externally imposed stigmatized identity of Aboriginals as weaker than non-Aboriginals. Chapter 5 on the stigmatized homeless in capitalist societies highlights the syndemic interactions that occur among mental illness, substance and interpersonal abuse, traumatizing loss, and other physical health problems in the vulnerable homeless population. Chapter 6 on HIV/AIDS and mental health syndemics in Kenya situates the stigmatized interactions that unfold in the social, political, economic, and historical contexts that form the framework of this syndemic. Chapter 1 discusses the stigmatization of drug users and the stark lack of available drug treatment, which leaves drug users vulnerable to syndemic disease clustering. Chapter 4 traces the social, behavioral, and biological pathways of depression and obesity stigma syndemics as mapped out on the bodies of people obtaining bariatric surgery, which is itself a stigmatized procedure. Chapter 3 examines the multiple pathways of interaction between depression and obesity, situating the resulting syndemic within ongoing structurally produced political and economic crises in Puerto Rico. All of the chapters critically discuss the myriad ways in which stigma synergistically interacts with the various health conditions and social inequalities. Many of these authors developed their proposed stigma-linked syndemics using original ethnographic data they collected under human subjects review processes that require the de-identification of participants. To meet these requirements, and following anthropological convention, in all chapters that include excerpts or participant quotes from original ethnographic data, participants are identified only by pseudonyms, or otherwise kept de-identified or anonymous.

Over the last three decades, syndemics theory has emerged and diffused across health-related disciplines because the concepts it introduced have helped researchers and providers to examine the actual health issues they find in the world of human social and disease suffering. This integrated set of chapters, and those in its companion volume, further this effort by carefully probing the special role of stigma in syndemic production and experience. Within the context of the HIV/AIDS epidemic in Haiti, Castro and Farmer (2005) have voiced concern that because stigma is often visible its presence has been used to give short shrift to other co-present powerful social inequalities that are harder to identify and conceptualize. A syndemics approach, by contrast, as illustrated in the framing of stigma within contexts of multiple and often reinforcing structural inequalities, allows the significance of stigma to be demonstrated while highlighting the multiple social forces perpetuating human social suffering.

REFERENCES

Brennan, Mark, Marlena Vega, Israel Garcia, Antonia Abad, and Michael B. Friedman. 2005. "Meeting the Mental Health Needs of Elderly Latinos Affected by Depression: Implications for Outreach and Service Provision." *Care Management Journals* 6(2): 98–106.

Bulled, Nicola, Merrill Singer, and Rebecca Dillingham. 2014. "The Syndemics of Childhood Diarrhea: A Biosocial Perspective on Efforts to Combat Global Inequities in Diarrhea-Related Morbidity and Mortality." *Global Public Health.* DOI:10.1080/17441692.2014.924022.

Castro, Arachu, and Paul Farmer. 2005. "Understanding and Addressing AIDS-Related Stigma: From Anthropological Theory to Clinical Practice in Haiti." *American Journal of Public Health* 95(1): 535–39.

Chukwuanukwu, R., C. Onyenekwe, L. Martinez-Pomares, R. Flynn, S. Singh, G. Amilo, N. Agbakoba, and J. Okoye. 2016. "Modulation of the Immune Response to Mycobacteriumtuberculosis during Malaria/M. Tuberculosis Co-infection." *Clinical and Experimental Immunology.* DOI: 10.1111/cei.12861. [Epub ahead of print]

Clark, Cindy. 2012. "Asthma Episodes: Stigma, Children, and Hollywood Films." *Medical Anthropology Quarterly* 26(1): 921–15.

Coulter, Robert, Suaanne Kinsky, Amy Herrick, Ron Stall, and José Bauermeister. 2015. "Evidence of Syndemics and Sexuality-Related Discrimination Among Young Sexual-Minority Women." *LGBT Health* 2507, DOI: 10.1089/lgbt.2014.

Dressler, William W. 2007. "Cultural Dimensions of the Stress Process: Measurement Issues in Fieldwork." In *Measuring Stress in Humans*, edited by Gillian Ice and Gary D. James, 275–79. Cambridge: Cambridge University Press.

Everett, Margaret. 2009. "Diabetes Among Oaxaca's Transnational Population: An Emerging Syndemic." *Annals of Anthropological Practice* 36(2): 295–311.

Forno, Erick, and Juan C. Celedón. 2009. "Asthma and Ethnic Minorities: Socioeconomic Status and Beyond." *Current Opinion in Allergy and Clinical Immunology* 9(2): 1541–60.

Goffman, Erving. 1963. *Stigma: Notes on the Management of Spoiled Identity*. New York: Simon and Schuster.

González-Guarda, Rosa, Aubrey Florom-Smith, and Tainayah Thomas. 2011. "A Syndemic Model of Substance Abuse, Intimate Partner Violence, HIV Infection, and Mental Health among Hispanics." *Public Health Nursing* 28(4): 3667–68.

Gudsnuk, Kathryn, Frances A. Champagne. 2912. "Epigenetic Influence of Stress and the Social Environment." *ILAR Journal* 53(3): 2792–88.

Hoenig, Leonard. 2012. "The Branding of African American Slaves." *JAMA Dermatology* 14(2): 271. DOI:10.1001/archdermatol.2011.2683.

Hopper, Susan. 1981. "Diabetes as a Stigmatized Condition: The Case of Low-Income Clinic Patients in the United States." *Social Sciences and Medicine* 15b(1): 111–9.

Jenkins, Janis H., and Elizabeth A. 2008. Carpenter-Song. "Stigma Despite Recovery: Strategies for Living in the Aftermath of Psychosis." *Medical Anthropology Quarterly* 22(4): 381–409.

Jessop, Donna, and D. Rutter. 2003. "Adherence to Asthma Medication: The Role of Illness Representations." *Psychology and Health* 18(5): 595–612.

Jha, Amishi, Jason Krompinger, and Michael J. Baime. 2007. "Mindfulness Training Modifies Subsystems of Attention." *Cognitive, Affective, & Behavioral Neuroscience* 7(2): 1091–99.

Leong, Albin B. 2006. "The Challenge of Asthma in Minority Populations." In *Bronchial Asthma: A Guide for Practical Understanding and Treatment*, edited by M. Eric Gershwin and Timothy E. Albertson, 357–83. Totowa, NJ: Humana Press.

Lewis, Robin, Valerian Derlega, E. Clarke, and Jenny Kuang. 2006. "Stigma Consciousness, Social Constraints, and Lesbian Well-Being." *Journal of Counselling Psychology* 53(1): 485–86.

Lick, David, Laura Durso, and Kerri Johnson. 2013. "Minority Stress and Physical Health Among Sexual Minorities." *Perspectives on Psychological Science* 8(5): 5215–48.

Link, Bruce, Jo Phelan. 2006. "Stigma and Its Public Health Implications." *The Lancet* 367(9509): 528–29.

Logie, Carmen H., Llana James, Wangari Tharao, and Mona R. Loutfy. 2012. "'We don't exist': A Qualitative Study of Marginalization Experienced by HIV-Positive Lesbian, Bisexual, Queer and Transgender Women in Toronto, Canada." *Journal of the International AIDS Society* 15(2). DOI: 10.7448/IAS.15.2.17392s.

McEwan, Bruce. 2000. "Allostasis and Allostatic Load." In *Encyclopedia of Stress*, edited by George Fink, 1454–59. San Diego, CA: Academic Press.

Mendenhall, Emily. 2012. *Syndemic Suffering: Social Distress, Depression, and Diabetes among Mexican Immigrant Women.* Walnut Creek, CA: Left Coast Press.

Ostrach, Bayla, and Merrill Singer. 2012. "At Special Risk: Biopolitical Vulnerability and HIV/STI Syndemics among Women." *Health Sociology Review* 21(3): 258–71.

Parker, Richard, and Peter Aggleton. 2003. "HIV and AIDS-Related Stigma and Discrimination: A Conceptual Framework and Implications for Action." *Social Science and Medicine* 57(1): 132–34.

Penza-Clyve, Susan, Catherine Mansell, and Elizabeth McQuaid. 2004. "Why Don't Children Take Their Asthma Medications? A Qualitative Analysis of Children's Perspectives on Adherence." *Journal of Asthma* 41(2): 1891–97.

Puhl, Rebecca M., and Chelsea A. Heuer. 2010. "Obesity Stigma: Important Considerations for Public Health." *American Journal of Public Health* 100(6): 1019–28.

Romanowski, Kamila, Edward Clark, Adeera Levin, Victoria Cook, and James Johnston. 2016. "Tuberculosis and Chronic Kidney Disease: An Emerging Global Syndemic." *Kidney International* 90(1): 34–40.

Rüsch, Nicola, Mario Müller, Barbara Lay, Patrick Corrigan, Roland Zahn, Thekla Schönenberger, Marco Rössler, Silke Lengler Christina Blank, and Wulf Rössler. 2014. "Emotional Reactions to Involuntary Psychiatric Hospitalization and Stigma-Related Stress Among People with Mental Illness." *European Archives of Psychiatry and Clinical Neuroscience* 264:35. DOI:10.1007/s004060-130-4125.

Singer, Merrill. 2013. "Respiratory Health and Ecosyndemics in a Time of Global Warming." *Health Sociology Review* 21(1): 98–111.

Singer, Merrill. 2010. "Pathogen-Pathogen Interaction: A Syndemic Model of Complex Biosocial Processes in Disease." *Virulence* 1(1): 10–18. DOI: 10.4161/viru.1.1.9933.

Singer, Merrill. 2009. *Introduction to Syndemics: A Critical Systems Approach to Public and Community Health*. San Francisco: Jossey-Bass.

Singer, Merrill. 1996. "A Dose of Drugs, A Touch of Violence, A Case of AIDS: Conceptualizing the SAVA Syndemic." *Free Inquiry in Creative Sociology* 24(2): 99–110.

Singer, Merrill, and Scott Clair. 2003. "Syndemics and Public Health: Reconceptualizing Disease in Bio-Social Context." *Medical Anthropology Quarterly* 17(4): 4234–41.

Stankiewicz, Adrian, Artur H. Swiergiel, and Pawel Kisowski. 2013. "Epigenetics of Stress Adaptations in the Brain." *Brain Research Bulletin* 98: 76–92.

Wright, Eric, Neal Carnes, and Matthew Colón-Diaz. 2016. "Understanding the HIV/AIDS Epidemic in the United States—the Role of Syndemics in Shaping Public Health." In *Understanding the HIV/AIDS Epidemic in the United States: The Role of Syndemics in the Production of Health Disparities*, edited by Eric Wright, Neal Carnes, 11–7. Cham, Switzerland: Springer.

Chapter One

The Role of Drug User Stigmatization in the Making of Drug-Related Syndemics

Merrill Singer and James Ziegler

INTRODUCTION TO DRUG USE AND STIGMA: THE ROLE OF STIGMA IN DRUG USER HEALTH

There is a leading cultural narrative about drug users in the United States and beyond, one that is imbued with rigid, stigmatizing and harmful stereotypes. It portrays illicit drug users as ultimate moral threats to society, a group to be feared and dreaded, an attitude that has motivated the passage of draconian laws designed to punish severely those arrested for drug-related offenses (see Singer and Page 2013). Exemplary is the Supreme Court decision of June 27, 1997 that imposed a mandatory sentence of life in prison without possibility of parole for those convicted of possessing more than 1.5 pounds of cocaine. In the view of the Supreme Court, possession of cocaine is the moral equivalent of the heinous crime of first-degree murder. A further illustration of the dominant "blame drug users" mindset, one that gained national attention several years ago, was the explanation given by elected officials for the looting that shocked the nation in the awful days after Hurricane Katrina devastated many parts of New Orleans in August 2005.

With many residents still stranded by polluted floodwaters, and others packed in woefully unhygienic conditions in the Superdome, the media began playing up sensational stories of widespread looting at local retail businesses. Dismayed, many television viewers were transfixed by footage showing people hauling away stolen appliances, electronic gear, and other non-survival goods. The Mayor of New Orleans at the time, Ray Nagin, during an interview on Air America Radio, was quick to blame drug users for the looting and other violence occurring in the shattered city (CNN.com 2005). Soon too, when interviewed on The Early Show, Louisiana Governor Kathleen Blanco claimed that drug addicts were the main perpetrators of looting. As the Drug Policy Alliance Network commented,

> This problem is, of course, not unique to New Orleans. All over the country substance abusers are routinely blamed for crime and other social ills—there is little discussion of the notion that prohibitionist drug policies themselves contribute to just these sorts of problems. It is far more politically popular to point to "drug addicts" as the bogeymen. (2005)

Social processes of marking and bounding groups by identifying distinctive badges of group membership (e.g., styles of dress, ways of talking, types of behavior, occupation of particular social spaces) and the erecting of often-impassable social barriers between groups are expressions of stigmatization (Fine 1994; Weis 1995). This concept generally is understood in terms of Goffman's (1963:5) seminal discussion as involving the social construction of "an undesired differentness" that engulfs the whole person and results in their discrediting and disempowerment relative to non-stigmatized individuals. Notable social markers of illicit drug users include various psychiatric labels, such as impulsivity or addictive personality disorder (e.g., Verdejo-Garcia, Lawrence, and Clark 2008), particular forms of public appearance (e.g., a shifty look, inexpensive or worn clothing, disheveled malnourished appearance, lack of self-care, nervous pacing), specific behaviors (e.g., involvement in criminal activity, hanging out in dangerous places, engaging in various crimes), and, often, being a member of an ethnic minority. As Bass and Kane-Williams asserted with regard to the last point, "The picture most Americans have of a typical drug dealer or user is that of a young black male and the impression is that drug use is rampant and universal in the black community" (1993:79).

The consequence of this imagery and understanding is frequently echoed in social descriptions of drug users as little more than human rubbish (Friedman 1998). This is the very term for drug users and other devalued patients that is employed by the health care providers described by Jeffery (1979) in his analysis of discrimination in hospital emergency rooms. He observed (1979) that "two broad categories were used to evaluate patients: good or interesting, and bad or rubbish." Various other demeaning labels are applied by health care workers to alcoholics and illicit drug users encountered as hospital patients. In the early 1980s, for example, Bryan Page heard emergency room staff at Jackson Hospital in Miami using the term "SHPOS" ("Sub-Human Piece of Shit") to refer to recidivistic alcoholics and heroin addicts who would present more than once during a three-month rotation (Singer and Page 2013). Other comparable labels include: "AALFD" ("Another Asshole Looking For Drugs"), "FD" ("Fucking drunk"), PG (Pharmaceutically Gifted), "SBOD"

("Stupid bitch/bastard on drugs"), and "SHS" ("Sullen, Hostile, Stupid," which often is used specifically refer to an inner-city drug/alcohol addict).

This kind of intense stigmatization of drug users begins with their construction as amoral or immoral beings capable of the most atrocious crimes imaginable. Such imagery remains despite many studies clearly demonstrating the regularity and normalization of drug use in particular populations, such as young adults (Blackman 2010; Parker, Aldridge, and Measham 1998; Parker, Williams, and Aldridge 2002). Moreover, it persists despite research showing that drug users do make rational decisions and do not mirror the established and widely broadcast popular understandings about them. Based on such research, Hart reports

> Over and over . . . drug users continued to defy conventional expectations. Not one of them crawled on the floor, picking up random white particles and trying to smoke them. Not one was ranting or raving. No one was begging for more, either—and absolutely none of the cocaine users I studied ever became violent. I was getting similar results with methamphetamine users. They, too, defied stereotypes. (2013:3)

Hart, like others, concluded that the effects of structural violence, including poverty, discrimination, and social marginalization, have been misrepresented as the effects of drug use.

Nonetheless, one notable expression of the harmfulness of stigmatizing marking and bounding processes is the limited availability of drug treatment. While lip service may be paid in public discourse to the need for more and better drug treatment, the directing of public funds to treatment (compared to the amount spent on interdiction, arrest, and incarceration of drug users), and the actual availability of and access to treatment, after care and social reintegration programs belies the existence of a strong social commitment to assisting recovery from drug use (Singer 2004). Socially, there is a widespread (if inaccurate) assumption that drug use treatment does not work and hence it is a waste of public resources on an undeserving, recalcitrant, and, indeed, threatening and repulsive population. This attitude was found, by Baker and Isaac (1973:245), for example, among the nurses, law students, and police they studied, people who "described drug abusers as immoral people committing an immoral act by taking drugs and as displaying criminal tendencies." Similarly, research in the Bushwick section of Brooklyn, New York by Mateu-Gelabert et al. (2005) found that the majority of 363 young adults surveyed:

> view drug users negatively, especially heroin and crack users, although many view marijuana as acceptable. Most (61%) . . . said they strongly dislike crack

> smokers, while 71 percent said they strongly dislike drug injectors. . . . Many residents use pejorative terms to refer to those who use heroin and/or crack (e.g., "tecato," "crack head," "dope head," "dope fiend," "junkie," "banger"), and often ascribe negative characteristics to drug users (e.g., weak character, stealing and/or constantly asking for money, ignorant, not being trustworthy, and willing to have sex for drugs or money). (Mateu-Gelabert et al. 2005:804)

What are the consequences for drug users of such stigmatization? Building on a materialist analysis of social processes of disgracing and ostracism, in this chapter we examine drug user stigmatization from a syndemics perspective. We argue that stigmatization puts drug users at severe risk for disease, disease clustering, and adverse disease interaction, with grave outcomes for their health and well-being, indeed for their very survival. To make this argument, the authors review the body of literature on drug-related syndemics to identify: (1) the key ways in which stigma has contributed to syndemics production, and, in turn, the ways that drug-related syndemics themselves are stigmatizing; (2) the array of health conditions ensnared in drug-related syndemics; (3) the various types or categories of drug-related syndemics investigated to date; (4) the contributions of drug research to overall syndemics theory; and (5) findings and recommendations in the literature and in our own experience on the prevention and treatment of drug-related syndemics.

Stigma and Syndemics Production

It is probably no coincidence that the first syndemic described in the literature was SAVA (a deadly disease interaction involving substance abuse, violence, and AIDS) among injection drug users living in the United States (Singer 1996). Subsequently, the issue of mental health was added to the research agendas of SAVA syndemics investigators because of findings suggesting this as an additional interacting health problem among drug using populations (Stall et al. 2007). Moreover, SAVA research subjects have come to include non-injection drug users, men who have sex with men (MSM), and various ethnic or gender minorities. Drug-related syndemics research has been carried out in various countries, suggesting the broad international occurrence of these disease interactions. The issues of concern in SAVA research include examination of the patterns and consequences of interface among several mental health conditions (e.g., depression, anxiety), various kinds of drug use, childhood and later exposure to physical and emotional violence, and involvement in risky behaviors that can lead to HIV and other infections. In this literature, overtly or at least suggestively, stigma has been identified as playing a significant role in creating social experiences and relationships that drive syndemic interaction, producing significant rates of morbidity and mortality in many drug-using populations.

Consequently, stigma has become an issue of increasing attention as a social source of health risk and as an effective barrier to health and social service utilization among people who use drugs (Latkin et al. 2010; Simmonds and Coomber 2009). The stigmatization of drug users is often complex and involves multiple components, including labeling and discrimination based on socially devalued ethnic status, gender, involvement in condemned behaviors (e.g., commercial sex), sexual minority status, and general health condition (Chan et al. 2007). Research by Rudolph et al. (2012) in Thai Ngugen, Vietnam, for example, found that illicit drug users who are HIV-positive suffer from "layered" or "double stigma" in which socially punishing treatment because of one's HIV/AIDS status is loaded on top of other pre-existing experiences of stigma based on their other socially perceived and denigrated characteristics as consumers of illicit drugs. This multiple stigmatization, which involves "labeling, stereotyping, separation, and discrimination" (Rudolph et al. 2012:240), creates a notable health-sensitive weight of adverse social experience. As one study participant stated, "When I was addicted the community hatred was 5 [on a scale of 11–0]. When I got HIV, the hatred was 12-times more" (Rudolph 2012:241). While the participants in this study suffered from community mistrust because of their use of illicit drugs, and the social stereotypes that adhere to this behavior, when it became known that they were HIV-positive, they report enduring the additional burdens of social isolation and open discrimination.

How does drug-user stigmatization of this sort facilitate syndemic production? While stigma is produced by social others, especially in contexts of inequality and differential power, those who are targeted as having socially devalued and stigmatized characteristics "may not only perceive or anticipate negative treatment by other people, but may also come to endorse the stigma associated with that status themselves" (Calabrese et al. 2015). In other words, when people are subjected to daily, structurally imposed and social experienced insults, indignities, and emotional injuries over a period of time, stigma can be internalized. Internalization occurs as the negative experiences and feelings produced by the ways people are treated in society push members of a pariah population to accept negative self-images and a sense of unworthiness.

Importantly, internalization has been identified as a pathway through which societal stigma may shape health status (Earnshaw et al. 2013). This has been demonstrated in research among drug users in St. Petersburg, Russia, for example, where the administration of instruments designed to test the independent health effects of internalized drug use stigma and internalized HIV infection stigma found that both were negatively associated with health status and health service utilization.

> At the bivariate level, both forms of internalized stigma were associated with poorer self-rated health, higher symptom count, lower likelihood of receiving regular HIV care, and lower likelihood of receiving drug treatment within the past year. Moreover, an interaction effect between internalized HIV stigma and internalized drug stigma was evident for three of four [measured] outcomes, such that high internalized HIV stigma was more strongly related to symptom count, HIV care, and drug treatment at high vs. low levels of internalized drug stigma. (Calabrese et al. 2015)

In other words, these findings affirm that internalized HIV stigma and internalized drug stigma were not simply additive in their adverse impacts on health, but syndemically interactive in their negative relationship with both health status and health care service utilization. While focusing on both physical and mental health symptoms, this research supports the work of Earnshaw and colleagues (2015), which examined and affirmed the syndemic interaction between internalized HIV and drug stigmas in the enhanced production of negative mental health symptoms among drug users in the United States.

These studies undergird the biosocial understanding at the heart of the syndemics perspective that "we all live and act in bodies that literally embody—biologically, across the lifecourse—our societal and ecological context" (Kreiger 2005:8). In effect,

> We carry our histories in our bodies. How would we not? . . . So when you measure things like people's cholesterol levels, for example, it's not just an innate property of people. It's a function of who people are and what they're exposed to in the world, what their opportunities are. You start to see biology as a biological expression of the social conditions in which we live. (Kreiger 2008:1)

Enduring stigma—including the internalization of stigma and self-blame—constitutes stressful social experience that has direct impact on biology in the form of disease symptoms (Phelen et al. 2015; Dressler 2004). As emphasized by The Center for Studies on Human Stress at the University of Montreal (2015), while humans have evolved as a species to respond well to short-term stressful events, repeated and enduring activation of the body's stress response system over a long period of time produces wear and tear on this system. The adverse effect of chronic stress can interfere with the body's stress hormone levels (e.g., corisol) returning to normal (Lupien et al. 2009). When this occurs, other body systems also remain in an elevated state of alert producing known health-related physical risks (e.g., high blood pressure, raised blood sugar). As Jules Harrell et al. (2003:247) report, based on their review of relevant clinical studies, being subject to discriminatory behavior can have the effect of both raising blood pressure and "permanently alter[ing] physiological functioning." Chronic stress also has significant impacts on mental health (Juster et al. 2011). Depression, anxiety, and emotional burnout frequently accompany each other and interact with chronic stress.

Stigma, in short, as a structural contributor to and chronic stressor of body systems, can contribute to multiple diseases (e.g., cardiovascular conditions, diabetes, depression) that have been found to be both frequent and syndemically interactive among illicit drug users. In their research among street injection drug users in Hartford, Singer and Clair (2003), for example, found that study participants reported a range of comorbid conditions, including HIV infection, endocarditis, diabetes, and mental health problems. Among the 988 participants in this study, 244 were infected with HIV (25 percent), reflecting the comparatively high rate of infection among drug injectors in the northeastern United States at the time. Of these HIV-infected individuals, 91 percent suffered from at least one other major disease. Forty-three percent of the HIV-infected individuals in the study reported suffering from three or more significant diseases besides HIV. As discussed below, it is this kind of disease clustering that is the basis for syndemic production, as co-morbid and sequential health conditions interact with adverse consequences.

While the stigmatization of drug users drives syndemics production, it is also true that drug-related syndemics are themselves stigmatizing. Fear of stigma and discrimination have been found to be key factors preventing people from being tested for HIV infection and from obtaining HIV/AIDS treatment once diagnosed (Ford et al. 2005; Earnshaw et al. 2012). As Parker and Aggleton (2002) note, there is a synergy between preexisting sources of stigma toward groups such as drug users and the stigmatization they suffer because of HIV/AIDS infection. Drug-related syndemics, in short, are a two-edged sword driven by and triggering stigmatization.

Health conditions Ensnared in Drug-Related Syndemics

As indicated earlier, recognition of syndemics began during and was a product of the AIDS pandemic as it impacted drug users. The association that exists between HIV/AIDS and various forms of drug use has given rise to the most commonly described set of syndemics among drug researchers. As the Centers for Disease Control and Prevention (2015) emphasizes: "Although injection drug use . . . is a direct route of [HIV] transmission, drinking, smoking, ingesting, or inhaling drugs such as alcohol, crack cocaine, methamphetamine ("meth"), and amyl nitrite ("poppers") are also associated with increased risk for HIV infection. These substances may increase HIV risk by reducing users' inhibitions to engage in risky sexual behavior." Moreover, in people already infected with HIV, drug use of various kinds can accelerate disease progression while adversely affecting adherence to treatment.

Among the populations at heightened risk for drug-related HIV infection are those suffering from a mental health disorder, especially depression and anxiety, and thus HIV and mental health disorders constitute the two most commonly investigated health conditions ensnared in drug-related syndemics globally. The syndemic interaction of drug abuse, HIV infection, and mental health disorders was explored, for example, by González-Guarda and colleagues (2011, 2011, 2013) among Hispanics. Based on a sample of 548 self-identified, sexually active Hispanic women between the ages of 18 and 50 years of age living in South Florida who were primarily recruited from a community-based organization providing social services to Hispanic immigrants, González-Guarda et al. (2013) found a significant correlation between the syndemically linked health conditions of drug use, mental health problems (depression), HIV risk (partner's risk for HIV and STI history), being subject to intimate partner violence, and "Hispanic Stress." The latter construction, measured through the Hispanic Stress Inventory (Cervantes et al. 1991), is, in part, a measure of ethnic stigmatization and includes Likert items like "I have felt unaccepted by others due to my Latino culture"; "Because of my poor English, people have treated me badly"; and "I have felt that I would never regain the status and respect that I had in my home country." Likewise, in a study of 290 women incarcerated in three Midwestern U.S. jails, Kelly et al. (2013) found that in addition to HIV risk, 62 percent of study participants had a lifetime history of mental health problems, over half (55.2 percent) were drug-dependent in the year before incarceration, most (64.5 percent) reported a history of physical or sexual abuse before age 16, and nearly half (46.4 percent) had experienced intimate partner violence in the year prior to incarceration. These health conditions also have been linked syndemically in several studies of men who have sex with men (Halkitis et al. 2013; Mustanski et al. 2007; Stall et al. 2007).

Three other significant diseases commonly enmeshed in drug-related syndemics are sexually transmitted infections (other than HIV), hepatitis (especially Hepatitis C), and tuberculosis. All of these diseases are highly interactive with each other and with HIV infection (Singer 2009b). In a study of methamphetamine use among club-patrons in two cities on the east coast of China, for example, Meizhen et al. (2014) found that the prevalences of syphilis (9.7 percent) and Hepatitis C (HCV) infection (3.7 percent) were "alarmingly high" compared to the general population and that study participants infected with syphilis were more likely to be infected with HCV.

Additionally, participants infected with HCV were more likely to have ever injected drugs and/or be infected with syphilis. These researchers described an emergent and worrisome syndemic in a population newly engaged both in drug use and sexual activity. In a study in the northeastern United States among low-income patients attending a public STD clinic, Senn, Carey and Vanable (2010) found that experiences of child sexual abuse and adult partner violence, depression, drug use (including binge drinking and marijuana consumption), and sexual risk behavior were prevalent in their sample. Participants who reported binge drinking or marijuana use had greater odds of having more than one sex partner in the past three months. Those who reported child sexual abuse, depression, or recent marijuana use were more likely to be diagnosed with an STD.

In their study of 435 crack cocaine users in Houston, Ross and colleagues (1999) report 13 percent of their participants tested positive for syphilis infection, 61 percent had a herpes infection, 52 percent had am HBV infection, 41 percent had an HCV infection, and 12 percent were infected with HIV. Significant multivariate predictors for HIV, HBV, and HCV were previous reporting an STD infection and injection drug use (including sharing needles). Similarly, using data from a mobile medical clinic in New Haven, Connecticut, Morano et al. (2013) found high HIV (8.0 percent of clinic enrollees) and HCV (10.1 percent) infection rates, with 26.1 percent of individuals with HCV being coinfected with HIV. Both monoinfection and coinfection were independently correlated with crack cocaine use in their sample.

This discussion suggests the importance of the syndemics of crack cocaine. In these syndemics, several identifiable pathways of disease interaction have been identified: 1) crack cocaine use prompts involvement in risky sexual practices that accelerated the spread of several STDS, and the consequent adverse interaction of STDs with each other, with HIV, and with non-STD infectious diseases like tuberculosis; 2) by reducing adherence to HIV treatment and by biochemically advancing HIV/AIDS disease progression, cocaine contributes to enhanced HIV viral loads and the acquisition of co-infections that further increase the health burden of affected populations; and 3) crack cocaine use complicates access to health care among individuals infected with tuberculosis, and may contribute to increased infectivity and susceptibility to infection, and supporting the adverse interaction of tuberculosis with other infectious diseases (Singer 2014).

The role of crack cocaine in tuberculosis stems from a set of pulmonary complications associated with inhaling cocaine. Signs and symptoms of this health condition, known as "crack lung," include shortness of breath, intensive cough that can involve producing blood, chest pain, filling of air spaces in the lung with fluids, and the collection of air in the pleural cavity (Mançano et al. 2008). Clinical concerns have been raised that suffering from crack lung increases susceptibility to tuberculosis infection upon exposure (Crane et al. 1991; Leonhardt et al. 1994). Story, Bothamley, and Hayward (2008), for example, examined approximately 1,000 pulmonary patients between 15 and 60 years of age who were undergoing treatment in London in July 2003. They compared crack cocaine users in their sample with users of other illicit drugs and with those who did not report drug use. They found that 86 percent of crack cocaine users were positive for tuberculosis (i.e., there were TB bacteria in their sputum) compared to 56 percent of other drug users, and 36 percent of those who did not report drug use. These researchers concluded that there is "a dangerous synergy between TB and crack cocaine" (Story et al. 2008:1468). Notably, researchers also have identified a relationship between cocaine use and asthma exacerbation (Rome et al. 2000; Rubin et al. 1990).

Another health problem found particularly among injection drug users that has become involved in drug-related syndemics is skin and soft tissue infection often leading to cutaneous abscesses and ulceration. An evaluation of approximately 350 injection drug users at Jackson Memorial Hospital in Miami, for example, found that 64 percent suffered from skin and soft tissue infections (Tookes et al. 2015). While these infections commonly are caused by both streptococci and anaerobes pathogens at the point of needle penetration, the frequency of abscesses among drug injectors has increased significantly since the emergence of the infectious agent known as community-associated methicillin-resistant Staphylococcus aureus (Jenkins et al. 2015). Sometimes these infection are related to the drugs themselves. Another disease disproportionately common among injection drug users is endocarditis, an infection of the inner lining of the heart. All of these infections have been described as components of drug-related syndemics (Singer and Clair 2003).

Other diseases that have been (less commonly) described as components of drug-related syndemics include malaria (Bastos et al. 1999), obstructive pulmonary disease (van Zyl et al. 2010), diabetes (Shelton and Quin 2005), and drug overdose (Gilbert et al. 2013). With regard to the latter, drug overdose, which has emerged as a factor in the deaths of more drug users than has HIV/AIDS, Gilbert and co-works (2013:56), observe that a growing body of evidence "suggests that opioid overdose and HIV infection are burgeoning intertwined epidemics among people who inject drugs . . . in Central Asia" (i.e., Kazakhstan, Kyrgyzstan, Tajikistan, Turkmenistan and Uzbekistan). More broadly, it is well established that "injecting drug use and HIV infection among [people who inject drugs] continue to spread globally" (Des Jarlais et al. 2013). In sum, taken together, there is a panoply of potential life threatening and debilitation diseases that are linked syndemically through drug use and enhanced by stigmatization of drug users and the diseases they disproportionally suffer from.

How Stigma Constructs Drug-Related Syndemics: Biosocial Interaction

In the construction of drug syndemics, stigma is an important player in a feedback loop that creates and intensifies syndemic interactions. Ethnic and class stigmatization, especially among African Americans and Latinos, create inner-city social pariah areas, which, in turn, fuel drug use and sales as a response to lack of opportunities and resources. The poverty and violence associated with these areas, combined with drug use contribute to concentrations of interacting diseases such as AIDS, STIs and TB which then serve as stigma magnifiers, increasing the stigmatization of an already stigmatized population.

Singer (2009) conceptualizes the class stigmatization that contributes to the ghettoization of the inner-city in terms of Wacquant's concept of the hyperghetto. The hyperghetto is the transformation of certain areas into "ethno-class prisons" (Singer 2009a: 145) where stigmatized lower class and minority populations become trapped by poverty, lack of opportunities and institutional racism. America's urban core has jettisoned working class jobs in the global neoliberal race to the bottom and the average poverty rate in inner cities is double that of suburbs (Singer 2009a). Singer and co-workers, for example, have described these patterns in a series of articles based on research in Hartford, Connecticut (Romero-Daza et al. 1998; Singer et al. 2006; Vivian et al. 2005).

Bourgois (2003) documents how Puerto Rican participants in his research on a crack cocaine dealing network shifted in and out of licit office work often many times over their lifetimes only to be pushed back into their impoverished East Harlem neighborhood and illicit drug sales by the racism and lack of respect they would routinely encounter in the licit job market. In our rapidly changing, and increasingly globalized, world, many of the jobs Bourgois' participants from East Harlem had aren't available anymore even if stigmatized inner city populations were willing to submit themselves to the indignity of the racial and class stereotypes he describes. Bourgois and Schonberg (2009) describe how this lumpenization of a discarded class whose labor is devalued leads to the explicit reproduction of structural and symbolic violence in the moral "gray zone" (Levi 1988) of their communities.

In addition to the rendering of invisible violence (see Zizek 2008) explicit through the process of lumpen abuse (Bourgois and Schonberg 2009), lack of opportunities and resources in marginalized inner city neighborhoods also more directly promotes violence (Singer 1994, 1996, 2009a). Drug use and sales associated with the same lack of opportunities add to the violence because of a lack of access to the standard legal and judicial system (Singer 2006, 2008). At the same time, experience of violence pushes already stigmatized populations to drug use as a means of coping with trauma (Singer 1994, 1996, 2009a).

The syndemic perspective offers a vantage for seeing the existence of multi-directional interaction among the psychosocial effects of stigma, the bodily and psychological effects of drug use, and a variety of illnesses including the harmful effects of experiencing the continuum of violence—normalized and hidden (see Bourgois 2009), or explicit—to which the urban poor are routinely subjected (Singer 1994, 1996, 2006).

SAVA provides a compelling example of the biosocial pathways through which stigma interacts with illness to produce a syndemic. As Singer points out (1994), AIDS isn't for everyone. The AIDS epidemic is extremely unequally distributed, affecting marginalized and stigmatized populations much more commonly than more mainstream groups and strata. Both of the first groups associated with HIV in the United States, MSM and injection drug users demonstrates this.

For the Hartford inner city, Singer (1996, 2006) described the relationship between violence and HIV for many of the residents he interacted with while conducting research. He noted:

> While violence was not a core variable in our initial research design, the frequency of violence and its painful impact on the lives of our study participants has become increasingly apparent. In life history interviews, study participants describe jarring tales of violence and suffering. (Singer 1996: 100)

Singer lays out several paths for potential interaction between violence and HIV/AIDS, including condom resistance, rape, sexual abuse, and drug use as a means of coping with marginalized existence and explicit violence.

Thus we argue that stigmatization can produce its own justification. In this instance, ethnic and class stigmatization have helped produce dense inner city clusters of potentially life threatening and debilitation diseases that, being present in many bodies, have become linked syndemically through the pathway of drug use, and, in turn, are enhanced by the harmful effects of the additional stigmatization of drug users and the diseases they disproportionally endure. Through this process, the bodies of inner city populations begin to mirror the stigmatizing images that populate the minds of dominant social groups.

Categories of Drug Syndemics

Most of the diseases ensnared in drug-related syndemics can be fit into the categories of infections, mental health problems, emotional traumas, and physical injuries.

Infectious Diseases

HIV/AIDS and HCV are two pillars of drug related infectious disease syndemics. Both have the initial interaction of being blood born virus, which can and often are spread by injection drug use. Connections have also become clearer between non-injection drug use and the spread of HIV—including alcohol use (Padilla, Guilamo-Ramos, and Godbole 2012; Pitpitan et al. 2013; Prakash et al. 2002; Russell, Eaton, and Petersen-Williams 2013; Sikkema et al. 2011) and methamphetamine use among MSM on the Internet (Specter 2005). Experience of violence can also play a role (Singer 1996, 2006). Mechanisms such as drug-related decreased inhibitions, fear of intimate partner violence, and drug acquisition strategies often lead to risky sexual behaviors (Gielen et al. 2007; González-Guarda, Florom-Smith, and Thomas 2011; Illangasekare et al. 2013). Lower assessment of life chances/life satisfaction can also contribute to decisions to engage in risk behaviors and drug use (Singer 1994; Bourgois 2003).

Other common drug related infectious disease syndemics include tuberculosis, malaria and other STI. Correlation has been established between tobacco smoking, TB, HIV, and chronic obstructive pulmonary disease with potential interaction (Reyes, et al. 1996; Rodwell, et al. 2010; Story, et al. 2008; Tran, et al. 2007; Van Zyl Smit et al. 2010). Use of contaminated syringes is associated with malaria infection which can have a syndemic interaction with HIV infection and injection drug use (Bastos, et al. 1999; Bulled and Singer 2011).

Mental Health

At the intersection of drug and mental health syndemics, studies have been carried out on syndemic interactions with depression, trauma, PTSD, and stress/anxiety. There are also a number of studies that, rather than looking at syndemics with any specific mental health issue present, broadly include any diagnosis of a mental health issue (Kelly et al. 2014; Eisenberg and Blank 2014a; Walkup et al. 2008; Moeller, Halkitis, and Surrence 2011a). In a Veterans Affairs sample, for example, Himelboch et al. (2007) found an interaction between schizophrenia and drug abuse associated with higher rates of HIV infection than among individuals with a diagnosis of schizophrenia not engaged in drug abuse. The latter group had rates of HIV infection that were lower than in the general VA population. Based on a review of the literature, Lori et al. (2008) report that studies in their sample suggest that about one-third of patients with major depressive disorder also have drug use disorders, and this is more than comorbidity as sufferers with both conditions had higher risk of suicide and greater social and personal impairment compared to those with just depressive symptomology. The body of literature affirms that there is likely a bidirectional interaction between drug abuse and mental health disorders, with drug use contributing to and exacerbating mental health problems and mental health problems promoting drug use (e.g., by individuals who self-medicate or because of impacts of mental health problems on judgment), resulting in increased risk of various kinds (e.g., for HIV/STI infection, for involvement in violence, for injurious accidents).

Violence

Violence has become a well-established element of drug-related syndemics (Stall et al. 2007; Halkitis et al. 2013b; Singer 1996). Violence can interact with different disease states through the many mechanisms previously discussed, including through a feedback loop that involves both drug use and street drug selling playing rolls in inciting trauma-inflicting violence, which, in turn, prompts drug use as a coping strategy (Singer 2006). Street drug users report intimate contact with various forms of violence, including witnessing street violence, involvement in partner violence, engagement in gang violence as perpetrator or victim, and suffering police violence targeted at drug users (Singer et al. 2001). Domestic violence, including both childhood sexual and other physical abuse and intimate partner violence in adulthood are commonly entwined with drug use. Violence experienced in childhood has been linked to the development of mental health problems, including anxiety, depression and food-related disorders, which, in turn, in victims of childhood violence have been shown to contribute to the eventual development of drug abuse. Similarly, suffering intimate partner violence is two to three times greater in women who use drugs than in the general population of women (Brewer et al. 1998). In a longitudinal study of women in methadone treatment, for example, El-Bassel et al. (2005) found that (1) women who reported frequent crack use were significantly more likely than non–drug using women to report subsequent intimate partner violence; (2) women who reported suffering intimate partner violence were significantly more likely than women who did not report enduring violence to indicate subsequent frequent heroin use; and 3) even frequent marijuana users were significantly more likely than non–drug users to report subsequent exposure to such violence. All of these syndemic connections were associated with more adverse outcomes. Among men who have sex with men, several factors have been found to increase HIV risk, including multiple drug use, childhood sexual abuse, and intimate partner violence (Stall et al. 2003). Moreover, drug-involved men who have sex with men are at greater risk of suicidality (Li 2015).

Injury

Drug related syndemics can ensnare various types of injuries including overdose, abscesses and direct harm/self-mutilation associated with a number of emergent drug trends. In central Asia, one metanalysis of existing literature estimates that approximately 21 to 24 percent of IDU in the region have experienced an opioid overdose, surpassing AIDS-related deaths (Gilbert et al. 2013). Biological links related to liver function or decreased CD4 white blood cell counts in people coinfected with HIV or HCV are suggested as well as relationships between sexual risk behaviors and overdose risk behaviors. Garcia's (2010) research in New Mexico, while it does not directly utilize a syndemic perspective, suggests another link between stigma, depression, and self-induced overdose as a method of suicide among heroin users.

Finally, emergent drug use trends like the use of "bath salts" in America and the use of krokodil in former Soviet states, both of which are linked to structural factors, have been widely reported to result in tragic injuries and body deformation (Grund, Latypov, and Harris 2013; Dorairaj et al. 2012; Murray, Murphy, and Beuhler 2012; Regunath et al. 2012). Pharmacologically, bath salts—so-called because they have been sold under that label to disguise their actual use as a mind-altering drug—usually contain some type of cathinone originally from the plant *Catha edulis* (khat) but now found in synthetic form. Bath salts are snorted, smoked, or injected by users, and their use has been linked to a range of health issues including self-injury (National Institute on Drug Abuse 2015). Krokodil, which is a homemade injectable opioid that contains tissue-damaging processing chemicals, has become prevalent in Russia and the Ukraine. This drug acquired its street name because of the excessive bodily damage its use can lead to, including ulcerations, discolored scale-like skin, and amputations due to drug-related gangrene (Grund, Latypov and Harris 2013; Hendricks et al. 2014).

Contributions of Drug Research to Stigma Syndemics Theory

Stigma is a multifaceted adverse social process involving prejudice, stereotypes, and active discrimination that can be experienced by targets as lived-experience, anticipated-experience, and internalized-experience (Latkin et al. 2012). As Phelan et al. (2008) maintain, there are distinct structural functions of stigma, including (1) exploitation/domination of subgroups; and (2) enforcement of social norms for all social members. As we have suggested, drug users endure stigma on multiple entwined levels, as ethnic minority members, as poor and working class individuals, as users of illicit drugs, and as sufferers of dreaded diseases. Overall, drug research has made significant contributions to stigma syndemics theory. From providing one component of the SAVA syndemic among street and other drug users (Meyer, Springer, and Altice 2011; Salas-Wright, Olate, and Vaughn 2015; Singer 1996, 2006) to research linking drugs use, mental health, and risky sexual behavior in MSM (Eisenberg and Blank 2014b; Halkitis et al. 2013; Hirshfield et al. 2015; Moeller, Halkitis, and Surrence 2011b; Parsons, Grov, and Golub 2012; Yu et al. 2013), drug use has proven to be a critical component in the emergence and spread of many syndemics in which stigma serves as a primary engine. In the study of drug users, it is possible to reveal how: (1) stigma as a lived-experience helps to create conditions of disease clustering as well as enhanced levels of violence/trauma; (2) stigma as both a lived and anticipated experience advances disease progression through stress-related reduction in immune functioning and by leading drug users to avoid treatment; and (3) stigma as an internalized experience contributes to mental health problems and risky behaviors, including violence.

While research on interactions between HIV/AIDS and drug use has moved beyond the simple biological connection of blood contact through sharing injection equipment, this disease pathway provided an entry point for the discussion of a multitude of other interactions and still serves as a model to explain key components of the syndemics approach to understanding the nature of disease as a factor in health. Many introductory discussions of disease interaction in social context use drug syndemics as examples, and often discuss SAVA as the first described syndemic (Baer, Singer, and Susser 2003; Singer 2005, 2009). In many ways, drug research opened the door for the development of the syndemic approach to disease conception, and provided a new and more holistic way of understanding HIV/AIDS and the litany of diseases that are both most common among the urban poor and other marginalized populations, and are heavily stigmatized. Moreover, a syndemics perspective reveals the true complexities and impacts of what is sometimes referred to as "the drug problem," a problem which is not driven by worthless people but by damaging policies, harmful social practices, and the role of social inequality in the making of disease. Stigmatization of marginalized populations on the basis of ethnicity, social class, sexual orientation, disease or other criteria, moreover, is a powerful force in driving drug use and drug-related syndemics. Similarly, the stigmatization of drug-users magnifies adverse outcomes, promoting continued drug consumption and exposure to a range of syndemically linked and often highly damaging or lethal threats to health.

REFERENCES

Baer, Hans A., Merrill Singer, and Ida Susser. 2003. *Medical Anthropology and the World System*. Greenwood Publishing Group.

Baker, Frank, and Frank Isaacs. 1973. "Attitudes of Community Caregivers Toward Drug Users." *The International Journal of the Addictions* 8(2): 243–252.

Bass, L. and Kane-Williams, E. 1993. "Stereotype or Reality: Another Look at Alcohol and Drug Use among African American Children." *Public Health Reports* 108 (Supplement 1): 78–84.

Bastos, F., C. Barcellos, C. M. Lowndes, and S. Friedman. 2009. "Co-infection with Malaria and HIV in Injecting Drug Users in Brazil: A New Challenge to Public Health?" *Addiction* 94(8): 11651–74.

Blackman, Shane. 2010. "Drug War Politics: Governing Culture through Prohibition, Intoxicants as Customary Practice and the Challenge of Drug Normalization." *Sociology Compass* 4(10): 841–55.

Bourgois, Philippe. 2003. *In Search of Respect: Selling Crack in El Barrio*. Cambridge University Press.

Bourgois, Philippe. 2009. "Recognizing Invisible Violence. A Thirty-Year Ethnographic Retrospective." *Global Health in Times of Violence*: 184–90.

Bourgois, Philippe I., and Jeffery Schonberg. 2009. *Righteous dopefiend*. University of California Press.

Brewer, Devon, Charles Fleming, Kevin Haggerty, and Richard Calalano. 1996. "Drug use predictors of partner violence in opiate-dependent women." *Violence Victimization* 13(2): 1071–15.

Bulled, Nicola, and Merrill Singer. 2011. "Syringe-Mediated Syndemics." *AIDS and Behavior* 15(7): 15391–545.

Calabrese, Sarah, Sara Burke, John Dovidio, Olga Levina, Anneli Uusku, Linda Niccolai, and Robert Heimer. 2015. "Internalized HIV and Drug Stigmas: Interacting Forces Threatening Health Status and Health Service Utilization Among People with HIV Who Inject Drugs in St. Petersburg, Russia." *AIDS & Behavior* (published online). DOI 10.1007/s104610-151-1004.

Centers for Disease Control and Prevention. 2015. "HIV and Substance Use in the United States." http://www.cdc.gov/hiv/riskbehaviors/substanceuese.html.

Cervantes, Richard, Amado Padilla, and Nelly de Snyder. 1991. "The Hispanic Stress Inventory: A Culturally Relevant Approach to Psychosocial Assessment." *Psychological Assessment* 3(3): 438–447.

Chan, K., Y. Yang, K. Zhang, and D. Reidpath. 2007. "Disentangling the Stigma of HIV/AIDS from the Stigmas of Drug Use, Commercial Sex, and Commercial Blood Donation—A Factorial Survey of Medical Students in China: A Qualitative Study." *International Journal of Nursing Studies* 47(1): 384–88.

CNN.com. 2005. "New Orleans Mayor Lashes Out at Feds." http://www.cnn.com/2005/US/09/02/katrina.nagin/index.html.

Crane, C., F. Wise, J. Reardon, W. Brunner, B. Dorfman, S. Coulter, and G. Rutherford. 1991. "Crack Cocaine Use Among Persons with Tuberculosis—Contra Costa Country, California, 1987–1990." *Morbidity and Mortality Weekly Report* 40: 485–488.

Davis, Loria, Akihito Uezato, Jason Newell, and Elizabeth Frazier. 2008. "Major depression and comorbid substance use disorders." *Current Opinion in Psychiatry* 21(1): 14–18.

Des Jarlais, Don, S. Pinkerton, H. Hagan, V. Guardino, J. Feelemyer, H. Cooper, A. Hatzatkis, and A. Uuskula. 2013. "30 Years on Selected Issues in the Prevention of HIV among Persons Who Inject Drugs." *Advances in Preventive Medicine*. DOI:10.1155/2013/346372.

Dorairaj, J. J., C. Healy, M. McMenamin, and P. A. Eadie. 2012. "The Untold Truth about 'Bath Salt' Highs: A Case Series Demonstrating Local Tissue Injury." *Journal of Plastic, Reconstructive & Aesthetic Surgery* 65(2): e37–e41.

Dressier, William. 2004. "Culture, Stress and Cardiovascular Disease." In *The Encyclopedia of Medical Anthropology*. Carol R. Ember and Melvin Ember, eds., 328–335. New Haven, CT: Human Relations Area Files.

Drug Policy Alliance Network. 2005. "Drug Users Demonized by Hurricane Coverage." http://www.drugpolicy.org/news/090905hurricane.cfm.

Earnshaw, V., L. Bogart, J. Dovidio, and D. Williams. 2013. "Stigma and Racial/Ethnic HIV Disparities: Moving Toward Resilience." *American Psychology* 68(4): 225–236.

Earnshaw, Valerie, Laramie Smith, Stephenie Chaudoir, I-Ching Lee and Michael M. Copenhaver. 2012. "Stereotypes About People Living with HIV: Implications for Perceptions of HIV Risk and Testing Frequency Among At-Risk Population." *AIDS Education and Prevention* 24(6): 574–581.

Earnshaw, V., L. Smith, C. Cunningham, and M. Copenhaver. 2015. "Intersectionality of Internalized HIV Stigma and Internalized Substance Use Stigma: Implications for Depressive Symptoms." *Journal of Health Psychology* 20(8): 1083–1089.

Eisenberg, Marlene M., and Michael B. Blank. 2014. "The Syndemic of the Triply Diagnosed: HIV Positives with Mental Illness and Substance Abuse or Dependence." *Clin Res HIV/AIDS* 1: 1006.

El-Bassel, Nabila, Louisa Gilber, Elwin Wu, Hyun Go, and Jennifer Hill. 2005. "Relationship Between Drug Abuse and Intimate Partner Violence: A Longitudinal Study Among Women Receiving Methadone." *American Journal of Public Health* 95(3): 465–470.

Fine, Michelle. 1994. "Working the Hyphens: Reinvention Self and Other in Qualitative Research." In *Handbook of Qualitative Research*. Norman Denzin and Yvonna Lincoln, eds., 70–82. Thousand Oaks, CA: Sage Publications.

Ford, Kathleen, Dewa Wirawan, Gusti Sumantera, Anak Sawitri, and Mandy Stahre. 2004. "Voluntary HIV Testing, Disclosure, and Stigma Among Injection Drug Users in Bali, Indonesia." *AIDS Education and Prevention* 16(6): 487–498.

Friedman, Samuel. 1998. "The Political Economy of Drug-user Scapegoating—and the Philosophy and Politics of Resistance." *Drugs: Education and Policy* 5(1): 15–32.

Garcia, Angela. 2010. *The Pastoral Clinic: Addiction and Dispossession Along the Rio Grande*. Los Angeles: University of California Press.

Gielen, A., R. Ghandour, J. Burke, P. Mahoney, K. McDonnell, and P. O'Campo. 2007. "HIV/AIDS and Intimate Partner Violence: Intersecting Women's Health Issues in the United States." *Trauma, Violence & Abuse* 8(2): 178–198. DOI:8/2/178 [pii].

Gilbert, L., S. Primbetova, D. Nikitin, T. Hunt, A. Terlikbayeva, A. Momenghalibaf, and N. El-Bassel. 2013. "Redressing the Epidemics of Opioid Overdose and HIV Among People Who Inject Drugs in Central Asia: The Need for a Syndemic Approach." *Drug and Alcohol Dependence* 132: 56–60.

Goffman, Eric. 1963. *Stigma: Notes on the Management of Spoiled Identity*. Englewood Cliffs, NJ: Prentice-Hall.

González-Guarda, Rosa, Aubrey Florom-Smith, and Tainayah Thomas. 2011. "A Syndemic Model of Substance Abuse, Intimate Partner Violence, HIV Infection, and Mental Health Among Hispanics." *Public Health Nursing* 28(4): 366–378.

González-Guarda, Rosa, Brian McCabe, Amber Vermeesch, Rosina Cianelli, Aubrey Florom-Smith, and Nilda Peragallo. 2013. "Cultural Phenomena and the Syndemic Factor: Substance Abuse, Violence, HIV and Depression Among Hispanic Women." *Annals of Anthropological Practice* 36(2): 212–231.

González-Guarda, Rosa, Brian McCabe, Aubrey Florom-Smith, Rosina Cianelli, and Nilda Peragallo. 2011. "Substance Abuse, Violence, HIV, and Depression: An Underlying Syndemic Factor Among Latinas." *Nursing Research* 60(3): 182–189.

Grund, Jean-Paul, Alisher Latypov, and Magdelena Harris. 2013. "Breaking Worse: The Emergence of Krokodil and Excessive Injuries Among People Who Inject Drugs in Eurasia." *International Journal of Drug Policy* 24(4): 265–274.

Halkitis Perry, Robert Moeller, Daniel Siconolfi, Erik Storholm, Todd Solomon, and Kristen Bub. 2013. "Measurement Model Exploring a Syndemic in Emerging Adult Gay and Bisexual Men." *AIDS and Behavior* 17 (2): 662–673.

Halkitis, Perry, Richard Wolitski, and Gregio Millett. 2013. "A Holistic Approach to Addressing HIV Infection Disparities in Gay, Bisexual, and Other Men Who Have Sex with Men." *American Psychologist* 68(4): 261–273.

Harrell, Jules, Sadiki Hall, and James Tallaferro. 2003. "Physiological Responses to Racism and Discrimination: An Assessment of the Evidence." *American Journal of Public Health* 93(2): 243–248.

Hart, Carl. 2013. *High Price: A Neuroscientist's Journey of Self-Discovery That Challenges Everything You Know About Drugs and Society*. New York: HarperCollins.

Hendricks, LaVelle, Delores Rice, Linda Ball, and Steve Ball. 2014. "Krokodil: A New Synthetic Drug Emerging. Substance Use Prevention in American High Schools." *International Journal of Education* 2(1).

Himelhoch, Seth, John McCarthy, Dara Ganoczy, Deborah Medoff, Lisa Dixon, and Frederic Blow. 2007. "Understanding Associations Between Serious Mental Illness and HIV Among Patients in the VA Health System." *Psychiatric Services* 58(9): 1165–1172.

Hirshfield, S., E. W. Schrimshaw, R. D. Stall, A. D. Margolis, M. J. Downing Jr., and M. A. Chiasson. 2015. "Drug Use, Sexual Risk, and Syndemic Production among Men Who have Sex with Men Who Engage in Group Sexual Encounters." *American Journal of Public Health* 105(9): 1849–1858.

Illangasekare, Samantha, Jessica Burke, Geetanjali Chander, and Andrea Gielen. 2013. "The Syndemic Effects of Intimate Partner Violence, HIV/AIDS, and Substance Abuse on Depression among Low-Income Urban Women." *Journal of Urban Health* 90(5): 934–947.

Jeffery, Roger. 1979. "Normal Rubbish: Deviant Patients in Casualty Departments." *Sociology of Health and Illness* 1(1): 90–107.

Jenkins, T., B. Knepper, S. Jason Moore, C. Saveli, S. Pawlowski, D. Perlman, B. McCollister, and W. Burman. 2015. "Microbiology and Initial Antibiotic Therapy for Injection Drug Users and Non-Injection Drug Users with Cutaneous Abscesses in the Era of Community-associated Methicillin-resistant Staphylococcus aureus." *Academic Emergency Medicine* 22(8): 992–997.

Juster, R., G. Bizik, M. Picard, G. Arsenault-Lapierre, S. Sindi, L. Trepanier, M. Marin, N. Wan, Z. Sekerovic, C. Lord, A. Fiocco, P. Plusquellec, B. McEwen, and S. Lupien, 2011. "A Transdisciplinary Perspective of Chronic Stress in Relation to Psychopathology Throughout Lifespan Development." *Development and Psychopathology* 23(3): 725–776.

Kelly, Patricia, An-Lin Cheng, Elaine Spencer-Carver, and Megha Ramaswamy. 2013. "Syndemic Model of Women Incarcerated in Community Jails." *Public Health Nursing* 31(2): 118–125.

Kreiger, N. 2008. "Unnatural Causes . . . Is Inequality Making Us Sick?" *California Newsreel.* http://www.unnaturalcauses.org/assets/uploads/file/krieger_interview.pdf.

Kreiger, Nancy. 2005. "Introduction." In *Health Disparities & the Body Politic*. Cambridge, MA: Harvard School of Public Health.

Latkin, C., A. Srikrishnan, C. Yang, S. Johnson, S. Solomon, S. Kumar et al. 2010. "The Relationship Between Drug Use Stigma and HIV Injection Risk Behaviors Among Injection Drug Users in Chennai, India." *Drug and Alcohol Dependency* 110(3): 221–227.

Leonhardt, K., F. Gentile, B. Gilbert, and M. Aiken. 1994. "A Cluster of Tuberculosis Among Crack House Contacts in San Mateo County, California." *American Journal of Public Health* 84: 1834–1836.

Li, R., Y. Cai, Y. Wang, Z. Sun, C. Zhu, Y. Tian, X. Jiang, and F. Gan. 2015. "Psychosocial Syndemic Associated With Increased Suicidal Ideation Among Men Who Have Sex With Men in Shanghai, China." *Health Psychology* PMID: 26462059.

Liao, M., D. Kang, X. Tao, C. Cox, Y. Qian, G. Wang, C. Yang, et al. 2014. "Syndemics of Syphilis, HCV Infection, and Methamphetamine use Along the East Coast of China." *BMC Public Health* 14.

Lupien, S., B. McEwen, M. Gunnar, and C. Heim. 2009. "Effects of Stress Throughout the Lifespan on the Brain, Behaviour and Cognition." *Nature Reviews—Neurosciences* 10(6): 434–445.

Mançano, A., E. Marchiori, G. Zanetti, D. Escuissato, B. Duarte, and A. Apolinário Lde. 2008. "Pulmonary Complications of Crack Cocaine Use: High-Resolution Computed Tomography of the Chest." *Jornal Brasiliero Pneumologia* 34: 323–327.

Mateu-Gelabert, C., C. Maslow, M. Flom, M. Sandoval, M. Bolyard, and S. Friedman. 2005. "Keeping It Together: Stigma, Response, and Perception of Risk in

Relationships Between Drug Injectors and Crack Smokers, and Other Community Residents. *AIDS Care* 17(7): 802–813.

Meizhen, Liao, Dianmin Kang, Xiaorun Tao, Catherine Cox, Yuesheng Qian, Guoyong Wang, Cui Yang, XiaoYan Zhu, Na Zhang. Bi Zhenqiang, and Yujiang Jia. 2014. "Syndemics of Syphilis, HCV Infection, and Methamphetamine Use Along the East Coast of China." *BMC Public Health* 14: 172. DOI:10.1186/14712-4581-41-72.

Meyer, Jaimie P., Sandra A. Springer, and Frederick L. Altice. 2011. "Substance Abuse, Violence, and HIV in Women: A Literature Review of the Syndemic." *Journal of Women's Health* 20(7): 991–1006.

Moeller, Robert W., Perry N. Halkitis, and Katie Surrence. 2011. "The Interplay of Syndemic Production and Serosorting in Drug-using Gay and Bisexual Men." *Journal of Gay & Lesbian Social Services* 23(1): 89–106.

Mohamed, A. Rafik, and Erik D. Fritsvold. 2010. *Dorm Room Dealers*. Boulder, CO: Lynne Rienner Publishers.

Morano, Jamie, Britton Gibson, and Fredrick Altice. 2013. "The Burgeoning HIV/HCV Syndemic in the Urban Northeast: HCV, HIV, and HIV/HCV Coinfection in an Urban Setting." *PloS ONE* 8(5): e64321.

Mustanski, Brian, Robert Garofalo, Amy Herrick, and Geri Donenberg. 2007. "Psychosocial Health Problems Increase Risk for HIV Among Urban Young Men Who Have Sex with Men: Preliminary Evidence of a Syndemic in Need of Attention." *Annals of Behavioral Medicine* 34(1): 37–45.

Murray, Brittany L., Christine M. Murphy, and Michael C. Beuhler. 2012. "Death Following Recreational use of Designer Drug 'Bath Salts' Containing 3, 4-Methylenedioxypyrovalerone (MDPV)." *Journal of Medical Toxicology* 8(1): 69–75.

National Institute on Drug Abuse. 2015. "Flakka (alpha-PVP). Emerging Trends." http://www.drugabuse.gov/drugs-abuse/emerging-trends.

Padilla, M. B., V. Guilamo-Ramos, and R. Godbole. 2012. "A Syndemic Analysis of Alcohol use and Sexual Risk Behavior among Tourism Employees in Sosua, Dominican Republic." *Qualitative Health Research* 22(1): 89–102.

Parker, Howard, Judith Aldridge, F. Measham. 1998. *Illegal Leisure: The Normalization of Adolescent Recreational Drug Use.* London: Routledge.

Parker, Howard, Lisa Williams, and Judith Aldridge. 2002. "The Normalization of 'Sensible' Recreational Drug Use: Further Evidence from the North West England Longitudinal Study." *Sociology* 36(4): 941–964.

Parsons, Jeffrey T., Christian Grov, and Sarit A. Golub. 2012. "Sexual Compulsivity, Co-Occurring Psychosocial Health Problems, and HIV Risk among Gay and Bisexual Men: Further Evidence of a Syndemic." *American Journal of Public Health* 102(1): 156–162.

Phelan, S., D. Burgess, R. Puhl, L. Dyrbye, J. Dovidio, M. Yeazel, J. Ridgeway, D. Nelson, S. Perry, J. Przedworski, S. Burke, R. Hardeman, and M. van Ryn. 2015. "The Adverse Effect of Weight Stigma on the Well-Being of Medical Students with Overweight or Obesity: Findings from a National Survey." *Journal of General Internal Medicine* 30(9): 1251–1258.

Phelan, J., B. Link, and J. Dovidio. 2008. "Stigma and Prejudice: One Animal or Two?" *Social Science and Medicine* 67(3): 358–367.

Pitpitan, Eileen V., Seth C. Kalichman, Lisa A. Eaton, Demetria Cain, Kathleen J. Sikkema, Melissa H. Watt, Donald Skinner, and Desiree Pieterse. 2013. "Co-Occurring Psychosocial Problems and HIV Risk Among Women Attending Drinking Venues in a South African Township: A Syndemic Approach." *Annals of Behavioral Medicine* 45(2): 153–162.

Prakash, Om, Andrew Mason, Ronald B. Luftig, and Abraham P. Bautista. 2002. "Hepatitis C Virus (HCV) and Human Immunodeficiency Virus Type 1 (HIV-1) Infections in Alcoholics." *Front Biosci* 7: e286–300.

Reyes, J. C., R. R. Robles, H. M. Colon, C. A. Marrero, X. Castillo, and M. Melendez. 1996. "Mycobacterium Tuberculosis Infection Among Crack and Injection Drug Users in San Juan, Puerto Rico." *Puerto Rico Health Sciences Journal* 15(3): 233–236.

Rodwell, T., R. Barnes, M. Moore, S. Strathdee, A. Raich, K. Moser, and R. Garfein. 2010. "HIV-Tuberculosis Coinfection in Southern California: Evaluating Disparities in Disease Burden." *American Journal of Public Health* 100 (Suppl 1): S178–85.

Rome, Lauren, Michael Lippmann, William Dalsey, Pamela Taggart, and Sherry Pomerantz. 2000. "Prevalence of Cocaine Use and Its Impact on Asthma Exacerbation in an Urban Population." *Chest* 117(5): 1324–1329.

Romero-Daza, Nancy, Margaret Weeks, and Merrill Singer. 1998. "Much More than HIV! The Reality of Life on the Streets for Drug-Using Sex Workers in Inner City Hartford." *International Quarterly of Community Health Education* 18(1): 107–119.

Ross, Michael, Lu-Yu Hwang, Lori Leonard, Ming Teng, and Lawrence Duncan. 1999. "Sexual Behaviour, STDs and Drug Use in a Crack House Population." *International Journal of STDs and AIDS* 10(4): 224–230.

Rubin, Rhonda, and Joel Neugarten. 1990. "Cocaine-Associated Asthma." *American Journal of Medicine* 88: 438–439.

Rudolph, A., W. Davis, V. Quan, T. Ha, N. Minh, A. Gregowski, M. Salter, D. Celentano, and V. Go. 2012. "Perceptions of Community- and Family-Level Injection Drug User (IDU)- and HIV-Related Stigma, Disclosure Decisions and Experiences with Layered Stigma Among HIV-Positive IDUs in Vietnam." *AIDS Care* 24(2): 239–244.

Russell, Beth S., Lisa A. Eaton, and Petal Petersen-Williams. 2013. "Intersecting Epidemics among Pregnant Women: Alcohol use, Interpersonal Violence, and HIV Infection in South Africa." *Current HIV/AIDS Reports* 10(1): 103–110.

Salas-Wright, Christopher, Rene Olate, and Michael G. Vaughn. 2015. "Substance use, Violence, and HIV Risk Behavior in El Salvador and the United States: Cross-National Profiles of the SAVA Syndemic." *Victims & Offenders* 10(1): 95–116.

Senn, Theresa, Michael Carey, and Peter Vanable. 2010. "The Intersection of Violence, Substance Use, Depression, and STDs: Testing of a Syndemic Pattern among Patients Attending an Urban STD Clinic." *Journal of the National Medical Association* 102(7): 614–620.

Shelton, B., and J. Quin. 2005. "Diabetes and Illicit Drug Use." *Practical Diabetes International* 22(6): 22–24.

Sikkema, K., M. Watt, C. Meade, K. Ranby, S. Kalichman, D. Skinner, and D. Pieterse. 2011. "Mental Health and HIV Sexual Risk Behavior Among Patrons of Alcohol Serving Venues in Cape Town, South Africa." *Journal of Acquired Immune Deficiency Syndromes* 57(3): 230–237.

Simmonds, L. and R. Coomber. 2009. "Injecting Drug Users: A Stigmatised and Stigmatising Population." *International Journal of Drug Policy* 20 (2):121–130.

Singer, Merrill. 1994. "AIDS and the Health Crisis of the US Urban Poor; the Perspective of Critical Medical Anthropology." *Social Science & Medicine* 39(7): 931–948.

Singer, Merrill. 1996. "A Dose of Drugs, A Touch of Violence, A Case of AIDS: Conceptualizing the SAVA Syndemic." *Free Inquiry in Creative Sociology* 24(2): 99–110.

Singer, Merrill. 2004. "Why Is It Easier to Get Drugs than Drug Treatment?" In Arachu Castro and Merrill Singer, eds. *Unhealthy Health Policy: A Critical Anthropological Examination*. Walnut Creek, CA: AltaMira Press, 287–303.

Singer, Merrill. 2005. *Something Dangerous: Emergent and Changing Illicit Drug use and Community Health*. Chicago: Waveland Press.

Singer, Merrill. 2007. *Drugging the Poor: Legal and Illegal Drugs and Social Inequality*. Chicago: Waveland Press.

Singer, Merrill. 2009a. "Desperate Measures: A Syndemic Approach to the Anthropology of Health in a Violent City." *Global Health in Times of Violence*. Santé Fe: School for Advanced Research Press, 137–156.

Singer, Merrill. 2009b. "Introduction to Syndemics: A Systems Approach to Public and Community Health." San Francisco, CA: Jossey-Bass.

Singer, Merrill. 2014. "The Infectious Disease Syndemics of Crack Cocaine." *The Journal of Equity in Health* 3(1): 32–44.

Singer, Merrill, and Scott Clair. 2003. "Syndemics and Public Health: Reconceptualizing Disease in Bio-Social Context." *Medical Anthropology Quarterly* 17(4): 423–441.

Singer, Merrill, and J. Bryan Page. 2013. *The Social Value of Drug Addicts: The Uses of the Useless.* Walnut Creek, CA: Left Coast Press.

Singer, Merrill, Pamela Erickson, Louise Badiane, Rosemary Diaz, Dugeidy Ortiz, Traci Abraham, and Anna Marie Nicolaysen. 2006. "Syndemics, Sex and the City: Understanding Sexually Transmitted Disease in Social and Cultural Context." *Social Science and Medicine* 63(8): 2010–2021.

Singer, Merrill, Janie Simmons, Michael Duke, and Lorie Broomhall. 2001. "The Challenges of Street Research on Drug Use, Violence, and AIDS Risk." *Addiction Research and Theory* 9(4): 365–402.

Specter, Michael. 2005. "Higher Risk." *The New Yorker*: 38–45.

Stall, Ron, Mark Friedman, and Joseph Catania. 2007. "Interacting Epidemics and Gay Men's Health: A Theory of Syndemic Production Among Urban Gay Men." In *Unequal Opportunity: Health Disparities Affecting Gay and Bisexual Men in the United States*, Richard Wolitski, Ron Stall, and Ronald O. Valdiserri, eds. Oxford: Oxford University Press.

Stall, Ron, Thomas Mills, John Williamson, Trevor Hart, Greg Greenwood, Jay Paul, Lance Pollack, Diane Binson, Dennis Osmond, and Joseph Catania. 2003. "Association of Co-Occurring Psychosocial Health Problems and Increased Vulnerability to HIV/AIDS Among Urban Men Who Have Sex with Men." *American Journal of Public Health* 93(6): 939–942.

Story, A., G. Bothamley, and A. Hayward. 2008. "Crack Cocaine and Infectious Tuberculosis." *Emerging Infectious Diseases* 14: 1466–1469.

The Center for Studies on Human Stress. 2015. "Types of Chronic Stress." http://www.humanstress.ca/stress/understand-your-stress/types-of-chronic-stress.html.

Tookes, H., C. Diaz, H. Li, R. Khalid, and S. Doblecki-Lewis. 2015. "A Cost Analysis of Hospitalizations for Infections Related to Injection Drug Use at a County Safety-Net Hospital in Miami, Florida." *PLoS ONE* 10(6): e0129360. DOI: 10.1371/journal.pone.0129360.

Tran, N. B., R. M. Houben, T. Q. Hoang, T. N. Nguyen, M. W. Borgdorff, and F. G. Cobelens. 2007. "HIV and Tuberculosis in Ho Chi Minh City, Vietnam, 1997–2002." *Emerging Infectious Diseases* 13(10): 1463–1469.

Valdiserri, Ronald, Jag Khalsa, Corinna Dan, Scott Holmberg, Jon Zibbell, Deborah Holtzman, Robert Lubran, and Wilson Compton. 2014. "Confronting the Emerging Epidemic of HCV Infection among Young Injection Drug Users." *American Journal of Public Health* 104(5): 816–821.

van Zyl Smit, R., M. Pai, W. Yew, C. Leung, A. Zumla, E. Bateman, and K. Dheda. 2010. "Global Lung Health: The Colliding Epidemics of Tuberculosis, Tobacco Smoking, HIV and COPD." *The European Respiratory Journal* 35(1): 27–33.

Verdejo-Garcia, Antonio, Lawrence, Andrew, and Luke Clark. 2008. "Impulsivity as a Vulnerability Marker for Substance-Use Disorders: Review of Findings from High-Risk Research, Problem Gamblers and Genetic Association Studies." *Neuroscience and Biobehavioral Reviews* 32(4): 777–810.

Vivian, Jim, Hassan Saleheen, Merrill Singer, Juhem Navarro, and Greg Mirhej. 2005. "Under the Counter: The Diffusion of Narcotic Analgesics to the Inner City Street." *Journal of Ethnicity and Substance Abuse* 4(2): 97–114.

Walkup, J., M. B. Blank, J. S. Gonzalez, S. Safren, R. Schwartz, L. Brown, I. Wilson, A. Knowlton, F. Lombard, C. Grossman, K. Lyda, and J. Schumacher. 2008. "The Impact of Mental Health and Substance Abuse Factors on HIV Prevention and Treatment." *Journal of Acquired Immune Deficiency Syndromes* 47(Suppl 1): S15–9.

Weis, Lois. 1995. "Identity Formation and the Processes of 'Othering': Unraveling Sexual Threads." *Educational Foundations* 9(1): 17–33.

Yu, F., E. J. Nehl, T. Zheng, N. He, C. J. Berg, A. F. Lemieux, L. Lin, A. Tran, P. S. Sullivan, and F. Y. Wong. 2015. "A Syndemic Including Cigarette Smoking and Sexual Risk Behaviors Among a Sample of MSM in Shanghai, China." *Drug & Alcohol Dependence* 132(1): 265–270.

Zizek, Slavoj. 2008. *Violence: Six Sideways Reflections*. New York: Picador.

Chapter Two

Perception and Discrimination

The Biomedical Foundations of a Syndemic of Substance Abuse, Violence, and Suicide Among Aboriginal People in Ontario, Canada

Gerald McKinley

In the mid-1980s the suicide rate among Aboriginal youth in Ontario, particularly in Northwestern Ontario, began increasing at a steady rate. Prior to 1985 suicide took place in the region at a rate of approximately one death per year. In 1985 this rate increased to ten deaths and climbed to twenty-two deaths by 1995 (Nodin 1996). Nodin Counselling Services, a First Nations run mental health program in the region, recorded a similar increase in self-harm during this time frame and steadily high rates of violence (Nodin 1996). This region of Ontario can still be considered remote for southerners. With the exception of a few winter roads across frozen lakes, there are no roads providing outside access to the communities spread across the boreal forest and lowland swamps (Long 2010). Access to the communities requires flying into dirt runways. The Aboriginal population in the regions consists mainly of Anishinaabek First Nations and Cree First Nations. The Anishinaabek term *Bimaadiziwin*, or *pimadaziwin* in A. Irving Hallowell's ethnographic writings, is used to describe the proper life one should lead or "life in the fullest sense" (Hallowell 1955, 290). In practice it means that individuals have a responsibility to demonstrate for younger generations the proper way to live a traditional life. As such it places the onus on youth to take responsibility for their actions and their development. *Bimaadiziwin* is not a synonym for health. Instead is can be considered as a holistic concept best understood as a verb, a way of living, rather than a state.

The population in the region is young and has grown 22 percent between 1996 and 2001 with birth rates double have of the general Canadian population (MacTavish et al. 2012, 209). The growing population has seen numerous changes to their social, political and economic structures within the life of older generations. Between 1906 and 1930, the signing of the international

Treaty Number Nine brought the area and its inhabitants officially into Canada (Long 2010). With the signing of the treaty southern involvement in the daily lives in the north increased. Education shifted from a traditional system of care within a family unit to residential schools for their kids, to schools run by First Nations but still far from the children's home communities. Economics structures that maintained independence shifted due to the decline in the fur trade and the closing of Hudson Bay Company posts to a system of dependence on social welfare and government program. Relocating family units away from traditional trap lines decreased local leadership, transferring power from *ogimaag* (or loosely Chiefs) to imposed political structure under the Indian Act (Baxter 2015; Long 2010). Prior to the outbreak of the current suicide epidemic in the region, the local health authority was concerned about epidemic levels of substance abuse and violence existing in the population as a result of structural violence which in turn drives further stigma against the community (Lynn 1973; Nodin 1996). Substance use included widespread drinking of homebrew, a powerful moonshine like drink, and solvent sniffing. Highlighting the importance of acknowledging the role of stigma in the development of biosocial health, in one study from the region indicated that nineteen Aboriginal blood samples averaged 48.1 micrograms (μg)/100ml (Davis 1973). Nine samples had values over 50 μg/100ml and the highest value reported was 86 μg/100ml and the lowest is 18 μg/100ml (Davis 1973). There is no safe limit for lead in the blood stream.

In terms of biomedical effects, lead is believed to contribute to an overexpression of the amyloid-β protein precursor (AβPP) and amyloid-β (Aβ) which is associated with late-life depression (Bihaqi et al. 2011). A further pathway of concern from in their study is a down-regulation (4-fold) of the 5-hydroxytryptamine 1B receptor (5-HT-1B) that resulted from lead exposure early in life (Bihaqi et al. 2011, 826). Down-regulation of the 5-HT-1B alters the release of neurotransmitters, including lower serotonin levels, increased impulsivity, changes drug pharmacodynamics, stress sensitivity, mood, anxiety, and aggression. All of these factors are associated with increased risk of suicide and suicidal ideation (Clark and Neumaier 2001). Senut et al. (2012) suspect that early childhood lead poisoning can contribute to epigenetic modification.

This example highlights how I explore how social conditions, created by and resulting from a racist colonial system, damaged *bimaadiziwim* and produced conditions where substance abuse, violence and suicide come together and interact in a form of syndemic. While I acknowledge that the SAVA syndemic is well studied (Singer 1994, 2009; Singer et al. 1996), with the absence of HIV/AIDS in the present study, the SAVA syndemic is inappropriate. For clarity, I refer to the syndemic outlined in this chapter as Suicide,

Substance Use, and Violence (SSV). This chapter's objective is to explore the biological interaction of three health factors and to demonstrate how these are caused by structural violence affecting the daily lives of Aboriginal communities in Ontario, Canada. Suicide, substance use, and violence use are not naturalized aspects of traditional Aboriginal cultures in the area, but were introduced through ongoing colonial pressures, including but not limited to the Indian Act, residential schools, poverty, social inequality and the forced adoption of Aboriginal youth. Terry Wotherspoon argues that this history has served to negatively differentiate Aboriginal peoples in Canada which in turn affects their ability access their rights and resources (Wothespoon 2007, 133).

This chapter also explores the role of social perspective in the development of a syndemic. In order to do this it is important to distinguish between disease as a biological outcome and illness as a social condition in order to explore the role that the social construction of social sigma plays in the maintenance of social conditions and biosocial health outcomes. As such, stigma creates the bidirectional social conditions, conceived as structural violence, which negatively burden a marginalized population, creating a state where allostatic loads are disproportionately present for those carrying the stigma allowing disease and illness to thrive and where the burden of disease is utilized to reify existing stigmas. In large part, because of this I will propose in this chapter that *bimaadiziwim* is becoming harder to live.

Material collected for this chapter comes from a number of sources. Statistical data has been gathered from the Office of the Chief Coroner for Ontario. This data includes age, community, sex, method of suicide, and date of death for Aboriginal suicides in the Province from 1991 to 2014. The author supplemented the statistical data with a file review of fifty-two suicides that took place in 2013 and 2014, and used the file reviews to confirm rates of interaction between suicide, substance use, and violence within the population. Original ethnographic data in this chapter came from two main sources. The first is ongoing field research with Aboriginal people in Northwestern Ontario including fieldwork in urban settings and in a fly-in community located in the far north of the province. The second source of ethnographic data comes from semi-structured interviews conducted with Aboriginal youth recruited at Western University in London, Ontario. All research was reviewed by Western University's Research Ethics Board prior to its commencement.[1]

DEFINING STIGMA

The definition of stigma I utilize comes from Erving Goffman who defines stigma as "an attribute that is deeply discrediting" (Goffman 1963, 3). Goffman continues to write "that a language of relationships, not attributes, is really needed" in the understanding of the concept of stigma (Goffman 1963, 3). Attributes contain socially constructed values but without those attributes being in a relationship with other values, stigma cannot marginalize the stigmatized population. Common stigmas attributed to Aboriginal people in Canada include being inferior to Western settlers, lazy, drunk, on social assistance or violent (Monture 2007, 207). Bruce Link and Jo Phelan's (2001) expansion of Goffman's definition in this chapter was deliberately chosen because their four elements of stigma provide a method of considering the process of stigmatization. As such, stigma exists when: (1) human differences are distinguished and labeled; (2) labeled persons are associated with undesirable characteristics; (3) labeled persons are Othered creating an "us" and "them" separation; and (4) the stigmatization process is dependent upon social, economic and political power which creates and maintains the separation of labeled persons (Link and Phelan 2001, 367).

This chapter expands on Link and Phelan's definition and the role of perspective, or perspectivism, in understanding how stigma contributes to increased suicide, substance use and violence among Aboriginal peoples in Canada (Viveiros 1998). Eduardo Viveiros de Castro defined perspectivism as "the conception, . . . according to which the world is inhabited by different sorts of subjects or persons, human and non-human, which apprehend reality from distinct points of view" (Viveiros 1998, 469). As an ontological position, perspectivism articulates well the worldview of the Anishinaabek people with whom I work. Their belief-world is in fact made up of multiple classes of persons who maintain their own unique perspective on events (Hallowell 1955). Viveiros' term "to see as" is important for the understanding of how a subject's perspective aids in the study of the relationship between mental illness and stigma (Viveiros 1998, 470). Perspective is a cultural mechanism through which society guides its members on how to see their world. Perspective plays an important role in Goffman's insistence on the importance of relationships, and in Link and Phelan's expanded definition, which includes othering and discrimination (Goffman 1963; Link and Phelan 2001). The invisibility of structural or institutional discrimination is made visible through the perspective lens of the stigmatized.

Many of the communities in Ontario most affected by the SSV syndemic are fly-in communities that are geographically remote and closed off to the vast majority of non-Aboriginal Canadians. A unique aspect of Canadian law allows the Crown, a metonymic term for the government which reflects Canada's colonial history, complete control over the daily lives of Aboriginal peoples. The Indian Act, first enacted in 1876 and still in place after numerous revisions, makes anyone who is registered with Indian status a ward of the Crown (Indian Act 1985). As such the dominant majority, through the Crown, is able to exercise unidirectional control over the daily lives of this stigmatized minority. With the exception of a few national or regional bodies a local community context is often voiceless and powerless to control modes of representation that are too often the only consistent connection between Aboriginal and non-Aboriginal communities. This includes government press releases, media representations and public discourse. Research by Brad Clark (2014) indicates that media coverage of Aboriginal peoples in Canada "consistently deploys stereotypes frames rooted in colonialism." He goes on to reflect that representation of Aboriginal peoples tends to be either invisible or hypervisible in this coverage that has its roots in negative historical colonial representations (Clark 2014).

STIGMA AND THE SOCIAL DETERMINANTS OF HEALTH

Link and Phelan identify structural discrimination as a key component of stigma in society (2001). Structural discrimination is defined as set of practices that "includes the policies of private and governmental institutions that intentionally restrict the opportunities" (Corrigan, Markowitz, and Watson 2004). Structural discrimination, uses as a synonym for structural violence in this chapter, allows us to consider disadvantage at a macro level by exploring how the system maintains disadvantage (Link and Phelan 2001, 372). The impact of structural discrimination on Aboriginal people in Canada is well documented and is applied in the chapter to understand how stigma and biosocial health create the SSV syndemic (Waldram, Herring and Young 2006). Because of structural discrimination, Aboriginal peoples are more likely to experience food insecurity relative to the non-Aboriginal population; have lower annual incomes and lower educational attainment relative to non-Aboriginal people; are four times more likely to live in over-crowded housing; have decreased life expectancies; and have higher rates of major depression (18 percent), problems with alcohol (27 percent) and experiences with sexual abuse during childhood (34 percent) (Mikkonen and Raphael 2010, 42–43; Waldram, Herring, and Young 2006). Several of these areas will be explored in greater detail later in this chapter.

On the role of stigmatization and social determinants of health in the development of the current suicide epidemic in First Nations communities, Kauta Kandhai wrote, "Aboriginal status was enmeshed with other social determinants of health to create a tsunami of stigmatization and discrimination leading to impoverishment, marginalization, incarceration, and suicide of youth and their culture" (Kandhai 2015, 61). Status as a ward of the Crown, as discussed above with the Indian Act, plays an important role in Kandhai's statement. Through the Indian Act the Crown maintains control over key aspects of social determinants of health in Aboriginal lives including housing, education, health care, political structure, family structure, and access to resources. The separation of "Us" from "Them" is written into the Canadian Constitution. It is also important to note that Aboriginal people also maintain this distinction to a degree as Aboriginal leaders call for nation to nation relationships between Canada and Aboriginal peoples while the Federal Crown maintains a paternalistic fiduciary relationship (Coulthard 2007, 438). However, the Aboriginal leadership's focus is on empowerment and balancing the relationship rather than maintaining social, economic and political power imbalances that maintain social inequity (Coulthard 2007).

THREE EPIDEMICS PRESENT IN SUICIDE FILES

The proposed SSV syndemic in Aboriginal populations in the Province of Ontario and the role that stigma plays in its maintenance is based on my review of official suicide files from the Office of the Chief Coroner, Ontario ($n = 52$).[2] During 2013 there were 40 recorded Aboriginal suicides in Ontario (Office of the Chief Coroner). The Aboriginal population in Ontario accounts for approximately 2 percent of the total population; Aboriginal suicide deaths accounted for approximately 15 percent of youth (under 25) suicides (Statistics Canada).

Of the 51 completely reviewed files, 27 were of female suicide victims and 24 male victims. The average age of females was 22 years and males averaged 28 years of age. Females ranged in age from 12 to 50 years while males' ages ranged from 13 to 43 years of age. For reasons that are still being researched, a higher or similar rate of completed female to male Aboriginal suicides has started to become the norm in Ontario over the past decade. This chapter explores how the SSV syndemic contributes to a similar method of suicide death in the decreasing of sex difference. This trend differs from the national non-Aboriginal average where males have a rate three times higher than females (Statistics Canada 2012). Thirty-six of the suicides took place on a First Nations Reserve and fifteen took place in an urban context. The method of suicide was hanging in 84 percent of the cases. Females were just as likely to complete suicide by hanging as males.

Substance use was measured after the fact using identifiers in the Coroner's narrative and the post-mortem report. The signifiers "substance (ab) use," "drug use," "alcohol (ab)use" and "history of" for any of the previous signifiers was considered to be evidence of the existence of substance use as a proximal factor in the suicides. Substance use includes gas sniffing, excessive alcohol consumption, illegal drug use and illegal use of prescription drugs. Cases where the individual was referred to as a "social drinker" were not included in the count. Eighty-two percent of the cases reviewed were deemed to have evidence of substance abuse. Substance use among Aboriginal peoples is a consistent stigma in their lives with a number of studies providing only conflicting answers to the problem (Waldram, Herring, and Young 2006, 112). Paul Whitehead and Michael Hayes warn that substance use in Aboriginal communities needs to be considered within their unique ecological, or social, context rather than contributing to discourse that separates "types" of people (Whitehead and Hayes 1998, xvi). Importantly, they reject that substance use is a problem in the population because Aboriginal people constitute a so called "fundamentally different type of people" (Whitehead and Hayes 1998, xvi). Mota et al. (2012) found that one-third of 1,125 First Nations youth surveyed in Manitoba, Canada, were substance users and had self-reported depressive symptoms within the past twelve months. Their study confirmed that depressive disorders and substance abuse are associated with suicide and suicidal ideation within First Nations populations in Canada. Mota et al. further note that substance use is a form of self-medication against the emotional pain suffered by youth and associated with mood disorders such as depression (Mota et al. 2012, 1359). The author argues that this reflects the connection between structural violence and SSV.

In order to find supporting evidence for SSV, the association of present suicides from data in the Coroner's files was measured using one of two identifiers. The first was a record of suicidal ideation or previous attempts by the individual. The second was a recent experience with suicide either by a close friend, family member or in a small, close knit community. Suicidal ideation and/or previous attempts are associated with an increase in completed suicides (Joiner 2005). Suicide was present as a factor in 67 percent ($n = 34$) of the 51 cases reviewed.

McKenzie et al. found that suicide deaths and suicidal ideation within communities can be the result of imitation and proximity up to twelve months after a suicide outbreak (McKenzie et al. 2005). Contagion-as-context, where the most recent suicide need not be in the proximate location or have direct contact with the originating suicide for the clustering to be developed, has also been identified a risk factor for the spread of suicide (Cheng et al. 2014).

The final proximal factor reviewed in the official record was measures of violence, indicated by signifiers for intimate partner violence, child abuse, self-harm and other forms of physical violence. Violence was present in 63 percent of the suicide files reviewed. Each of these forms of violence is associated with suicide and substance use by increasing an individual's chances of developing depression (Fazel et al. 2015; Brockie et al. 2015). Kang et al. (2015) have identified a strong connection between violence, substance use, suicide and depression in adolescents. In addition, a dysregulation of the sympathetic nervous system and the hypothalamic-pituitary-adrenal axis (HPA axis) has been located in suicidal patients who suffer from major depression (McGirr 2010). Ben-Efrain et al. (2011) identified gene-environment interactions in female victims of sexual violence that affected gene expression associated with the HPA axis.

The combination of suicide, substance use, and violence was present in 41 percent of the cases reviewed. These cases were distributed as 30 percent female suicides and 54 percent of male suicides. By comparison, Brockie et al. recorded a higher rate of physical violence in males versus females in their study of the relationship between adverse childhood events, depression, PTSD, drug use and suicides in on-reserve Native American populations (Brockie et al. 2015, 416). That study, along with narratives collected during my fieldwork in a number of Aboriginal communities, helps confirm a relationship between suicide, substance use and violence. What is becoming similarly clear from reviewing these suicide files is that Aboriginal individuals seemingly self-medicate to deal with the interpersonal violence and suicides in their communities. Increased violence is driving an increase in suicide rates and substance use; and, the suicides within these communities are contributing to increased substance use which is also associated with increased violence.

SSV SYNDEMIC

The syndemic relationship between substance abuse and various forms of interpersonal violence has long been established in existing literature, since the identification of the first syndemic by Merrill Singer (Singer 1996). Singer's early work on SAVA demonstrates the important contribution that ethnographic fieldwork can make in public health research as violence was not a core variable in his initial research (Singer 1996, 100). The author's ethnographic field research and statistical data confirm that suicide also shares a syndemic relationship with substance use and violence. The correlation between substance use, depression and suicide is well known (Kang et al. 2015). A continuing challenge, and my intention in this chapter, is to identify how the three components interact to not only increase the existence of the others but to also delineate precisely what biological mechanisms drive their existence and interactions. The relationship between substance use, self-reported suicidality, and changes within the brain has been established elsewhere (Kokkevi et al. 2012; Kang et al. 2015; Ben-Efrain 2011). The author considers depression the connecting pathway in SSV as it is associated with all three. Despite being stigmatized as merely a "bad mood," significant evidence exists confirming depression to be a biomedical condition caused by chemical reactions and gene-environment interactions which alter brain function (Hostinar et al. 2014). Additionally, depression is already associated with suicidal ideation, suicide attempts, aggressive behavior and substance use among adolescents and is highly correlated with social conditions such as structural violence (Kang et al. 2015, 15; Ben-Efrain 2011; McGirr 2010).

Despite the challenge of identifying depression using coroner's files, it is important in ongoing syndemic research to consider the role that depression plays SSV. Berman, Jobes and Silverman cite a number of studies indicating an increase in depressive symptoms in adults and adolescents presenting with suicidality (Berman, Jobes, and Silverman 2006, 103–104). Ali et al. (2013) demonstrated how alcohol affects brain function in relation to suicide. Increased emotional state, aggressiveness and self-destructive behavior are associated with alcohol's effect on the limbic system. Changes to the cerebral cortex are associated with impaired thinking, judgement and lowered inhibitions (Ali et al. 2013, 23). All of these physical responses to alcohol are associated with increased suicidality and completed suicides.

In the context of working with Aboriginal partners, the line between stigma and racism is challenging to define, and many of the key concepts from each definition blur the boundaries between the others. Certainly racism and racist policies cannot gain the invisibility they need to exist in a so-called progressive state without the aid of stigma. Both represent a signification of differences across power relationships where "we" are normative and "they" are Other. Both stigmatization and racialization are "a dialectical process of human differentiation" where the former focuses on social valuation of labels and the latter depends on perceived biological and physical characteristics (Hier 2007, 28).

Racism continues to interact with colonialism in Canada by maintaining structural differences between Aboriginal and non-Aboriginal peoples. Patricia A. Monture contends that the characterization of Aboriginal peoples as inferior was essential for colonial policy as it justified child welfare and educational policies that take children from their families and place them in state care in alarmingly high numbers (Monture 2007, 207). These "ostensibly benevolent interventions" imposed normative ideologies on the lives of Aboriginal communities under the guise of "child protection" (Maxwell 2014, 409). The over-representation of Aboriginal children in the child welfare system has become a large enough problem that the First Nations

Child and Family Caring Society of Canada and the Assembly of First Nations have filed a human rights complaint against the Federal Government due to systematic discrimination in funding of on-reserve programs (Sinha et al. 2013, 823). Unfortunately physical and sexual abuse, neglect, racism, substance use and suicide are common in the lives of those children who end up in the system (Kirmayer, Tait, and Simpson 2009, 10–11). The author's suicide file reviews contained confirmation of Children's Aid Society (CAS) involvement in six of the thirteen suicide victims aged 18 or under. Of these all but one confirmed the presence of suicide, substance use, and violence in the youth life. As CAS files are not recorded for adult suicides additional information is not available.

Structural violence involves multiple social institutions including schools, newspapers, welfare agencies, businesses, municipal services and the criminal justice system (Hedican 2013, 227). The exploration of three social determinants of health in greater detail helps shed light on how policy based on systemic or institutional discrimination contributed to the SSV syndemic by establishing how structure creates the conditions where the three elements can interact. Based on field research in Northern Ontario, this section explores education, food insecurity and social support networks to understand the daily circumstances faced by the Aboriginal population in the region. Education and schools continues to be a problem for Aboriginal people in Canada despite the closing of the residential schools in 1996. A 2009 report produced by the First Nations Education Council contends that "while First Nations have taken on greater administrative responsibility and control over education services since then, official funding has not yet been established that would enable First Nations education systems to provide second- and third-level services at a level comparable to that offered by provincial education systems across Canada" (FNEC 2009, 28).

Discussions with participants during ethnographic research in Northern Ontario have repeatedly returned to the topic of education as a special concern, largely focusing on Aboriginal youth needing to leave their home community to attend school. As a social determinant of health, education is traditionally associated with increased health at the individual and community level (Yamashita and Kenkel 2015). However, Kirmayer, Brass and Tait note that First Nations youth from remote communities obtaining a high school education in Quebec face decreasing or negative health outcomes (Kirmayer, Brass, and Tait 2000). Here, in terms of health outcomes, Aboriginal youth, particularly women, were better off dropping out after grade 8 or ensure that they reached the post-secondary level. Individuals from the community I am working with believe these outcomes to be true. On this topic several members of the community have raised concerns over the current educational structure. The community school runs grades Junior Kindergarten to eight. After grade eight students are expected to travel approximately 280 miles (450 km) to Thunder Bay, Ontario, to attend the Northern Nishnawbe Education Council run school. As there are no roads to and from their community transportation is only available through expensive air travel. The school itself makes every effort to ensure that the curriculum meets the needs of the students. Some live with family members, others are boarded. One community member noted that when he attended residential school he was never given the chance to get into real trouble. Youth today, he noted, are met when they arrive by gang members who promise friendship and support but soon teach the kids how to do drugs and get involved in gang activity.

Both the former residential school and current system share a structural limitation that forces youth to be removed from their homes in order to participate in education. This significant factor of displacement, as in other settings is associated with a change in health behaviors associated with increased drug use and violence. Remaining in school provides youth with access to counselling services and support. However, local narratives recounting high drop-out rates mean that a majority of youth are likely losing access to these supports. Not finishing high school has long-term effects on an individual's income and access to employment. It is also evident that the educational structure can increase the likelihood of individual youth becoming involved with increased risk-taking behavior as a result of the system helping them locate a peer group within a marginalized, and perhaps criminal, organization. For any youth dropping out of school also increases the risk of becoming homeless.

Education in Northern Ontario has seen a number of changes over the past sixty years. One Aboriginal Elder reflected on never having attended a school but told me a story about what it was like watching the float plane take her kids away to residential school. She mentioned the old float plane dock and how the community would sit there the whole day and cry after the children were taken. Because of the structure of the current education system, families today still face the flight of children south. One community member raised a concern over Ontario government policy stating that children move forward with their chronological age cohort regardless of how prepared they are for high school. The result is children who are not emotionally or intellectually ready for high school are experiencing the move south.

Structural violence has resulted in high levels of food insecurity for Aboriginal people in Canada. Remote or fly-in communities are the most affected. Recent work in the region where I conducted my fieldwork has recorded food insecurity rates at 70 percent of households with 17 percent of community households self-reporting themselves as severely food insecure (Skinner, Hanning, and Tsaji 2013, 31). A positive relationship between food insecurity and depression has been identified in recent years (Leung et al. 2015). In their study marginal food insecurity resulted in 7.7 percent of the population having some form of depressive symptoms, high food insecurity resulted in 11.1 percent and very high food insecurity resulted in 19.6 percent of the study population having symptoms. In all 38.4 percent of their study population experienced depressive symptoms associated with food insecurity. Depression is believed to partner with perceived stress and anxiety as food becomes less secure (Laraia et al. 2009). Food insecurity in the region is the result of poverty, unreliable food supplies, high cost of food, environmental contamination of local food sources, and the loss of traditional practices for procuring food (Skinner et al. 2014, 2). Over the past 60 years the community's food supplies in Northern Ontario have changed from local country food consisting of fish, beaver, moose, caribou, ducks, geese to a diet largely based on store-bought foods.

A 2014 report from the Council of Canadian Academies' Expert Panel on the State of Knowledge of Food Security in Northern Canada investigated the loss of country food option and inadequate, expensive store options, which increases the risk for acute myocardial infarction mortality, increased rates of obesity and other cardiovascular disease (CVD), and increased risk of diabetes. From a mental health perspective, the report also states that food insecurity is related to increased risk of depression, substance use and suicide (Council of Canadian Academies 2014, xix). The report offers a strong connection between structural violence and SSV through the pathway of depression. In addition, Kmetic, Reading, and Estey (2008) demonstrated how children who experience food insecurity also experience significantly increased risks of negative health outcomes across their life courses. Early childhood food insecurity is associated with an increased risk of depression, poor school performance and drug addiction across the life course (Chilton et al. 2015). They also located a positive relationship between food insecurity and increased household violence, risk of diabetes, CVD, anxiety and early mortality.

Change to food acquisition strategies affects more than just nutrition. The long-term effects on the changes to intra-community relationships must also be considered. Food procurement has played an important role in the development of the cultural systems of the Anishinaabek and Cree peoples who reside in Northern Ontario (Hallowell 1955). Changes to the procurement process altered important social structure that facilitated the integration of youth into the community. Partnered with the out-schooling of youth away from the community, the changes to community-level social support networks are significant. Theories on social support networks work with the assumption that stronger networks provide a buffering effect for individuals. Hostinar,

Sullivan and Gunner (2014) reported that the social support networks provided a form of modulation of individual responses to potentially stressful events, which may dampen the response of the HPA axis, which, as discussed above, is associated with increased risk of suicide, substance use and violence in adolescents. Rosal et al. (2004) have also described a decreased salivary cortisol level in individuals with stronger social support networks.

LIVED EXPERIENCE OF STIGMA IN THE DAILY LIVES OF ABORIGINAL PEOPLES

I argue that the social conditions that create and maintain the biological pathways which contribute to the SSV syndemic exist because of the legal framework created by the Indian Act and the historical and ongoing marginalization of Aboriginal peoples are maintained by their stigmatization. In order to understand the internalization or embodiment of stigma, I have been conducting interviews with Aboriginal youth over the past two years with the purpose of understanding how they see themselves and their community within the Canadian context. On the topic of stereotypes one interviewee responded by saying:

> They stereotype natives and that's really bad. Um. I'm sure some people fit those stereotypes but also there isn't any insight as or trying to understand . . . there's no empathy towards the issue of the residential schools . . . it's like get over it and they just look at the culture so negatively like oh why don't you have to pay taxes? This that like . . . so many things and its just like get over it basically . . . and I don't know . . . how the culture is suppose to get over it . . . it's very broken in my opinion . . . so that's like telling people in the holocaust to get over it. But it's just a different race and some something and it happened in a different way . . . but it's the same thing. (Aboriginal Youth, London, Morning, March 17, 2015)

A semi-structured interview allowed youth to speak openly on a variety of topics. The above individual reflected on a lack of empathy for real events in Aboriginal community histories and the focusing of attention on misunderstood tax laws. The ongoing legacy of residential schools contributes negatively to the psychological and physical health of communities. Using the Beck Depression Inventory Short Form, Amy Bombay, Kimberly Matheson and Hymie Anisman identified increased depressive symptoms in the second generation offspring of residential school survivors relative to community members without the residential school connection (Bombay, Matheson and Anisman 2011, 375). Additionally, suicidal ideation is increased (37.2

percent of participants) among individuals who had a least one parent attend residential school when compared to those who did not (25.7 percent of Aboriginal participants) according to the First Nations Regional Longitudinal Survey (Bombay, Matheson, and Anisman 2014, 324). Unfortunately, the youths that I'm working with feel that the important health impact of the residential schools is ignored because of the erroneous belief that Aboriginal people in Canada do not pay taxes. In short, they feel that the stigma over perceived taxation privileges, which they do not actually enjoy, is used to hide the damages done by the ongoing colonization of their traditional territories.

The youth expressed a concern over social stresses and marginalization associated with stigma that was most often experienced in the education system. One youth stated:

> I feel very almost marginalized because I just . . . people don't understand the history and I think that's a big missing piece and I really do believe that in every Canadian institute that it should be mandatory to take an indigenous course because a lot of people are ignorant and don't understand and being a minority of that culture people often . . . not necessarily degrade but there're not . . . they are ignorant towards us and it's unfortunate and I've had some falling outs already this year in that and it's really frustrating. (First Nations Youth, London, Afternoon, March 17, 2015)

The social stresses reported by the youth have been associated with increased production of pro-inflammatory cytokines in animals and humans. Social rejection, a component of stigma, has been shown to increase cytokine production in the areas of the brain associated with depression while social connectedness decreases it (Audet et al. 2014, 1–2). According to Hedican (2013), the intolerance that enables the stigma and partnered social rejection to exist runs through all aspects of life for Aboriginal people living in Ontario.

PERSPECTIVE, DISCRIMINATION, STIGMA AND SSV

Link and Phelan differentiate between individual discrimination where person A discriminates against person B, and structural discrimination, where institutional practices contain the means of discriminating against entire communities (Link and Phelan 2001, 372). The author's focus in this chapter is on the bidirectional role of structural violence as it produces stigma and the relationship of such stigma to what I term a SSV syndemic facing Aboriginal people in Northwestern Ontario. The author also frames this syndemic as a key to understanding the role that perspective plays in the relationship between stigma, discrimination and health outcomes. Perspective frames events and allows for the formation of narratives based on those events.

As discussed above, the discriminatory practice of sending Aboriginal children to residential schools to teach them to be Christians and more European in behavior was seen as a positive action by the Crown and the Churches who ran the schools and were based in still existent stigma and stereotypes maintaining a key separation between Settler and Indigenous populations. At the same time the same actions were seen as a violent, discriminatory practice by those who suffered physical, sexual, and emotional abuse in the schools. As such, the narratives of residential schools have become embodied in the identity of many Aboriginal peoples in Canada. Ronald Niezen's (2013) discussion of how these events and their narratives form a collective identity is particularly important and is central to how related concepts like historical trauma are understood. One youth's statement exemplary of others: "the residential schools broke people. They broke the people. It left a really big mess and there is a lot to clean up there and to help and the residential schools . . . I know my mother was affected by that absolutely and in my upbringing it was shown" (First Nations Youth, London, Morning, March 17, 2015). Another simply responded with "when you say historical trauma it reminds me of residential schools" (First Nations Youth, London, Afternoon, March 18, 2015)

Perspective plays an important role in the evaluation of discrimination which leads to behavioral and biological adaptations to events and actions (Bombay, Matheson, and Ainsman 2014, 75). The perception of structural discrimination as stressful can lead to increased substance use as a form of self-medication to the stress. Increased baseline stress hormones affect brain function and the size of regions of the brain associated with stress responses such as the HPA axis. The result of consistent overstimulation of the HPA is a reprogramming of the system, which makes the individual hyper-vigilant and reactive in stressful situations. Early life stress has been demonstrated to reduce the growth of the pituitary gland in adolescents making these youth more susceptible to the onset of depression (Ganella et al. 2015). Assuming a stigma driven connection between depression and SSV, and clustering patterns for Aboriginal health outcomes, SSV will also potentially increase if they already exist within an individual's life circumstances. With depression being highly associated with the elements of SSV, and it is not a surprise to see the interaction of the three in the cases noted above.

CONCLUSION

In 1993, Nodin Mental Health Services gave a presentation to the medical community about the recent increase in suicides in the region. The reasons provided for the outbreak included family dysfunction and violence, substance use and the increase in suicides themselves which put communities in "crisis" (Nodin 1993). Among the causes of the "heaviness" or stress that the youth feel Nodin listed racism and discrimination (Nodin 1993, 5). Aboriginal people in the Province face challenges that the non-Aboriginal population does not. These differences are a result of systemic violence, which has been fueled by racism and maintained by socially accepted stigmas about Aboriginal people. The social conditions create a pathway that increases community level stress. Chronic stress affects brain function by over stimulating the body's stress response system and increasing levels of cytokine and stress hormones in the blood and brain. Over stimulation leads to sensitivity to stress and increased risk of depression and mood disorders. Depression is highly correlated with increased rates of suicide, substance use, and violence. Clustering of suicide among at-risk youth spreads the syndemic. Once in a, community suicide, substance use, and violence contribute to their own growth. In response, non-Aboriginal new media reifies pre-existing stigma with new coverage that reflects the dominants society's views on Aboriginal people.

Several of the youth that I interviewed made reference to the people being broken by their history of interaction with the Canadian State. Residential schools caused considerable damage. However, a single cause does not fuel the syndemic proposed in this chapter. The education system, high levels of food insecurity, breakdown of community level, positive social support networks, and media and non-Aboriginal bias all contributed to an institutional system of discrimination which promoted the biological pathways of syndemic interaction and promote the stigmas delineate above.

NOTES

1. I use the term Aboriginal throughout this chapter. In Canada Aboriginal is a legal definition contained within the Canadian Constitution signifying First Nations, Metis and Inuit peoples. The author uses individual signifiers such as First Nations when the context warrants a local identifier.

2. Detailed data was recorded on a pre-prepared excel spreadsheet for six known risk factors for Aboriginal suicide: substance use, violence, previous suicide attempts or ideation, proximity to suicide deaths, involvement in the criminal justice system, and identified mental illness. The reviewed files comprise all currently reported Aboriginal suicides from 2014 and a significant portion for 2013 making the files the best reflection of the current suicide problem. One file was removed from the analysis because of a lack of detailed information in the file. Data were collected from the Coroner's Narrative, the Post-Mortem, and any police or Children's Aid Society Reports contained in the files. The author reviewed all files at the Office of the Chief Coroner for Ontario in Toronto, Ontario during the summer of 2015.

REFERENCES

Ali, Shahid, Milankumar Nathani, Shahgufta Jabeen, Ijlal Yuzdani, Charles Mouton, Rahn Bailey, Mona Mahr, Rebecca Pate, and Wayne Riley. "Alcohol: The Lubricant to Suicidality." *Innovations in Clinical Neuroscience* 10, no. 1 (2013): 20–29.

Audet, Marie-Claude, Robyn J. McQuaid, Zal Merali, and Hymie Anisman. "Cytokine Variations and Mood Disorders: Influence of Social Stressors and Social Support." *Frontiers in Neuroscience* 8 (2014): 1–12.

Baller, Robert D and Kelly K Richardson. "The 'Dark Side' of the Strength of Weak Ties: The Diffusion of Suicidal Thoughts." *Journal of Health and Social Behavior* 50, no. 3 (2009): 261–276.

Berman, Alan, David A. Jobes, and Morton M. Silverman. *Adolescent Suicide: Assessment and Intervention*. Washington, DC: American Psychological Association, 2006.

Bihaqi, Syen Waseem, Hui Huang, Jinfang Wu, and Nasser H. Zawia. "Infant Exposure to Lead (Pb) and Epigenetic Modification in the Aging Primate Brain: Implications for Azheimer's Disease." *Journal of Alzheimer's Disease* 27 (2011): 819–833.

Bombay, Amy, Kimberly Matheson, and Hymie Anisman. "The Impact of Stressors on Second Generation Indian Residential School Survivors." *Transcultural Psychiatry* 48, no. 4 (2011): 367–391.

———. "Appraisals of Discriminatory Events Among Adult Offspring of Indian Residential School Survivors: The Influences of Identity Centrality and Past Perceptions of Discrimination." *Cultural Diversity and Ethnic Minority Psychology* 20, no. 1 (2014a): 75–86.

———. "The Intergenerational Effect of Indian Residential Schools: Implications for the Concept of Historical Trauma." *Transcultural Psychiatry* 51, no. 3 (2014b): 320–338.

Brochie, Teresa, Gail Dana-Sacco, Gwenyth Wallen, Holly Wilcox, and Jacquelyn Campbell. "The Relationship of Adverse Childhood Experiences to PTSD, Depression, Poly-Drug Use and Suicide Attempts in Reservation-Based Native American Adolescents and Young Adults." *American Journal of Community Psychology* 55 (2015): 411–421.

Cheng, Qijin, Hong Li, Vincent Silenzio, and Eric D. Caine. "Suicide Contagion: A Systematic Review of Definitions and Research Utility." *PLOS ONE* 9, no. 9 (2014): e108724.

Chilton, Mariana, Molly Knowles, Jenny Rabinowich, and Kimberly T. Arnold. "The Relationship Between Childhood Adversity and Food Insecurity: 'It's Like a Bird Nesting in Your Head.'" *Public Health Nutrition* (2015): 1–11.

Clark, M.S. and J.F. Neumaier. "The 5-HT-1B Receptor: Behavioral Implications." *Psychopharmocology Bulletin* 35, no. 4 (2001): 170–185.

Corrigan, Patrick W, Fred E Markowitz, and Amy C. Watson. 2004. "Structural Levels of Mental Illness Stigma and Discrimination." *Schizophrenia Bulletin* 30, no. 3 (2004):4814–91.

Council of Canadian Academies. Aboriginal Food Security in Northern Canada: An Assessment of the State of Knowledge. Ottawa, 2014.

Davies, John W. October 23, 1973. [letter to W. G. Goldthorpe]. Faculty of Medicine, Sioux Lookout. Program. A1997–0012. Box 004, file 28. University of Toronto Archives, Toronto, Ontario.

Fazel, Seena, Ackim Wolf, Zheng Chang, Henrik Larsson, Guy Goodwin, and Paul Lichtenstein. "Depression and Violence: A Swedish Population Study." *Lancet Psychiatry* 2 (2015): 224–232.

First Nations Education Council. 2009. "Paper on First Nations Education Funding."

Ganella, Despina, Nicholas B Allen, Julian G Skinner, Orti Schwartz, Jee Hyun Kim, Lisa Sheeber and Sarah Whittle. "Early Life Stress Alters Pituitary Growth During Adolescence: A Longitudinal Study." *Psychoneuroendorinology* 53 (2015): 185–194.

Goffman, Erving. *Stigma: Notes on the Management of Spoiled Identity*. New York: Simon and Schuster, 1963.

Hallowell, A. Irving. *Culture and Exp*erience. Philadelphia: University of Pennsylvania Press, 1955.

Health Canada. 2011. Accessed February 15, 2016. http://www.hc-sc.gc.ca/fniah-spnia/pubs/aborig-autoch/stats-profil-atlant/index-eng.php#a611.

Hedican, Edward J. *Ipperwash: The Tragic Failure of Canada's Aboriginal Policy*. Toronto: University of Toronto Press, 2013.

Heir, Sean P. 2007. "Studying Race and Racism in 21st-Century Canada." In *Race and Racism in 21st Century Canada: Continuity, Complexity and Change*, Sean P. Hier and Singh Bolaria, eds., 19–34. Peterborough, Canada: Broadview Press, 2007.

Hostinar, Camelia, Regina Sullivan, and Megan Gunnar. "Psychobiological Mechanisms Underlying the Social Buffering of the HPA Axis: A Review of Animal Models and Human Studies Across Development." *Psychological Bulletin*, 140, no. 1 (2014). DOI:10.1037/a0032671.

Indian Act. R.S.C., 1985, c. I-5.

Jiwani, Yasmin. "Doubling Discourse and the Veiled Other: Mediations of Race and Gender in Canadian Media." In *States of Race: Critical Race Feminism for the 21st Century*. Sherene Razack, Malinda Smith, and Sunera Thobani, eds., 59–86. Toronto: Between the Lines, 2010.

Joiner, Thomas. *Why People Die by Suicide*. Cambridge: Harvard University Press, 2007.

Kandhai, Kavita. "Aboriginal Social Injustice: Canada's Dirty Secret Leads to Suicide." In *Inviting Hope*, Kavita Kandhai, ed., 55–70. Winnipeg: Aboriginal Issues Press, 2015.

Kang, Tamara, Jennifer Eno Louden, Elijah Ricks and Rachell Jones. "Aggression, Substance Use Disorder, and Presence of a Prior Suicide Attempt Among Juvenile Offenders with Subclinical Depression." *Law and Human Behavior* 39, no. 6 (2015): 593–601.

Kirmayer, Laurence, Gregory Brass, and Caroline Tait. "The Mental Health of Aboriginal Peoples: The Transformation of Identity and Community." *Canadian Journal of Psychiatry* 45, no. 7 (2000): 607–616.

Kirmayer, Laurence, Caroline Tait, and Cori Simpson. "The Mental Health of Aboriginal Peoples in Canada: Transformations of Identity and Community." *Healing Traditions: The Mental Health of Aboriginal Peoples in Canada*, Gail Guthrie Valaskakis and Laurence J. Kirmayer, eds., 3–35. Vancouver and Toronto: UBC Press, 2009.

Kleinman, Arthur, and Rachel Hall-Clifford. "Stigma: A Social, Cultural and Moral Process." *Journal of Epidemiology & Community Health* 63, no. 6 (2009): 418–419.

Kmetic, Andrew, Jeffery Reading, and Elizabeth Estey. "Taking a Life Course Perspective on Cardiovascular Disease and Diabetes in First Nations Peoples." *Canadian Journal of Nursing and Research* 40, no. 3 (2008): 58–78.

Kokkevi, Anna, Clive Richardson, Deborah Olszewski, Joao Matias, Karin Monshouwer, and Thoroddun Bjarnason. "Multiple Substance Use and Self-Reported Suicide Attempts by Adolescents in 16 European Countries." *European Child and Adolescent Psychiatry* 21, no. 8 (2012): 443–450.

Laraia, Barbara A., Judith B. Borja, and Margaret E. Bently. "Grandmothers, Fathers, and Depression Symptoms Are Associated with Food Insecurity among Lower-Income First-Time African American Mothers in North Carolina." *Journal of the American Dietetic Association* 109, no. 6 (2009): 1042–1047.

Leung, Cindy W, Ellissa S. Epel, and Walter C. Willett. "Household Food Insecurity is Positively Associated with Depression Among Low-Income Supplemental Nutrition Assistance Program Participants and Income Eligible Non-Participants." *Journal of Nutrition* 145, no. 3 (2015): 622–627.

Link, Bruce G., and Jo Phelan. "Conceptualizing Stigma." *Annual Review of Sociology* 27 (2001): 363–385.

Long, John S. *Treaty No. 9: Making Agreement to Share the Land in Far Northern Ontario in 1905*. Montreal and Kingston: McGill-Queen's University Press, 2010.

Lynn, Helen. "Gasoline Sniffing and Lead Poisoning Among Young People in an Ojibway Indian Village." Faculty of Medicine, Sioux Lookout Program. A1997-0012. Box 004, file 28. University of Toronto Archives, Toronto, Ontario, 1973.

Maxwell, Krista. "Historicizing Historical Trauma Theory: Troubling The Trans-Generational Transmission Paradigm." *Transcultural Psychiatry* 51, no. 3 (2014): 407–435.

McKenzie, Nigel, Sabine Landan, Nauneet Kapur, Janet Meehan, Jo Robinson, Harriet Bickley, Rebecca Parsons, and Louis Appleby. "Clustering of Suicides Among People with Mental Illness." *British Journal of Psychiatry* 187 (2005): 476–480.

McQuaid, Robyn Jane, Amy Bombay, Opal Arilla McInnis, Kimberly Matheson, and Hymie Anisman. "Childhood Adversity, Perceived Discrimination and Coping Strategies in Relation to Depressive Symptoms Among First Nations Adults in Canada: The Moderating Roles of Unsupportive Interactions from Ingroup and Outgroup Members." *Cultural Diversity and Ethnic Minority Psychology* 21, no. 3 (2005): 326–336.

McTavish, Tracy, Marie-Odile Marceau, Michael Optis, Kara Shaw, Peter Stephenson, and Peter Wild. "A Participatory Process for the Design of Housing for a First Nation Community." *Journal of Housing and the Built Environment* 27, no. 2 (2012): 207–224.

Meyer, Jaimie, Sandra A. Springer, and Frederich L. Altice. "Substance Abuse, Violence and HIV in Women: A Literature Review of the Syndemic." *Journal of Women's Health* 20, no. 7 (2011): 991–1006.

Mikkonen, Juha and Dennis Raphael. *Social Determinants of Health: The Canadian Facts*. Toronto: York University School of Health Policy and Management, 2010.

Monture, Patricia A. "Racing and Erasing: Law and Gender in White Settler Societies." *Race and Racism in 21st-Century Canada: Continuity, Complexity and Change*. Sean P. Hier and Singh Bolaria, 197–216. Peterborough: Broadview Press, 2007.

Mota, Natalie, Brenda Elias, Bruce Tefft, Maria Medved, Garry Munro, and Jitender Sareen. "Correlates of Suicidality: Investigation of a Representative Sample of Manitoba First Nations Adolescents." *American Journal of Public Health* 102, no. 7 (2007): 1353–1361.

Muhlbauer, Susan. "Experience of Stigma by Families with Mentally Ill Members." *Journal of the American Psychiatric Nurses Association* 8, no. 3 (2002): 76–8.

Niezen, Ronald. *Truth and Indignation: Canada's Truth and Reconciliation Commission on Indian Residential Schools*. Toronto: University of Toronto Press, 2013.

Nodin Services. "Root Causes of Suicide." Faculty of Medicine, Sioux Lookout Program. A1997–0012. (Box 004, file 28). Toronto, Canada: University of Toronto Archives, 1993.

Rosal, Milagros, Jean King, Yancheng Ma and George W. Reed. 2004. "Stress, Social Support and Cortisol: Inverse Relationships?" Behavioural Medicine 30(1): 11–22.

Senut, Marie-Claud, Pable Cingolani, Arko Sen, Adele Kruger, Asra Shaik, Melmut Hirsch, Steven T. Suhr, and Douglas Ruden. "Epigenetics of Early-Life Lead Exposure and Effects on Brain Development." Epigenetics 4, 6 (2012): 665–674. DOI:10.2217/epi.12.58.

Singer, Merrill. "Aids and the Health Crisis of the Us Urban Poor: The Perspective of Critical Medical Anthropology." *Social Science and Medicine* 39, no. 7 (1994): 931–48.

———. "A Dose of Drugs, A Touch of Violence, A Case of AIDS: Conceptualizing the SAVA Syndemic." *Free Inquiry—Special Issue: Gangs, Drugs and Violence* 24, no. 2 (1996): 99–110.

———. *Introduction to Syndemics: A Critical Systems Approach to Public and Community Health*. San Francisco: Jossey-Bass, 2009.

Sinha, Vandua, Nico Trocme, Barbara Fallon, and Bruce MacLaurin. "Understanding the Investigation-Stage Overrepresentation of First Nations Children in the Child Welfare System: An Analysis of the First Nations Component of the Canadian Incidence Study of Reported Child Abuse and Neglect 2008." *Child Abuse and Neglect* 37 (2013): 821–831.

Skinner, Kelly, Rhona Hanning, J. Metatawabin, and Leonard J. S. Tsuji. "Implementation of a Community Greenhouse in a Remote, Sub-Arctic First Nations Community in Ontario, Canada: A Descriptive Case Study." *Rural and Remote Health* 14 (2014): 2545–2563.

———. "Prevalence and Severity of Household Food Insecurity of First Nations People Living in an On-Reserve, Sub-Arctic Community Within the Mushkegowuk Territory." *Public Health Nutrition* 17, no. 1 (2013): 31–39.

Statistics Canada. "Suicide Rates: An Overview" Ottawa: Government of Canada, #82-624-X, 2012.

Telzer, Eva, Andrew J. Feligni, Matthew D. Lieberman, Michelle E. Miernichi, and Adriana Galvin. "The Quality of Adolescents' Peer Relationships Modulates Neural Sensitivity to Risk Taking." *SCAN* 10 (2015): 389–398.

Thornberg, Robert. "School Bullying as a Collective Action: Stigma Process and Identity Struggling." *Children and Society* 29 (2015): 310–320.

Waldram, James B., D. Ann Herring, and T. Kue Young. *Aboriginal Health in Canada: Historical, Cultural, and Epidemiological Perspectives, Second Edition.* Toronto: University of Toronto Press, 2006.

Wotherspoon. Terry. 2007. "Incorporation of Aboriginal Labour." In *Race and Racism in 21st-Century Canada: Continuity, Complexity and Change*, Sean P. Hier and Singh Bolaria, eds., 131–150. Peterborough: Broadview Press, 2007.

Viveiros de Castro, Eduardo. 1998. "Cosmological Deixis and Amerindian Perspectivism." *Journal of the Royal Anthropological Institute* 4, no. 3 (1998): 469–488.

Whitehead, Paul C., and Michael J. Hayes. 1998. *The Insanity of Alcohol: Social Problems in Canadian First Nations Communities*. Toronto: Canadian Scholars' Press, 1998.

Yamashita, Takashi, and Suzanne Kunkel. "An International Comparison of the Association Among Literacy, Education and Health Across the United States, Canada, Switzerland, Italy, Norway and Bermuda: Implications for Health Disparities." *Journal of Health Communication* 20 (2015): 406–415.

Chapter Three

Disordered Minds and Disordered Bodies

Stigma, Depression, and Obesity Syndemic in Puerto Rico

Shir Lerman

Obesity and depression are syndemically interconnected and stigmatized illnesses with underlying structural factors, such as poverty, sexism, and racism (Diaz et al. 2001; Stevens-Watkins et al. 2014; Williams et al. 2007). Owing to the inherent visibility of obesity and ensuing societal and internalized shaming due to assumed laziness and lack of will power, individuals with obesity are at risk for developing depression (Fettich and Chen 2012). The experiences of being stigmatized causes affected individuals to "internalize perceived prejudices and develop negative feelings about themselves . . . which is manifested by decreased self-esteem and increased depression" (Latalova et al. 2014:1399). Conversely, depression stigma contributes to obesity via the overconsumption of high-carb foods as a coping mechanism (Bornstein et al. 2006).

Obesity and depression are both highly prevalent in Puerto Rico. Puerto Rico, as a U.S. Commonwealth, is a politically liminal territory without the full rights of U.S. states, which in turn contributes to the island's high rates of poverty and violence due to limited funding, the U.S. monopoly over trade rights, and competition for jobs. Depression is prevalent on the island due to prolonged stress over political uncertainty, colonization, poverty, and unemployment. Depression is stigmatized on the island due to an assumption of its connection with lack of self-control and the consumption of Western media and *telenovelas*, which emphasize a slender body ideal (Rodriguez-Soto 2013). Obesity is prevalent in Puerto Rico, due to a high-fat, high-carbohydrate diet that is historically and culturally tied to Puerto Rico's status as first a Spanish territory and subsequently, since 1898, its marginalization by the United States (Colón-López et al. 2014; Ortiz Cuadra 2013).

Based on data collected over almost a year of ethnographic research between 2012 and 2014, I argue that not only are obesity and depression both highly stigmatized on the island, but also that together they interact to form a syndemic relationship within the context of Puerto Rico's intractable and stigmatizing sociopolitical liminality, which in turn perpetuates the high rates of obesity and depression on the island.

SYNDEMICS

The author frames her research within syndemics theory, which expands upon earlier models of illness to address the sociopolitical and biological influences on illness interconnections and interactions (Singer et al. 2015). Syndemic illnesses are the result of deleterious interactions and consequences, through socio-physiological, biopolitical, and psychosocial pathways that produce disease burdens worse than the mere additive effects of two or more simultaneous diseases (Singer 2009). As with other conditions that occur largely in conditions of structural inequality, obesity and depression are more likely to occur for populations in certain marginalizing sociopolitical conditions, such as poverty, crime, unemployment, domestic violence, racism, sexism, and political immobility (Belle and Doucet 2003; Hanandita and Tampubolon 2014; Weaver and Mendenhall 2014). The biological and sociopolitical interconnections of depression and obesity interact with one another deleteriously. For these reasons, in this chapter, I foreground the biological and structural interactions between these two conditions, to highlight the role of stigma in producing deleterious health complications known as syndemics.

Stigma

Among the early Greeks and Romans, a stigma was a physical indication of deviance or marginal social status, a mark upon the body signifying that an individual was not a full member of society (Goffman 1963; Jones and Corrigan 2014). Since then, stigma has also come to encompass social marks of abhorrent behavior (Jones and Corrigan 2014). Erving Goffman (1963:3) defines stigma as "an attribute that is deeply discrediting," and which would cause an individual to be socially rejected. Goffman categorized stigma into three types: abominations of the body (physical deformities), blemishes of the individual character that are "perceived as weak will," and negative racial, national, and religious tribal identities (Goffman 1963:4). Stigma delineates the social distance between people in power, who stigmatize others and draw power from the process, and those who are stigmatized as outsiders (Link and Phelan 2001; Schabert et al. 2013). Stigmatizing others is a "tactical response to perceived threats, real dangers, and fear of the unknown" (Jenkins and Carpenter-Song 2008:382) that delegitimizes not only the stigmatized conditions but also the person and his or her experiences and interpretations.

Depression and obesity in particular are highly stigmatized; obesity is an abomination of the body and depression is a blemish of the individual character (Puhl and Brownell 2003; Quinn and Chaudoir 2009; Sartorius 2007). Depression stigma contributes to isolation from friends, family, and coworkers, due in part to the perceived shame and stigma of having depression; the isolation, in turn, propagates depression (Harpham et al 2007; Keeler et al. 2014). Obesity stigma, due in great part to the visibility of obesity, is often disguised within the pretext of concerns over the health consequences of obesity (Huizinga et al. 2009).

DEPRESSION

Major chronic depression (henceforth depression), a common mental illness, defines a collection of symptoms, such as sleepiness, consistently disheartened moods, and feelings of worthlessness, that affect approximately 350 million people worldwide; by 2020, depression is projected to impose the second-largest burden of ill health worldwide (National Alliance on Mental Illness 2013; National Institutes of Mental Health 2012). Research indicates that depression is strongly correlated with other illnesses, including obesity (Brewis 2011; Murphy et al. 2009). This correlation suggests the possibility of syndemic interaction between these two significant threats to health, an issue examined in this chapter.

Inequality, particularly in the forms of poverty, discrimination, sexism, and racism, is a major contributing factor to the onset of depression (Belle and Doucet 2003; Galea et al. 2007; Ro 2014; Williams et al. 2007). Chronic depression associated with sustained poverty increases the production of the hormone cortisol, which decreases stress-induced cellular inflammation. While short-term cellular inflammation reduction is beneficial, cortisol's long-term efforts to reduce inflammation suppresses the immune system, which puts individuals more at risk for developing other diseases (Brindley and Rolland 1989; Chiodini et al. 2007; Everson et al. 2002). The poverty, discrimination, and violence that predict depression include inadequate financial or educational opportunities and a lack of a strong and buffering social support network that enables some people to cope with the insults and injuries of poverty, homophobia, sexism, and racism (Diaz et al. 2001; Stevens-Watkins et al. 2014; Sutton et al. 2011). Fifteen percent of

Americans living below the U.S. federal poverty line report having depression, compared with 6.2 percent of Americans living at or above the federal poverty line (Pratt and Brody 2014). As one stark example of the applied implications of these statistics, childhood exposure to maternal depression detrimentally affects development: 28 percent of poor mothers report having depression compared to 17 percent of non-poor mothers, which is found to have adverse outcomes for child linguistic, cognitive, social, and motor development (Petterson and Albers 2001).

Depression is highly stigmatized; depression stigma insidiously affects social interactions, employment opportunities, self-esteem, and feelings of demoralization (Corrigan and Kosyluk 2014). Mental illness stigma reaches back to 5000 BCE, when Neolithic peoples would trepan the skulls of people whom they believed to be acting strangely and possessed by evil spirits (Foerschner 2010). In ancient Mesopotamia and Persia, mental illnesses were also seen as signs of demonic possession, and priests would treat the mentally ill in religious ceremonies (Alexander and Selesnick 1966). While ancient Greek physicians Hippocrates and Galen insisted that mental illnesses were natural processes and not spiritual diseases, the myth of mental illness as a sign of moral degeneracy persisted, and priests would often perform exorcisms on the mentally ill. With the advent of psychiatric institutions in the 13th century following the establishment of the Bethlem Royal Hospital in England (known colloquially and notoriously as Bedlam), living conditions for the mentally ill were often hellish: institution staff regularly abused, raped, and starved their patients (Porter 2002). Despite deinstitutionalization in the 1960s, people with mental illnesses are still viewed with suspicion and mistrust (Puhl and Heuer 2009). The social stigma attached to depression prevents sufferers from seeking help, and decreases their overall health and quality of life (Quinn and Chaudoir 2009; Sartorius 2007).

OBESITY

Obesity, a condition characterized by excessive adipose (fat) tissue, has gradually transformed from an expression of wealth and beauty in many cultures into an indicator of ill health and poverty (Farrell 2011; Greenhalgh 2015). In food-scarce societies, bodies with extra fat were often seen as desirable and an indication of wealth and social class in times when the over-abundance of food was an extreme rarity. Wealthy individuals in Europe and East Asia of the Middle Ages and Renaissance displayed obesity as 'badges of office,' therein announcing their ability to procure large quantities of rich foods (Bloomgarden 2003). Mechanical innovations during the Industrial Revolution in the late nineteenth century made cheaply produced, nutritionally poor foods widely accessible, and coupled with increased sedentism brought on by television consumption, obesity became more common (Caballero 2007).

Currently, slightly over one-third (35.7 percent) of Americans are obese (National Institute of Diabetes and Digestive and Kidney Disorders 2015). Obesity is a risk factor for other health concerns, including those examined in this chapter: diabetes and depression (Hayes et al. 2015; Shakher and Barnett 2009; Wagner et al. 2013; Whitmore 2010). It is also a heavy economic burden, due to the direct costs of treatment and the indirect costs of morbidity and mortality (such as missed workdays, higher healthcare insurance premiums, and lower wages due to obesity stigma) (Hammond and Levine 2010). The economic burden of obesity in the United States in 2008 was $147 billion, with adults with obesity spending 42 percent more on healthcare than adults without obesity, while researchers estimate that by 2030, these costs will rise by $48–66 million per year (Cawley and Meyerhoefer 2012; Padula et al. 2013; Wang et al. 2011).

Poverty is a major contributor to obesity (Brewis 2011; Brown and Konner 1987; Moffat 2010), more so among women than men (Bellisari 2016). Women who grew up in lower-income families tend to develop obesity as adults, and women with obesity are more likely to live in poverty, regardless of childhood economic status (Pudrovska et al. 2014). Furthermore, working long hours, urban slums, limited access to healthcare, a breakdown in social support, and the mechanization of labor-intensive jobs with an ensuing decrease in physical activity each contribute to the development of obesity (Mendenhall 2012). Low-income and ethnic minority families are also more frequently exposed to obesogenic advertising, such as sodas, fast food, and video games (Kumanyika and Grier 2006; Yancey et al. 2009), which propagate norms about culturally acceptable foods and standard body size, and perpetuate the inaccessibility of healthy foods for those communities.

The obese body is intensely politicized and highly stigmatized in Western developed nations, and its stigmatization is sometimes called the last socially acceptable form of discrimination (Vartanian and Smyth 2013). Obese individuals are thought by many to be lazy, unintelligent, uninterested in their own appearances, and lacking in self-discipline, and are less likely to be hired for jobs or to qualify for health insurance than individuals without obesity (Puhl and Brownell 2001; Wang et al. 2007). Beginning with the Industrial Revolution and continuing through the Cold War, large-scale military competition with the Soviet Union to produce the "healthiest citizens" underlined a shift from obesity as an indication of wealth to a moral marker of perceived laziness and unwillingness to serve one's country with one's body (Popkin 2009). This is particularly true for women, who joined the workforce in greater numbers between the 1880s and the 1920s; their more public roles as labor market employees made them vulnerable to appearance-based public scrutiny (Bellisari 2016). Indeed, women with obesity report decreased wages, earlier job termination, teasing, and lower self-esteem twice as frequently as men with obesity (Brewis 2014; Fettich and Chen 2012; Puhl and Heuer 2009). While both men and women feel the economic burden of obesity, women's estimated economic costs for obesity ($4,879/year are nearly twice as much) as are men's ($2,646/year), most of which is due to lower wages (Khazan 2014).

THE SYNDEMIC OF DEPRESSION AND OBESITY

Depression and obesity interact in a syndemic relationship, particularly in the context of poverty. Individuals with obesity are 20 times more likely than individuals without obesity to suffer from an episode of depression lasting for more than a year, and are five times more likely to gain additional weight than are individuals without depression (Brewis 2011; Murphy et al. 2009). The social stigma of obesity often contributes to the depression of individuals with obesity and contributes to the chronic psychological and physical chronic stress of obesity (Puhl and Heuer 2009). Obesity stigma contributes to self-imposed or socially sanctioned isolation, which leaves peopleightens the likelihood that people with obesity will suffer from depression (Puhl and Brownell 2006; Puhl and Heuer 2009).

Depression and obesity share several cyclical symptoms and health consequences, such as irregular sleeping and eating patterns (Gong et al. 2013), which make it easier for health care providers to overlook depression by attributing these factors solely to obesity. Depression causes the sufferer to either lose interest in eating and lose weight as a result, or to over-consume high-carbohydrate, high-sugar, high-fat foods and gain weight as a result (Sánchez-Villegas et al. 2012; Westover and Marganell 2002; Wurtman and Wurtman 1995). Foods with large quantities of carbohydrates, sugars, and fats are energy-dense, and the human body evolutionarily craves and stores these foods in order to save energy in case of food shortages (Bellisari 2016; Ulijaszek and Lofink 2006). Sweet, high-carbohydrate, high-fat foods trigger the production of serotonin, a hormone responsible for both happiness and suppressed appetite, by allowing the production of tryptophan, the building block of serotonin, at the expense of other hormones competing for access to the brain (Gibson 2006; Spring et al. 2008; Wurtman and Wurtman 1995).

While individuals with depression may gain psychopharmacological advantages by consuming food that triggers pleasant memories and the production of serotonin, those same foods also contain a lot of fat and cause substantial weight gain if consumed in large quantities (Wurtman and Wurtman 1995). Additionally, leptin, an adipose-produced hormone that controls fat distribution and food intake and is a key physiological indicator of obesity, is also correlated with depression. Despite elevated levels of the hormone due to increased amounts of adipose, increased leptin resistance contributes to difficulty recognizing satiety (Bornstein et al. 2006; Carter et al. 2013; Milaneschi et al. 2012). Leptin also regulates the Hypothalamic-Pituitary-Adrenal (HPA) axis, a set of direct feedback responses that loops between the hypothalamus, pituitary gland, and adrenal gland and which controls digestion, moods, reactions to stress (Bornstein et al. 2006; Gong et al. 2013). Increased levels of leptin have been found to over-stimulate the HPA axis, which places the body in a state of prolonged stress and depression (Carter et al. 2013; Gong et al. 2013), further exacerbating the cycle.

However, the exact cause-and-effect biological relationship of obesity and depression has yet to be explained in full. It is uncertain whether depression as an illness is present prior to the individual developing obesity, or vice versa (Patten et al. 2009; Serretti and Mandelli 2010).

PUERTO RICO, A STRUCTURAL SETTING FOR SYNDEMICS

Obesity and depression do not interact in a social vacuum. They build on one another synergistically and draw on their social environments. Puerto Rico provides a rich environment for depression and obesity to form a syndemic relationship, due to the island's status as a U.S. colony. Puerto Rico's proximity to the mainland United States and its current subordinate status as a U.S. commonwealth are strong factors influencing the complex identity of the island's people as simultaneously *Borinquen*, Caribbean, and American (Morris 1995; Thomas 2010). In 1917, President Woodrow Wilson signed the Jones-Shafroth Act, which "collectively made Puerto Ricans [restricted] United States citizens"; Puerto Ricans could thenceforth use U.S. passports and be conscripted for U.S. military service, but could not vote in presidential elections nor have congressional representation, instead having only a non-voting Resident Commissioner to represent the island in the U.S. House of Representatives. The island's status is liminal; Puerto Rico, according to the U.S. Congress in 1901, "belonging to . . . but not a part of" the United States. The U.S. Congress' policy has led to what Jorge Duany (2011) calls a "legally domestic, but culturally foreign" attitude toward Puerto Ricans that has done little to mitigate the felt effects of colonization. Puerto Rico's subaltern status (Grosfoguel 2003; Negrón-Portillo 1997) is based in American fear over adding a Hispanic state amid tensions over undocumented immigration from the wider world of Hispanic nations. This fear, in turn, draws on the inherent racism built into the United States' continuing occupation of Puerto Rico (Duany 2002; Grosfoguel 2003).

Puerto Rico's subaltern status is reflected in its economy. The 2008 economic crisis contributed to a per capita income of $15,200—half of Mississippi's (the poorest state in the Union) and a 2015 poverty rate of 46.2 percent—triple that of the national U.S. average (Alvarez 2014; Bishaw and Fontenot 2014; Chappatta 2016). Puerto Rico is $72 billion in debt to the United States and its "limited-state" status prohibits it from declaring bankruptcy, but with its 11.5 percent sales tax a discouragement to tourists (the bulk of Puerto Rico's industry), Puerto Rico's economy will not recover anytime soon (Alvarez 2014; Beyer 2015).

As this chapter will demonstrate, the political-economic climate contributes to increased obesity rates on the island, as well as to high rates of depression, as Puerto Ricans strive to redefine their relationship with the United States. Puerto Rico has a high adult obesity prevalence rate, with estimates ranging from 27.9 percent (CDC 2015a) to 40.8 percent (González et al. 2015; Pérez et al. 2013). In comparison, the adult obesity prevalence rate on the U.S. mainland is 34.9 percent for the overall population and 42.5 percent for the adult Hispanic population (CDC 2015b). A growing presence of mainland-based chain fast food restaurants, increasingly promoted by the commercial media, have established a permanent foothold on the island in recent decades as well, influencing the types of foods that are economically and geographically available to Puerto Ricans.

Puerto Rico's relationship with the United States exacerbates the high obesity rate on the island (Lerman 2016). The Jones Act, which dictates that only ships flying the U.S. flag may dock in Puerto Rico, contributes to economic and food dependency on the mainland: all foreign ships must dock at mainland U.S. ports first, even if they are carrying goods intended for Puerto Rico, and Puerto Ricans are required to pay additional taxes to compensate for the transportation of those goods, which account for 80 percent of all of the island's consumer goods (Duany 2002; Thomas 2010; Yost 2013). The high cost of food transportation and high taxes make it difficult to afford healthy foods.

With processed foods economically and energetically cheaper than home-grown and home-cooked foods (Gottlieb and Joshi 2010; Nestle 2007), Puerto Ricans on the island are rapidly transitioning into a population that consumes non-traditionally prepared soy and corn processed foods in lieu of local, home-cooked foods (Ortiz Cuadra 2013). This is particularly salient, as Puerto Rico has transformed from a primarily agricultural society under

Spanish rule, to a tourism-dependent urbanized society with limited agriculture and that consumes more and more processed foods (Colón-López et al. 2013; Ortíz Cuadra 2013). Moreover, 75 percent of Puerto Rico's population lives in the highly urbanized San Juan metropolitan area, which has limited space for growing produce at home (Garza et al. 2011; Ortiz Cuadra 2013). Due to decreased federal funding, public schools on the island have cut recess, which leaves children without the opportunity for the daily exercise and sports training they need to lead healthy lives, further exacerbating obesity rates on the island (Acosta-Pérez et al. 2012; Duany 2002). With nearly half of Puerto Rico's population living below the poverty line and with the increase of imported American foods on the island, particularly in the urban areas such as San Juan, obesity is the norm (Colon et al. 2013; Fitzgerald 2010; González et al. 2015).

To develop this chapter, I draw on extensive ethnographic data collected at a diabetes clinic in San Juan, Puerto Rico between May and August 2012.[1] Given the high prevalence rate of diabetes in Puerto Rico (Lerman 2016), and the near-universal co-occurrence of diabetes and obesity in the final sample ($n = 60$; 60 percent co-occurrence), the diabetes clinic proved a strategic site for collecting ethnographic data on the health issues of concern in this chapter. The data that inform the conceptual syndemic model and theoretical argument at the heart of this chapter include demographics and qualitative findings from semi-structured interviews on depression, obesity, and Puerto Rican identity.

ETHNOGRAPHIC PATHWAYS OF INTERACTION

Depression

Participants perceived depression symptoms psychosomatically: changes in appetite were the most commonly cited depression side effect ($n = 11$), followed by tiredness ($n = 9$), not wanting to get out of bed ($n = 8$), and changes in mood (particularly increased irritability, sensitivity, and crying) ($n = 8$). Because depression primarily affects mood, there was no perception of physiological inevitability about developing depression; blame for the illness' etiology is placed firmly on the individual, regardless of extenuating and contextualizing circumstances.

Depression stigma also contributed to a profound lack of open discussion about the illness. Fear of exposure was a concern for participants with depression, particularly since depression is a concealable state. Once depression was reported, it was no longer concealed and exposed the individual to more active forms of stigma directed specifically at that individual. Due to the fear of stigmatization, individuals with depression infrequently seek therapeutic help, and avoid disclosing their depression to their friends and family (Corrigan and Kosyluk 2014; Shidhaye and Kermode 2013). There are no public announcements about depression in Puerto Rico beyond the occasional television commercial for antidepressants. Furthermore, participants thought of depression as a personal process, oftentimes not telling anyone beyond a spouse about their depression. One participant, "Anabel Jiménez Ortiz"[2] was uncharacteristically open about the silence surrounding depression:

> I think maybe my mother had [depression], but we didn't talk about it. I was a kid, you know? Parents don't tell their kids about it, kids don't need to know that kind of stuff about their parents. I don't even know if she told my dad. I'm not sure what caused it for her. We don't hear about depression on the news, no one talks about it.

Anabel was an undergraduate Spanish literature major at the University of Puerto Rico and worked at her coffee shop in Viejo San Juan for three years to support herself. Even though she lived at home, she never discussed depression with her mother, and while she herself suffered from depression, did not seek help for it:

> No, I don't have the time for [help]. I work at a coffee shop, so I'm always busy working or studying. Besides, if I went to a doctor, it would go on my record. I don't want my future job potentially finding out about it, they wouldn't trust me. I want to be a professor, or maybe a politician. If I go into politics and they find out about my depression, that's it. My career in politics will be over. It's not fair, but what can I do? I try to meditate and go for walks.

"Gustavo Ruíz Molina," an accountant, also downplayed his depression, stating it was no one else's business:

> No, I haven't told anyone about having depression. Why should I? I don't need to make a big deal about it, because it's nobody else's business. I take a pill and that's it. Only my wife knows. We Puerto Ricans like to talk, but no one talks about depression because it's seen as not being very strong, especially not manly. There are just people floating around, pretending to be fine, but no one supports one another for this kind of thing. I almost didn't tell *you*, except that who are you going to tell? You don't know anyone I know, and you'll return home.

The lack of open communication about depression, both in public and between family members, highlighted how negatively depression is seen. Gustavo suspected that his uncle and sister both had depression, but due to the lack of communication surrounding depression, no one discussed it. Gustavo's uncle would later die due to undisclosed reasons; his parents would only say that his uncle had died because *la vida se lo trató mal* (life treated him badly).

Participants reported that there were few established social support networks for individuals with depression to use in building a sympathetic community, since forming one would involve publicly acknowledge having depression, and would indicate either a weak character or not being fully in control of one's reactions. Because of this, feelings of loneliness that were already part of depression were exacerbated, intensifying the depression experience and making it more difficult for participants to recover. For example, "Zaina Vásquez Colón" described her reluctance to discuss depression:

> No one talks about depression, you know? It's not like diabetes, where you hear about it all the time on the news. No one wants to admit to having depression. You don't talk to others to see how they're dealing with it. I wouldn't even know where to look for other people with depression. It makes depression worse, being so isolated.

Zaina lived in a large public housing project that had a reputation of being so dangerous and riddled with drugs and crime that the San Juan Metropolitan Police refused to enter the area. She told me that while the area wasn't *quite* as bad as the rumors suggested, it still had its dangerous moments, and that when she first moved to her apartment, she heard gunshots every night for a month before learning to ignore them. This living environment contributed both to Zaina's depression and to her reluctance to discuss her depression, for, as she told me, "Any sign of weakness can get you killed if you're not careful. People are always in each other's personal business." The combination of unsafe living conditions, the fear that these living conditions caused, and the fear of being exposed as having depression, all contributed to or exacerbated Zaina's depression.

Zaina's interview highlights both the role of stigma in depression perpetuation and the other factors that participants linked to the development of depression, including unemployment, the economy, fear of being the victim of crime, caring for family members, divorce, negative relationships with children and partners, and abuse. Not only does unemployment and employment insecurity contribute to depression, depression itself has severe implications for employment: with depression putting sufferers at risk for losing work due to depression-related missed work days (World Health Organization 2007). People living in poverty are at further risk for having prolonged symptoms because they are unable to afford proper treatment. Structural factors, manifested through high rates of poverty, unemployment, crime, and abuse, were the most frequently cited causes of ill health. Depression is known to syndemically interact with both neighborhood and individual poverty (Galea et al. 2007; Hanandita and Tampubolon 2014; Lund et al. 2010) and with being the target of intimate partner violence (Beydoun et al. 2012; Johnson et al. 2014; Ludermir et al. 2010). The interview with "Magdalena," a quiet woman in her mid-50s who works as a janitor for the University of Puerto Rico, took place in her apartment on her day off from work, over coffee. Magdalena contextualized her depression within the stresses of family and the myriad problems of living in Puerto Rico, particularly the financial strain of affording medical treatment:

> I was a victim of psychological abuse from my husband—he mistreated me for many years because he lost his job and was upset about being stuck at home, and finally I had to divorce him because I couldn't continue living with him, he hurt me very much. I still have symptoms: sometimes I'm afraid to leave the house, and I feel bad having fun—it's taking me time to heal.

"Luis," an electrician and boys' afterschool soccer coach, separately elaborated on the same point,

> With the economy and crime as they are, there are a lot of problems here, and people can't understand why. They don't want to talk about it: they don't go to the doctor to talk, and politicians don't want to do anything. Everyone's depressed as a result.

Luis' wife had died of breast cancer 19 months before our interview, leaving him with three children, a large stack of hospital bills, and a spiraling depression that he could not control. He credited his children and coaching his boys' soccer team with giving him a sense of purpose and a reason to leave the house. Even so, Luis worried about the environment in which his children were living, telling me that the high crime and poverty in San Juan were bad influences on them and that he worried about how they would live once they reached adulthood.

"María García," a seamstress and music teacher who picked up work wherever she could, explained:

> Well, stress caused my depression. My mother has Alzheimer's, and it's very difficult for me to take care of her. My daughter has a baby but the baby's father left and doesn't want to help her take care of him, so I need to help her take care of the baby as well. It's very difficult to live in Puerto Rico; there are no jobs, and the economy's bad. Also, my health insurance doesn't pay the full bill to see a psychologist, and psychologists cost a lot of money.

Bernardo owned a local convenience store and talked to many of the customers who passed through his store. He told me that while none of his customers explicitly admitted to having depression, many of them would hang out in his store and talk for lack of a better place to go. Many of his customers discussed the problems they were having without acknowledging that depression was the cause:

> Depression is a big problem in Puerto Rico, although not everyone calls it that. They'll talk about the problems they're having, though. There's a lot of problems, child abuse, men abusing their wives, a lot of fighting. We all have the same problem here, with the economy and problems with the family, and there's a lot of crime. I don't feel very safe living here, but it's my home.

María, Bernardo, Luis, and Magdalena's accounts were emblematic of interactions between depression and structural and interpersonal violence endemic to Puerto Rico and similar settings. The fighting and domestic abuse that participants reported, were a manifestation of the anger and fear that many felt after the economic crash, which the government was unable to prevent. The fighting and domestic violence were attempts to regain control over life, particularly over known factors: family members (Rabbani et al. 2008; Swan and Snow 2006; Umberson et al. 1998). Participants reported losing hope that their situations would improve, which they feel contributes to the higher depression rates. The economic crash and ensuing fewer resources also contributed to the high crime rates, particularly among the younger generations that could not find jobs and did not have any money saved. Ultimately, depression was seen as a result of life's stressors, particularly interpersonal stressors that could not be easily fixed. However, while the stressors were significant, and oftentimes long lasting, many participants emphasized not changing the stressors themselves, but rather how they themselves responded to the stressors. Depression was thus seen as a lapse in someone's control over his or her reactions, and it was each person's responsibility to get the help they needed. Placing the blame directly on the individual is a common feature in depression stigma (Angermeyer and Matschinger 2003; Phelan et al. 2013). The stigma surrounding depression prevented participants from seeking help: 80 percent of the participants either admitted to not seeking help when they needed it for depression, or stating that they would not seek help for it if they did have depression. This alarming statistic highlights the pressing need for increased community outreach programs on depression and the need to combat depression stigma.

Obesity

Unlike with depression, participants needed no coaxing to discuss obesity, obesity stigma, and food access; indeed, these were favorite topics among the participants, and many broached the topics before I had the opportunity to do so. Access to healthy food was a common problem in Puerto Rico and one that all of the participants shared. Many participants bonded with their friends and neighbors over the difficulty of buying healthy, affordable food on a regular basis, and particularly the difficulty that this presented in preparing food for their families and friends. Feeding others was an expression of love in Puerto Rico (Ortiz Cuadra 2013; Saldaña and Felix 2011), and participants were frustrated that they were unable to feed their loved ones as they wanted. Plump bodies are historically valued in Puerto Rico as being "embedded in a social network and . . . connected in a community of caring that has kept one well-fed" (Poponoe 2004:5; Rodriguez-Soto 2013). However, with the economic crisis causing Puerto Ricans to move to the United States in search of employment and the ensuing fracturing of tightly knit social networks, the participants are unable to afford healthy food, and plump bodies as the representations of communal love loses meaning. The simultaneous consumption of Western media in Puerto Rico has increased the desire for slender bodies and the burgeoning stigmatization of plump bodies.

I met with Zaina in her apartment, where we drank *café con leche*, ate *besitos de coco*,[3] and talked about health and politics. Zaina told me:

> My daughter is heavy. She's really smart—a pharmacist—but she has so much trouble getting a job! No one wants a fat pharmacist, they ask why they should take advice from someone who can't take care of her own weight. Everyone else here is fat, so is everyone lazy, too?

Zaina's concerns about obesity stigma in both the health and the lay environments resonated in other participants' interviews. Luis Pacheco Rivera took a broader view. He often fixed televisions as part of his job as an electrician, and he told me how his customers would discuss their favorite television programs with him while he worked. The television program that his customers watched most frequently, Luis explained, was the *telenovela*, an observation that I had noticed in the constant stream of *telenovelas* playing in the clinic where she worked. *Telenovelas*, Luis opined, represented the body issues that so many Puerto Ricans have developed in the last three or four decades:

> Obesity is relatively new in Puerto Rico, at least as a problem. Girls want to be skinny because of what they see on TV, and they make fun of the overweight girls. These girls who are teased, they try to become skinny, but they eat bad food, and they grow up with huge self-esteem issues. So they're depressed, and they try to push their own daughters to be really skinny. It never stops.

Luis' astute observation ties into gendered experiences of obesity. While both men and women in Puerto Rico and worldwide have obesity, women are more likely than men to experience stigma for having obesity: women are judged much more harshly on the basis of their appearance than are men, and as mentioned earlier, obese women have reported bullying, earlier job termination, and lower mental health outcomes twice as frequently as men with obesity (Brewis 2014; Fettich and Chan 2012; Puhl and Heuer 2009). In Puerto Rico, body size ideals are becoming smaller just as both obesity *and* obesity stigma are on the rise (Brewis et al. 2011), due to a combination of exposure to Westernized foods, changing family norms, and a consumption of Western media (Rodriguez-Soto 2013). Olga Ocasio Pagán, a legal aide, pointed out people and foods to me as we sat at a café enjoying *tres leches.*[4]

> We show love through food, and we feed skinny babies so they'll grow. It's normal in Puerto Rico. But now the doctors tell us that we're all fat, that we must lose weight, that we should eat healthier foods. They shame their patients into feeling guilty about enjoying life and eating good food with their families. . . . I'm not saying that being really heavy is healthy, mind you. I see some of the really heavy people, and they have trouble walking. But we don't need to be really skinny, either! We can enjoy *tres leches* and *flan* on occasion.

Olga's comments evoke "nostalgic gastronomy," a means of remaining connected to the home culture in the face of gastronomic changes while eating mainstream foods is a way to easily, visibly assimilate (Aranda 2007; Mankekar 2005). Food preparation and consumption reveal a lot about how people identify their cultural groups, their political, religious, and socioeconomic identifications, and the lens through which they interpret the world (Ortíz Cuadra 2013). These processes allow people to 'partake each day of the national past' (Barthes 2013:27) and unite them under the banner of nationality that offers cultural continuity in the face of change. They also offer insight into how people interact with and perceive others (Ortíz Cuadra 2013). In terms of obesity in Puerto Rico, it is insufficient to contextualize food access solely within the socioeconomic milieu. This chapter frames obesity and depression within the struggle to break away from American colonialism and create a unique Puerto Rican national identity by consuming the traditional Puerto Rican diet in the face of biomedical health practitioners' warnings to the contrary and the changes in physical activity that originally underlined the need for high-calorie diets. Processed foods (e.g., soda, candy, and fast food), which have become part and parcel of the globalized food market, have also become part of the standard Puerto Rican diet: energy-dense home-cooked foods that dominate traditional Puerto Rican cuisine, such as *plátanos*,[5] *arroz con habichuelas*,[6] and *alcapurrias.*[7] High rates of poverty and the cheapness of processed unhealthy foods combine and contribute to an inability to maintain a healthy diet. While this is also true for many Americans in poverty

(Czyzewski 2011; Labonté and Schrecker 2007; Langellier et al. 2012), it is particularly so for Puerto Ricans when they need to buy produce instead of growing it as they have in the past because of the structural inequality produced by the colonial relationship with the United States that makes it more difficult and expensive for Islanders to either produce *or* import food. Healthy food has become financially inaccessible and its trade increasingly regulated, contributing to growing social discontent. Juan Santiago López explained,

> A lot of people [in Puerto Rico] are heavy—it has to do with habits and food, and to do with working a lot and being in a hurry, and the eating Fast Food: we work a lot, we don't have time to cook, we can't rest and enjoy life and do exercise. Everyone used to walk, but now we have cars—it's the time we live in. Healthy food is very expensive—we can't always buy food like that.

Participants defined healthy foods as fruits, vegetables, salads, chicken, and fish, and water as the healthiest beverage. They also considered home-prepared food to be healthy. However, they admitted to eating what they considered to be unhealthier food, such as fried food, due to a lack of time, energy, and finances to constantly prepare healthy food, and to predilections for fast food.

Participants frequently discussed food access and food preparation as precursors to obesity, especially a lack of time to prepare healthier food at home and a plethora of fast food restaurants and junk food. Not everyone lived close to a supermarket with healthy food options, and even for those that did live close[8] to such supermarkets, healthy food was economically inaccessible. A bad economy resulted in difficulty purchasing healthy food, and contributed to food deserts. Ezequiel phrased it bluntly,

> Look, to eat healthy food, we need to be able to buy healthy food. Supermarkets have healthy food, but they're located mostly in the touristy areas, which are expensive. You can buy the fruits off the side of the street [from vendors], but there aren't always quantities to prepare food for your family. The bus system in San Juan is crap, and nonexistent in the rest of Puerto Rico. No one likes carrying heavy food home every day. We need cars, and not everyone can afford one. The healthy food is expensive, too. Canola oil is maybe \$3, and olive oil is maybe \$10. If you have a large family to feed on a small income, which are you going to buy? Sometimes it's cheaper to take your family to McDonald's, where you can buy a meal for \$2. Canola oil, even for \$3, isn't a full meal; it's just oil. I'm a big supporter of *la comida criolla*, but sometimes it's impractical. We're poor and unhealthy and really fat.

Marisol Tirado Torres discussed food access during a longer conversation about her family, stating,

> I have five children. I would rather buy a big bag of rice that feeds us for four or five days, then buy a bag of apples that would last a day, if the kids even ate the apples. The apples might spoil because the kids wouldn't want apples. I'd pay more money for less food and wasting some food. I work two jobs, and don't always have time to go to the supermarket. The closest supermarket is a twenty-minute drive in rush-hour traffic, and I need to then go home and cook all of it before my night job. It's exhausting. My husband works two jobs and comes home too exhausted to go grocery shopping. We barely make enough to do all of this, much less buy all the healthy food the doctors tell us we need to eat. Sometimes I think that it's easier to just be fat, even if it's unhealthier.

The difficulties of healthy food access, ready availability of unhealthy but heavily advertised food options, and diminishing patterns of exercise, manifested as obesity, and while participants were cognizant of the ramifications of obesity, they felt they were unable to make the changes needed.

Depression and Obesity

Depression and obesity interacted syndemically in this participant cohort. Obesity, rooted in the conflict between desire for traditional foods and food inaccessibility, is the consequence of depression and Puerto Rican political changes. Food holds emotional meaning: people eat comfort foods to feel better, especially if those comfort foods are linked to happier times (Barthes 2013; Gibson 2006). Participants emphasized long-term unhealthy food consumption as both prerequisite to obesity and correlated with depression. In particular, participants perceived individuals with depression to be more likely to eat without paying attention to what they were eating. Hector Ayala Pérez, reflecting a pattern of individual blaming, described the obesity-depression relationship as mindless eating, laziness, and disinterest in the world:

> A depressed person doesn't care what he or she is doing, what he or she is eating; the person just eats and gains weight. They don't want to leave the house, they don't do anything but cry, they don't move their bodies. Fat people suffer from having fewer friends, from body pain, from being able to do less with their bodies, so they become depressed.

Elena Santiago del Valle also emphasized the laziness stereotype:

> Fat people have depression, they don't want to leave the house, they don't exercise, they don't like their bodies, they complain. Also, depressed people eat by themselves so they can eat whatever they want. They don't have a lot of friends, anyway.

Hector and Elena's assertions express the stigma surrounding the syndemic depression-obesity relationship, namely that individuals could either develop depression, eat a lot due to apathy and develop obesity, and then sink deeper into depression as a result of the weight gain and associated stigma, or they could consume large quantities of food as a result of other factors, gain weight, and then develop depression as a result. All participants drew connections between obesity and depression, interpreting depression as both a consequence of and a contributor to obesity. As Luis mentioned, much of the obesity stigma that he and others have noticed stemmed from observing body sizes on TV, which are noticeably thinner than body sizes in the general population (Harrison 2000; Ferguson et al. 2011). There is demonstrated research linking obesity, body surveillance, body shame, and disordered eating, particularly among adolescent girls (Neumark-Sztainer et al. 2006; Tiggemann and Kuring 2004). Adolescent girls who experience obesity stigma are more likely to engage in disordered eating, such as binge eating, vomiting, and abusing diet pills (Puhl and Latner 2007). Adolescent girls are also more likely to experience depression on account of experiencing obesity stigma, and depression is independently correlated with disordered eating, especially anorexia nervosa and bulimia nervosa (Neumark-Sztainer et al. 2006; Thompson 1992). In Puerto Rico, the desire to be thin exists concurrently with depression as more and more people struggle with obesity but idealize the thin body type that they regularly see on TV.

SOCIOSTRUCTURAL FACTORS AND DIETARY SHIFT

Depression also developed as a result of the attempted changes made to the Puerto Rican diet and identity. Participants emphasized unhealthy food consumption as both the prerequisite to and perpetuation of obesity, and perceived it was correlated with their own and others' depression. In particular, individuals with depression were thought to be more likely to eat without paying attention to what they were eating (Ogden et al. 2013; Wansink 2010).

The laziness stereotype, and depression as the perceived concurrent cause and side effect, that the participants used to frame obesity is a common perception of people with obesity, including as documented by other authors in this volume (Brewis 2014; Brewis and Wutich 2015; McLennan and Ulijaszek 2015; Puhl and Heuer 2009). However, the laziness stereotype does not address the underlying syndemic intersections of depression and obesity, particularly as these are exacerbated by the proliferation of foods with high-fructose corn syrup and addictive properties such as sugar and fat (Gottlieb and Joshi 2010; Jackson 2013; Nestle 2007). However, Gabriel Lebrón

Mercado had a different perspective on structural factors in the depression-obesity link. A bus driver, history buff, and active union member, Gabriel cut to the core of what he saw as the primary reason behind the high obesity and depression rates in Puerto Rico:

> If the person is relatively young and has unhealthy *alimentación*, that person can suffer from depression as an adult. When I was a boy, there weren't so many restaurants as there are today—it was more expensive to eat in restaurants, including fast food. Now, young people eat in fast food restaurants because they're less expensive, and obesity is much more common in young people these days. Obesity was not a big problem when I was a boy.

Zaina was more heated:

> You know the USDA area in the [Luis Muñoz Marín International] airport? It's interesting that they only make us go through USDA when traveling to the United States, like they don't trust us. I didn't need to go through USDA when I flew to the Dominican Republic. That's the whole attitude that the United States has about Puerto Rico: distrust. They don't trust us to be Puerto Rican, so they send down American restaurants and American stores and we get diabetes from the American food because it's cheaper than buying fresh, which the American government makes more expensive. You were asking me about depression earlier. This is why everyone's depressed.

Zaina's observations are emblematic of the complicated relationships that Puerto Rico has with the mainland United States. The U.S. colonialism and subsequent structural factors that contribute to the linked realities of expensive produce, government corruption, and overall negative health outcomes on the island also affect islanders' mental health and overall outlook. In particular, due to the aforementioned Jones Act, elevated food prices due to import fees dictate food prices on the island, and the comparative cheapness of American fast food chains means that available healthy foods are limited. Participants were well aware of the politics of this and of the ensuing impact on the elevated obesity and diabetes rates in Puerto Rico, and it caused them significant mental distress.

The frequency and addictive qualities of fast foods add to the burden of combating obesity, particularly among people with depression who may already be predisposed to eat high quantities of foods high in sugars, fats, and carbohydrates. Sweet, high-carbohydrate, high-fat foods trigger the production of serotonin, a hormone responsible for both increased mood and suppressed appetite, by allowing the production of tryptophan, the building block of serotonin, at the expense of other hormones competing for access to the brain (Gibson 2006; Popkin 2009; Spring et al. 2008; Wurtman and Wurtman 1995). There is research looking at the relationship between depression and fructose malabsorption, a disorder in which the small intestine does not process fructose as well as it should, contributing to high levels of undigested fructose in the body and subsequent bloating, cramping, and diarrhea. Research suggests that fructose reacts with and reduces levels of tryptophan in women with fructose malabsorption, making them more vulnerable to developing depression (Deans 2011; Ledochowski et al. 2000; Varea et al. 2005). The over-consumption of cheap foods rich in carbs, fats, and sugars worsen the obesity-depression relationship both by increasing the rates of fructose and fats in the blood (Deans 2011; Varea et al. 2005) and by being marketed specifically for people who already live in poverty and are unable to afford the healthier, more expensive food items (Gottlieb and Joshi 2010; Nestle 2007). Mainland-based fast food restaurants established a permanent foothold on the island in the late 1950s (Rosa 2005), influencing the types of foods that are economically and geographically available to Puerto Ricans. With the plethora of high-carb, high-fat, high-sugar foods available in restaurants and supermarkets in Puerto Rico, Puerto Ricans are at high risk of developing both obesity and depression which reinforce and exacerbate each other and worsen the health consequences of each, in this structural setting.

Puerto Rican Political-Economy

The first interview topic to reach data saturation was whether participants trusted their government, to which the answer was a resounding 'no.' Participants did not trust either the Puerto Rican or the U.S. federal government, regardless of who was in power in which government. Adrian Correa Madera resignedly described Puerto Rican politics to me:

> We always vote for people we hope will do a better job, although we're all pretty fatalistic about the entire process. Fortuño didn't do a good job, and neither does Padilla now. [The author conducted these interviews in 2012 and 2014, during the tenures of Fortuño and Padilla, respectively.] Obama says he'll do whatever we choose, and we try, but . . . nothing. Regardless of what you want to happen to Puerto Rico, we've all given up a bit, as nothing ever changes. It's depressing. We eat and we drink and we don't work, because honestly, what else can we do?

María expressed her frustration over loving Puerto Rico but seeing the island mired in problems and watching friends and family move to the mainland:

> There are a lot of people here that suffer from depression. The economy's bad, there's no work, everyone wants to leave Puerto Rico for the United States to look for work, but they don't find work in the U.S., so they return, and then

> they're depressed again. It's a beautiful island with a lot of problems, an ugly paradise. My friends and family who have looked for work in the U.S. have told me that *they* were told that there are already too many Puerto Ricans in the U.S. and they don't need *more*. And that's despite our being legally able to work anywhere in the U.S., too.

Anabel was poetic:

> A lot of other Hispanics hate us because we're a U.S. Territory, they don't think that we're Hispanic because we get the privileges. How do we explain to our kids that they should be proud of being P.R. but that when they go to get a passport, they need to get a U.S. passport instead of a P.R. one? Everyone's very frustrated because the U.S. has been like this for a long time. They don't hate US citizens, but they hate the government. We can't keep going with our current status. I so wish we could have full independence, but we won't get any better. Statehood would help us with the economy, at least.

Anabel had worked at her coffee shop in Viejo San Juan for three years to support herself through college and was active in local protests and union meetings. Anabel was careful to distinguish between the U.S. government and regular Americans, acknowledging that, like in Puerto Rico, private citizens are not the same as the government that represents them.

María, Anabel, and Adrian's comments reveal an understanding of Puerto Ricanness as a stigmatized identity. Being Puerto Rican, seen by other Hispanic groups as "not sufficiently Hispanic" due to Puerto Rico's "owned status" and seen by the United States government as not fully part of the United States, leaves Puerto Ricans as a stigmatized "other" no matter how Puerto Ricans identify themselves (Negrón-Muntaner 2007; Ramos-Zayas 2003). The fact that so many Puerto Ricans live below the federal poverty line contributes to the stigma surrounding the island. Poverty is a stigmatized state (Reutter et al. 2009; Tabuchi et al. 2012; Wutich et al. 2014); despite the high poverty rate in Puerto Rico, the United States government continues to ignore Puerto Rico's living conditions, which affords the United States the economic benefits of having a territory (e.g., less money dedicated to federal programs such as Medicaid) without needing to dirty its hands with a poverty-stricken island (Alvarez and Goodnough 2015).

In particular, the Cabotage Law severely impacts Puerto Rico's economy, as tourists from places with higher taxes will visit more affordable locations. Many participants lost their jobs and were unable to afford healthy food, and the unemployment rates and tough economic climate contributed to participants experiencing a loss of control over their lives, which, in turn, led to increased domestic problems as families attempted to make do with fewer resources.

CONCLUSIONS AND RECOMMENDATIONS

Obesity and depression are both stigmatized states—as is Puerto Rico itself. The associated stigma mediates the relationship between the two illnesses, with obesity stigma increasing the risk for depression by creating social isolation and decreasing job and romantic prospects. In turn, depression stigma also creates social isolation and constant stress and triggers the development of obesity through comfort eating and the overproduction of cortisol, which is responsible for increased storage of abdominal body fat. Stigma reflects the positionality of power and inequality (Link and Phelan 2001; Schabert et al. 2013). It delineates between those in power, who stigmatize others and draw power from the process, and those who are stigmatized as outsiders. In the case of Puerto Rico, not only are depression and obesity stigmatized illnesses, but being Puerto Rican is also a stigmatized state that overlays the damaging structural syndemic factors of both depression and obesity. Children and adolescents with obesity did not do as well in school due to bullying and low self-esteem, and adults with obesity had more difficulty finding employment than their non-obese peers, which contributed to feelings of low self-worth and low mood (Latner et al. 2012; Puhl and Heuer 2010). In turn, the isolation and loneliness that develop with depression frequently motivate individuals to eat to "feel better" and gain weight as a result (Goodman and Whitaker 2002). The reality of being Puerto Rican led to suffering under high, imposed taxes on imported produce and to limited funding for physical activity programs, colonialist attitudes toward islanders, CDC aerial spraying without Puerto Rican permission, and the severe economic crisis that underlies outrageously high unemployment, crime rates, and related high rates of depression and obesity.

Participants suggested that structural changes, such as poverty, violence, and unemployment and associated lifestyle challenges are influential in their prevalence of obesity and depression. High rates of poverty and unemployment ensure that not only are obesity and depression prevalent in Puerto Rico, but that the illnesses feed into one another in a synergistic downward spiral. Due to the high unemployment rate, many cannot afford healthy food leading to an over-consumption of cheap, unhealthy food. This is exacerbated by living in unsafe neighborhoods and the negative impact of this on exercise and play. As a result of these structural and dietary changes, more people became at higher risk of developing obesity. The economic and occupational instability also contribute to increased risk for developing depression. Having depression has, in turn, contributed to a worsened diet, a lack of a stable and consistent social support network, and missed medical appointments, all of which worsen the risk and the side effects of obesity.

This syndemic develops and is worsened via institutionally produced economic instability, social fear, and artificially exacerbated nutritional pathways, which interact through the violence, crime, and political subalternity that plague Puerto Rico as a result of its historical and ongoing relationship to the United States. Contributing to the increased obesity rates on the island, as well as to the high rates of depression as Puerto Ricans strove to redefine their relationship with the United States, U.S. Cabotage laws and Puerto Rico's geographic distance from the mainland cause Puerto Ricans to pay more in fees and taxes for food shipped from the United States. Due to high and chronic levels of poverty, unemployment, crime, and violence in Puerto Rico under the economic crisis at the time, many of the participants were afraid to leave their houses for fear of their safety, and did not have steady employment. As a result, their physical activity levels were low—combined with the cheap, unhealthy foods they could afford to eat and could actually acquire on the island, this contributed to high rates of obesity. Participants also saw food (overconsumption) as the mediating factor between diabetes and depression, and as representative of Puerto Rico's political subalternity. The "traditional" Puerto Rican diet, as a result of long-term colonization, is high in carbohydrates and fats and relatively low in fresh fruits and vegetables. Participants cooked primarily Puerto Rican foods at home and struggled with maintaining the traditional diet in the face of both decreased levels physical activity and increasing food prices, while also facing diabetes and obesity diagnoses their providers likely told them were worsened by their culturally comforting food customs.

Puerto Rico's political status profoundly affects Puerto Rico's economic crisis, highlighting the island's multilayered dependency on the mainland and the need for immediate action. Puerto Rico's economic crisis crippled its workforce, is a major impetus for increased migration to the mainland in search of work, and prevents people from *returning* to the island (Gillespie 2015; Krogstad 2015). Because of the United States' continued resistance to making Puerto Rico a full state or granting it independence, the island cannot file for bankruptcy or otherwise change its own laws to improve its economy. Furthermore, the current Zika virus epidemic strongly affects Puerto Rico: with 5,500 confirmed cases (including 672 pregnant women) as of mid-2016 and the CDC estimating thousands more are infected each day, tourists have been warned to stay away from the island, further worsening the island's economy (McNeil 2016). Aerial spraying of NALED, a chemical toxic to bees, birds, and fish, to combat the virus has also caused thousands of Puerto Ricans to march against both the spraying and purported testing of these chemicals on Puerto Ricans, furthering the rift between Puerto Ricans and the U.S. federal government (McNeil 2016).

For this population, Puerto Rico is at an untenable crossroads. The island is caught between historically devastating structural factors and trying to escape from a black hole in which the structural factors and their associated health problems form a syndemic. Puerto Rico's political status makes it difficult for Puerto Rico to receive sufficient resources to address the structural problems that are the foundation of this (and likely other) syndemics that exist on the island. Having diabetes contributes to and worsens the presence of depression and vice versa. Both illnesses are grounded in the consumption of unhealthy food, which, in turn, is based on limited access to healthy food and a reliance on motorized transportation. Obesity increases depression and self-blame for diabetes. Abuse and high crime and unemployment also contribute to earlier onset depression, which, in turn, contributes to earlier onset diabetes.

The syndemic relationship between obesity and depression is mediated, produced, and exacerbated by structural factors such as poverty, racism, and colonization, all of which are inherent to the relationship between the United States and Puerto Rico. The participants' discussions of living with obesity and depression in Puerto Rico reveal that the two illnesses interact syndemically in their own and their loved ones' lives. Both depression and obesity stigma are emblematic of and closely tied to ongoing structural issues in Puerto Rico. Obesity stigma is representative of Puerto Rico's liminal status, of being caught between traditional Puerto Rican foods and changing social norms surrounding body size despite more and more Puerto Ricans developing obesity. Depression develops as a result of the fear generated by rampant crime, the experience of interpersonal violence, frustration with political inaction, struggles with unemployment, and enduring poverty in Puerto Rico, but due to the attendant stigma, people do not feel comfortable asking for help.

This research has several implications, particularly for interventions. The diabetes clinic does not employ mental health specialists, although the healthcare practitioners do refer their patients to off-site mental health professionals. Given the high depression rate among individuals with diabetes, it would behoove the clinic to bring in mental health professionals (e.g., psychologists) to give presentations to all of the clinic's patients and staff on how to prevent or treat mental illnesses, in order to not single out any patients with a mental illness. These presentations could either be given separately or as part of the preexisting nutrition courses to ensure attendance, as patients might not attend a session solely on mental health. The mental health professionals running the sessions could provide some guidance and provide names of mental health specialist referrals if needed. In order to maintain their patients' privacy, doctors can tell their patients about the mental health aspect of the classes during checkups.

Patients should be actively involved in the healing process. Creating a patient network will allow patients to facilitate carpooling to supermarkets and perhaps pooling financial resources to purchase healthier food. Getting to know other individuals with diabetes in the same neighborhood might also offer the opportunity to create opportunities for walks together so that people do not need to walk outside by themselves. This might also offer people the opportunity to share healthy food recipes. Supermarkets could also be offered tax incentives to open branches in neighborhoods with limited access to healthy food so that the neighborhood inhabitants will be able to travel to supermarkets more easily.

By focusing on Puerto Rico and its political status, in this chapter I demonstrate the relationship between health and politics and highlight the urgent need to address Puerto Rico's political status, in order to alleviate the illness production I identified while researching health on the island. Participants reported multilayered, complex relationships with their identities as Puerto Ricans, Hispanics, and Americans, viewed through the colonial lens. In investigating the nexus of Puerto Rican politics and the numerous health problems on the island, I join a small but thriving community of scholars who also research the numerous junctions of health and politics in Puerto Rico (Dietrich 2013; Loue 2011; Mulligan 2010, 2014; Pérez-Perdomo et al. 2003).

NOTES

1. Data collection consisted of interviews about diabetes, obesity, depression, eating habits, perceptions of health, experiences of migration between the island and the mainland, and Puerto Rican experiences of identity and illness, disease, and food, with sixty adult participants at the *Centro de Diabetes Para Puerto Rico*, a diabetes clinic at the University of Puerto Rico's Medical Sciences Campus in San Juan. During that time I engaged in regular, ongoing participant-observation in the Center and with clinic staff, as well as in the surrounding community. Questions on disease-specific stigmas were included in the question set for each disease. The author manually coded and analyzed the data, which yielded 58 inter-related codes. In addition, to develop a conceptual model of the syndemic proposed here, I also reviewed and analyzed relevant social science literature on obesity, depression, mental health stigma, and both obesity and depression syndemics.

2. A pseudonym, as are all names used to identify original study participants quoted in this chapter.

3. A popular dessert in Puerto Rico: coconut macaroons.

4. A sponge cake soaked in three different kinds of milk: evaporated milk, condensed milk, and heavy cream.

5. Plantains, which Puerto Ricans prepare in a variety of ways.

6. Rice and beans.

7. Fritters, generally filled with chicken or beef.

8. The participants defined "close" as either a ten-minute walk or a twenty-minute drive or bus ride.

REFERENCES

Abadía-Barrero, César Ernesto, and Arachu Castro. "Experiences of Stigma and Access to HAART in Children and Adolescents Living with Hiv/Aids in Brazil." *Social Science and Medicine* 62 (2006): 1219–228.

Acosta-Pérez, Edna, Glorisa Canino, Rafael Ramírez, Michael Prelip, Molly Martin, Alexander N. Ortega. "Do Puerto Rican Youth with Asthma and Obesity Have Higher Odds for Mental Health Disorders?" *Psychosomatics* 53, no. 2 (2012): 1627–71.

Alegria Drury, Christine Aramburu, and Margaret Louis. "Exploring the Association between Body Weight, Stigma of Obesity, and Health Care Avoidance." *Journal of the American Academy of Nurse Practitioners* 14, no. 12 (2002): 554–661.

Alexander, Franz G., and Sheldon T. Selesnick. *The History of Psychiatry: An Evaluation of Psychiatric Thought and Practice from Prehistoric Times to the Present.* New York: Harper and Row Publishers, 1966.

Alvarez, Lizette. "Economy and Crime Spur New Puerto Rican Exodus." *The New York Times*, A1. 2014. http://www.nytimes.com/2014/02/09/us/economy-and-crime-spur-new-puerto-rican-exodus.html?_r=0.

Alvarez, Lizette, and Abby Goodnough. "Puerto Ricans Brace for Crisis in Health Care." *The New York Times*. August 2, 2015. http://www.nytimes.com/2015/08/03/us/health-providers-brace-for-more-cuts-to-medicare-in-puerto-rico.html.

American Psychological Association. "Data on Behavioral Health in the United States." 2014. http://www.apa.org/helpcenter/data-behavioral-health.aspx.

Angermeyer, Matthias C., and Herbert Matschinger. "Public Beliefs About Schizophrenia and Depression: Similarities and Differences." *Social Psychiatry and Psychiatric Epidemiology* 38 (2003): 526–34.

Aranda, Elizabeth M. *Emotional Bridges to Puerto Rico: Migration, Return Migration, and the Struggles of Incorporation*. Plymouth, UK: Rowman & Littlefield Publishers, 2007.

Barney, Lisa J., Kathleen M. Griffiths, Anthony F. Jorm, and Helen Christensen. "Stigma About Depression and Its Impact on Help-Seeking Intentions." *Australia and New Zealand Journal of Psychiatry* 40, no. 1 (2006): 515–54.

Barthes, Ronald. "Towards a Psychosociology of Contemporary Food Consumption." In *Food and Culture: A Reader*, edited by Carole Counihan and Penny Van Esterik, 2333–0. New York, NY: Routledge, 2013.

Belle, Deborah, and Joanne Doucet. "Poverty, Inequality, and Discrimination as Sources of Depression among U.S. Women." *Psychology of Women Quarterly* 27, no. 2 (2003): 10–13.

Bellisari, Anna. *The Anthropology of Obesity in the United States*. New York: Routledge, 2016.

Beyer, Scott. "Puerto Rico, at 11.5 Percent, Has America's Highest Sales Tax." Forbes Business, August 17, 2015. http://www.forbes.com/sites/scottbeyer/2015/08/17/puerto-rico-at-1155-has-americas-highest-sales-tax/.

Bishaw, Alemayehu, Kayla Fontenot. "Poverty: 2012 and 2013." United States Census Bureau, 2014. https://www.census.gov/content/dam/Census/library/publications/2014/acs/acsbr1300-1.pdf.

Blazer, Dan G. *The Age of Melancholy: "Major Depression" and Its Social Origin* New York: Routledge, 2005.

Bloomgarden, Zachary T. "Prevention of Obesity and Diabetes." *Diabetes Care* 26, no. 11 (2003): 31727–78.

Bornstein, S. R., A. Schuppenies, M.-L. Wong, and J. Licinio. "Approaching the Shared Biology of Obesity and Depression: The Stress Axis as the Locus of Gene–Environment Interactions." *Molecular Psychiatry* 11 (2006): 892–902.

Brewis, Alexandra A. "Stigma and the Perpetuation of Obesity." *Social Science and Medicine* 118 (2014): 152–158.

———. *Obesity: Cultural and Biocultural Perspectives*. New Brunswick: Rutgers University Press, 2011.

Brewis, Alexandra A., and Amber Wutich. "A World of Suffering? Biocultural Approaches to Fat Stigma in the Global Contexts of the Obesity Epidemic." *Annals of Anthropological Practice* 38, no. 2 (2014): 269–283.

Brown, Peter J., and Melvin Konnor. "An Anthropological Perspective on Obesity." *Annals of the New York Academy of Sciences* 499 (1987): 294–346.

Caballero, Benjamin. "The Global Epidemic of Obesity: An Overview." *Epidemiologic Review* 29, no. 1 (2007): 155.

Carter, Sophie, Alexandre Caron, Denis Richard, and Frédéric Picard. "Role of Leptin Resistance in the Development of Obesity in Older Patients." *Clinical Interventions in Aging* 8 (2013): 829–844.

Cawley, John, and Chad Meyerhoefer. "The Medical Care Costs of Obesity: An Instrumental Variables Approach." *Journal of Health Economics* 31, no. 1 (2012): 219–330.

Center for Disease Control and Prevention. Obesity Prevalence Maps. (2015a). http://www.cdc.gov/obesity/data/prevalence-maps.html.

———. Adult Obesity Facts. (2015b). http://www.cdc.gov/obesity/data/adult.html.

Chappatta, Brian. "Puerto Rico Economy Worsens with Crisis, Most Anywhere You Look." (2016). http://www.bloomberg.com/politics/articles/201600-422-5/puerto-rico-economy-worsens-with-crisis-most-anywhere-you-look.

Collado-Schwarz, Angel. *Decolonization Models for America's Last Colony: Puerto Rico*. Syracuse: Syracuse University Press, 2012.

Colon, Eduardo, Aida Giachello, LaShawn McIver, Guadalupe Pacheco, Leonel Vela. "Diabetes and Depression in the Hispanic/Latino Community." *Clinical Diabetes* 31, no. 1 (2013): 434–45.

Colón-López, Vivian, Geetanjoli Banerjee, Alida María Gertz, Ana Patricia Ortiz, William Calo, Lila J. Finney-Rutten, Uriyoán Colón-Ramos, Bradford W. Hesse, and Guillermo Tortolero. "Behavioral Correlates of Fruit and Vegetable Intake in

Puerto Rico: Results from the Health Information National Trends Survey." *Puerto Rican Health Studies Journal* 32, no. 4 (2013): 194–99.

Corrigan Patrick W., and Kristin A. Kosyluk. "Mental Illness Stigma: Types, Constructs, and Vehicles for Change." In *The Stigma of Disease and Disability: Understanding Causes and Overcoming Injustices*, edited by Patrick W. Corrigan, 3555–6. Washington, DC: American Psychological Association, 2014.

Deans, Emily. "Could Soda and Sugar Be Causing Your Depression?" *Psychology Today*. (2011). https://www.psychologytoday.com/blog/evolutionary-psychiatry/201105/could-soda-and-sugar-be-causing-your-depression.

Diaz, Rafael M., George Ayala, Edward Bein, Jeff Henne, and Barbara V. Marin. "The Impact of Homophobia, Poverty, and Racism on the Mental Health of Gay and Bisexual Latino Men: Findings from 3 Us Cities." *American Journal of Public Health* 91, no. 6 (2001): 927–33.

Duany, Jorge. *Blurred Boundaries: Transnational Migration between the Hispanic Caribbean and the United States*. Chapel Hill: The University of North Carolina Press, 2011.

———. *The Puerto Rican Nation on the Move: Identities on the Island and in the United States*. Chapel Hill: The University of North Carolina Press, 2002.

Eknoyan, Garabed. "A History of Obesity, or How What Was Good Became Ugly and Then Bad." *Advances in Chronic Kidney Disease* 13, no. 4 (2006): 421–27.

Erdman Farrell, Amy. *Fat Shame: Stigma and the Fat Body in American Culture*. New York: New York University Press, 2011.

Ferrari, Alize J., Fiona J. Charlson, Rosana E. Norman, Scott B. Patten, Greg Freedman, Christopher J. L. Murray, Theo Vos, and Harvey A. Whiteford. "Burden of Depressive Disorders by Country, Sex, Age, and Year: Findings from the Global Burden of Disease Study 2010." *PLoS Medicine* 10, no. 11 (2013): e1001547.

Fettich, Karla C., and Eunice Y. Chen. "Coping with Obesity Stigma Affects Depressed Mood in African-American and White Candidates for Bariatric Surgery." *Obesity* 20, no. 5 (2012): 1118–21.

Fitzgerald, Nurgül. "Acculturation, Socioeconomic Status, and Health among Hispanics." *NAPA Bulletin* 34 (2010): 28–46.

Flores, Elena, Jeanne M. Tschann, Juanita M. Dimas, Elizabeth A. Bachen, Lauri A. Pasch, and Cynthia L. de Groat. "Perceived Discrimination, Perceived Stress, and Mental and Physical Health among Mexican-Origin Adults." *Hispanic Journal of Behavioral Sciences* 30, no. 4 (2008): 401–24.

Foerschner, Alison. "The History of Mental Illness: From Skull Drills to Happy Pills." *Inquiry* 2, no. 9 (2010). http://www.inquiriesjournal.com/articles/283/the-history-of-mental-illness-from-skull-drills-to-happy-pills.

Galea, Sandro, Jennifer Ahern, Arjit Nandi, Melissa Tracy, John Beard, and David Vlahov. "Urban Neighborhood Poverty and the Incidence of Depression in a Population-Based Cohort Study." *Annals of Epidemiology* 17, no. 3 (2007): 171–79.

Garza, Jeremiah R., Edna Acosta Pérez, Michael Prelip, William J. McCarthy, Jonathan M. Feldman, Glorisa Canino, and Alexander N. Ortega. "Occurrence and Correlates of Overweight and Obesity Among Puerto Rican Youth." *Ethnicity and Disease* 21 (2011): 163–69.

Gibson, Edward Leigh. "Emotional Influences on Food Choice: Sensory, Physiological and Psychological Pathways." *Physiology & Behavior* 89, no. 1 (2006): 5366–1.

Gillespie, James. "Puerto Rico's Terrible Economy Is Causing a Population Exodus." (2015). http://money.cnn.com/2015/06/15/news/economy/puerto-rico-debt/.

Goffman, Erving. *Stigma: Notes on the Management of Spoiled Identity*. New York: Simon and Schuster, 1963.

Gong, Yanhong, Dafang Wang, Xiulan Zhang, Zhiyong Qu, Pozi Liu, and Hong Zou. "The Potential Biological Mechanisms of Obesity Effects on Depression: A Systematic Review of the Literature and Knowledge Mining." *Health* 5, no. 11 (2013): 1811–18.

González, Lilliana, Grisel Ramos-Trautmann, Giselle M. Díaz-Luquis, Cynthia M. Pérez, and Cristina Palacios. "Vitamin D Status Is Inversely Associated with Obesity in a Clinic-Based Sample in Puerto Rico." *Nutrition Research* 35, no. 4 (2015): 287–93.

Gottlieb, Robert and Anupama Joshi. *Food Justice*. Cambridge, MA: The MIT Press, 2010.

Grosfoguel, Ramón. *Colonial Subjects: Puerto Ricans in a Global Perspective*. Berkeley and Los Angeles: University of California Press, 2003.

Hammond, Ross A. and Ruth Levine. "The Economic Impact of Obesity in the United States." *Diabetes, Metabolic Syndrome and Obesity: Targets and Therapy* 3 (2010): 285–95.

Hanandita, Wulung and Gindo Tampubolon. "Does Poverty Reduce Mental Health? An Instrumental Variable Analysis." *Social Science and Medicine* 113 (2014): 59–67.

Hayes, Sharon, Nina Stoeckel, Melissa A. Napolitano, Charlotte Collins, G. Craig Wood, Jamie Seiler, Heidi E. Grunwald, Gary D. Foster, and Christopher D. Still. "Examination of the Beck Depression Inventory-Ii Factor Structure Among Bariatric Surgery Candidates." *Obesity Surgery* 25, no. 7 (2015): 1155–60.

Hossain, Parvez, Bisher Kawar, and Meguid El Nahas. "Obesity and Diabetes in the Developing World—a Growing Challenge." *New England Journal of Medicine* 356, no. 3 (2007): 213–15.

Huizinga, Mary Margaret, Lisa A. Cooper, Sara N. Bleich, Jeanne M. Clark, and Mary Catherine Beach. "Physician Respect for Patients with Obesity." *Journal of General Internal Medicine* 24, no. 11 (2009): 1236–39.

Jackson, Lucas. "Battle of the Bulge: US Food Corporations Fueling Obesity Epidemic with Addictive Ingredients." (2013). https://www.rt.com/usa/food-obesity-health-us-776/.

Janjua, Naveed Zafar, Bushra Mahmood, M. Aminul Islam, and Robert L. Goldenberg. "Maternal and Early Childhood Risk Factors for Overweight and Obesity among Low-Income Predominantly Black Children at Age Five Years: A Prospective Cohort Study." *Journal of Obesity* (2012): 199.

Jones, Nev, and Patrick W. Corrigan. "Understanding Stigma." In *The Stigma of Disease and Disability: Understanding Causes and Overcoming Injuries*, edited by Patrick W. Corrigan, 933–34. Washington, DC: American Psychological Association, 2014.

Khazan, Olga. "Why Rich Women Don't Get Fat." *The Atlantic* (2014). http://www.theatlantic.com/magazine/archive/2014/04/why-rich-women-dont-get-fat/358643/.

Krogstad, Jens Manuel. "Puerto Ricans Leave in Record Numbers for Mainland U.S." PewResearch Center. (2015). http://www.pewresearch.org/fact-tank/2015/10/14/puerto-ricans-leave-in-record-numbers-for-mainland-u-s/.

Latalova, Klara, Dana Kamaradova, and Jan Prasko. "Perspectives on Perceived Stigma and Self-Stigma in Adult Male Patients with Depression." *Neuropsychiatric Disease and Treatment* 10 (2014): 1399–405.

Leddy, Meaghan A., Michael L. Power, and Jay Schulkin. "The Impact of Maternal Obesity on Maternal and Fetal Health." *Reviews in Obstetrics & Gynecology* 1, no. 4 (2008): 170–78.

Ledochowski, M., B. Widner, B Sperner-Unterweger, T. Propst, W. Vogel, and D. Fuchs. "Carbohydrate Malabsorption Syndromes and Early Signs of Mental Depression in Females." *Digestive Diseases and Sciences* 45, no. 7 (2000): 125–59.

Lerman, Shir. "'Un Pueblo Tan Dulce': Diabetes, Depression, and Obesity Syndemics in Puerto Rico." Dissertation, University of Connecticut, 2016.

Lichtenstein, Bronwen. "Stigma as a Barrier to Treatment of Sexually Transmitted Infection in the American Deep South: Issues of Race, Gender and Poverty." *Social Science and Medicine* 57 (2003): 243–45.

Link, Bruce G., Jo C. Phelan, Michaeline Bresnahan, Ann Stueve, and Bernice A. Pescosolido. "Public Conceptions of Mental Illness: Labels, Causes, Dangerousness, and Social Distance." *American Journal of Public Health* 89, no. 9 (1999): 132–33.

Ludermir, Ana Bernarda, Glyn Lewis, Sandra Alves Valongueiro, Thália Velho Barreto de Araújo, and Ricardo Araya. "Violence against Women by Their Intimate Partner During Pregnancy and Postnatal Depression: A Prospective Cohort Study." *The Lancet* 376, no. 9744 (2010): 903–910.

Lund, Crick, Alison Breen, Alan J. Flisher, Ritsuko Kakuma, Joanne Corrigall, John A. Joska, Leslie Swartz, and Vikram Patel. "Poverty and Common Mental Disorders in Low and Middle Income Countries: A Systematic Review." *Social Science and Medicine* 71, no. 3 (2010): 517–28.

Mankekar, Purnima. "'India Shopping': Indian Grocery Stores and Transnational Configurations of Belonging." In *The Cultural Politics of Food and Eating: A Reader*, edited by James L. Watson, Melissa L. Caldwell, 19722–14. Malden, MA: Blackwell Publishing, 2005.

Marsella, Anthony J., Norman Sartorius, Assen Jablensky, and Fred R. Fenton. "Cross-Cultural Studies of Depressive Disorders: An Overview." In *Culture and Depression: Studies in the Anthropology and Cross-Cultural Psychiatry of Affect and Disorder*, edited by Arthur Kleinman, Byron Good, 299–324. Berkeley: University of California Press, 1985.

Martínez-Pincay, Igda E. and Peter J. Guarnaccia. "It's Like Going Through an Earthquake': Anthropological Perspectives on Depression Among Latino Immigrants." *Journal of Immigrant & Minority Health* 9, no. 1 (2007): 172–28.

McLennan, Amy K., and Stanley J. Ulijaszek. "Obesity Emergence in the Pacific Islands: Why Understanding Colonial History and Social Change Is Important." *Public Health Nutrition* 18, no. 8 (2015): 1499–505.

McNeil, Jr., Donald G. "Zika Cases in Puerto Rico Are Skyrocketing." *The New York Times*, July 31, 2016. http://www.nytimes.com/2016/07/31/health/zika-virus-puerto-rico.html.

Mendenhall, Emily. *Syndemic Suffering: Social Distress, Depression, and Diabetes among Mexican Immigrant Women.* Walnut Creek, CA: Left Coast Press, 2012.

Milaneschi, Yuri, Eleanor M. Simonsick, Nicole Vogelzangs, Elsa S. Strotmeyer, Kristine Yaffe, Tamara B. Harris, Magdalena I. Tolea, Luigi Ferrucci, and Brenda W. Penninx. "Leptin, Abdominal Obesity and Onset of Depression in Older Men and Women." *Journal of Clinical Psychiatry* 73, no. 9 (2012): 1205–11.

Miller, Gregory E. and Edith Chen. "The Biological Residue of Childhood Poverty." *Child Development Perspectives* 7, no. 2 (2013): 67–73.

Moffat, Tina. "The 'Childhood Obesity Epidemic': Health Crisis or Social Construction?" *Medical Anthropology Quarterly* 24, no. 1 (2010): 122–21.

Morbidity and Mortality Weekly Report (MMWR). "Attitudes Toward Mental Illness—35 States, District of Columbia, and Puerto Rico, 2007." Centers for Disease Control and Prevention (2010). http://www.cdc.gov/mmwr/preview/mmwrhtml/mm5920a3.htm.

Morris, Nancy. *Puerto Rico: Culture, Politics, and Identity*. Westport, CT: Praeger Publishers, 1995.

Murphy, J. M., N. J. Horton, J. D. Burke Jr., R. R. Monson, N. M. Laid, and A. M. Sobol. "Obesity and Weight Gain in Relation to Depression: Findings from the Stirling County Study." *International Journal of Obesity* 33, no. 3 (2009): 335–41.

National Institute of Diabetes and Digestive and Kidney Disorders. "Overweight and Obesity Statistics." (2015). http://www.niddk.nih.gov/health-information/health-statistics/Pages/overweight-obesity-statistics.aspx.

Negrón-Muntaner, Frances. "Looking Good." In *A Companion to Latina/O Studies*, edited by Juan Flores, Renato Rosaldo, 427–40. Malden, MA: Blackwell Publishing, 2007.

Negrón-Portillo, Mariano. "Puerto Rico: Surviving Colonialism and Nationalism." In *Puerto Rican Jam: Rethinking Colonialism and Nationalism*, edited by Frances Negrón-Muntaner, Ramón Grosfoguel, 39–56. Minneapolis: University of Minnesota Press, 1997.

Nestle, Marion. *Food Politics: How the Food Industry Influences Nutrition and Health*. Berkeley: The University of California Press, 2007.

Ogden, Jane, Nicola Coop, Charlotte Cousins, Rebecca Crump, Laura Field, Sarah Hughes, and Nigel Woodger. "Distraction, the Desire to Eat and Food Intake. Towards an Expanded Model of Mindless Eating." *Appetite* 62 (2013): 119–26.

Ortíz Cuadra, Cruz Miguel. *Eating Puerto Rico: A History of Food, Culture, and Identity*. Translated by Russ Davidson. Chapel Hill: University of North Carolina Press, 2013.

Padula, William V., Richard R. Allen, and Kavita Nair. "Determining the Cost of Obesity and Its Common Comorbidities from a Commercial Claims Database." *Clinical Obesity* 4 (2013): 53–58.

Patten, Scott B., Jeanne V. A. Williams, Dina H. Lavorato, Lauren Brown, Lindsay McLaren, and Michael Eliasziw. "Major Depression, Antidepressant Medication and the Risk of Obesity." *Psychotherapy and Psychosomatics* 78, no. 3 (2009): 182–86.

Pérez, Cynthia M., Hesmy Sánchez, and Ana P. Ortiz. "Prevalence of Overweight and Obesity and Their Cardiometabolic Comorbidities in Hispanic Adults Living in Puerto Rico." *Journal of Community Health* 38, no. 6 (2013): 1140–46.

Petterson, Stephen M., and Alison Burke Albers. "Effects of Poverty and Maternal Depression on Early Child Development." *Child Development* 72, no. 6 (2001): 1794–813.

Phelan, Sean M., Joan M. Griffin, George L. Jackson, S. Yousuf Zahar, Wendy Hellerstedt, Mandy Stahre, David Nelson, Leah L. Zullig, Diana J. Burgess, and Michelle van Ryn. "Stigma, Perceived Blame, Self-Blame, and Depressive Symptoms in Men with Colorectal Cancer." *Psycho-Oncology* 22 (2013): 65–73.

Popkin, Barry M. *The World Is Fat: The Fads, Trends, Policies, and Products That Are Fattening the Human Race*. New York: Penguin Group, 2009.

Poponoe, Rebecca. *Feeding Desire: Fatness, Beauty and Sexuality Among a Saharan People*. New York: Routledge, 2004.

Porter, Roy. *Madness: A Brief History*. New York: Oxford University Press, 2002.

Pratt, Laura A., and Debra J. Brody. "Depression in the U.S. Household Population, 2009–2012." Centers for Disease Control and Prevention, 2014. http://www.cdc.gov/nchs/data/databriefs/db172.pdf.

Puhl, Rebecca M. and Kelly D. Brownell. "Confronting and Coping with Weight Stigma: An Investigation of Overweight and Obese Adults." *Obesity* 14, no. 10 (2006): 180–211.

———. "Bias, Discrimination, and Obesity." *Obesity Research* 9, no. 12 (2001): 788–805.

Puhl, Rebecca M., and Chelsea A. Heuer. "The Stigma of Obesity: A Review and Update." *Obesity* 17, no. 5 (2009): 941–64.

Pudrovska, Tetyana, Eric N. Reither, Ellis S. Logan, and Kyler J. Sherman-Wilkins. "Gender and Reinforcing Associations Between Socioeconomic Disadvantage and Body Mass over the Life Course." *Journal of Health and Social Behavior* 55, no. 3 (2014): 283–301.

Quinn, Diane M., and Stephenie R. Chaudoir. "Living with a Concealed Stigmatized Identity: The Impact of Anticipated Stigma, Centrality, Salience, and Cultural Stigma on Psychological Distress and Health." *Journal of Personality and Social Psychology* 97, no. 4 (2009): 634–51.

Rabbani, F., F. Qureshi, and N. Rizvi. "Perspectives on Domestic Violence: Case Study from Karachi, Pakistan." *Eastern Mediterranean Health Journal* 14, no. 2 (2008): 415–26.

Ramos-Zayas, Ana Y. *National Performances: The Politics of Class, Race, and Space in Puerto Rican Chicago*. Chicago: The University of Chicago Press, 2003.

Rao, Deepa, Dellanira Valencia-Garcia. "Stigma Across Cultures." In *The Stigma of Disease and Disability: Understanding Causes and Overcoming Injustices*, edited by Patrick W. Corrigan. Washington, DC: American Psychological Association, 2014.

Reutter, Linda I., Miriam J. Stewart, Gerry Veenstra, Rhonda Love, Dennis Raphael, and Edward Makwarimba. "'Who Do They Think We Are, Anyway?': Perceptions of and Responses to Poverty Stigma." *Qualitative Health Research* 19, no. 3 (2009): 297–311.

Ritenbaugh, Cheryl. "Obesity as a Culture-Bound Syndrome." *Culture, Medicine, and Psychiatry* 6 (1982): 347–61.

Ro, Annie. "Occupational Mobility and Depression Among the Foreign-Born in the United States." *Journal of Immigrant & Minority Health* 16, no. 6 (2014): 1149–56.

Rodriguez-Soto, Isa. "Intergenerational Variation in Cultural Models of Body Size in Puerto Rico." PhD diss., Arizona State University, 2013.

Rosa, Taina. "The Fast-Food Industry." *Puerto Rico Herald* 9, no. 2 (2005). June 28, 2005. http://www.puertorico-herald.org/issues2/2005/vol09n30/CBFastFood.html.

Saldaña, Jr., Ruben, George Felix. "Orale! Food and Identity Amongst Latinos." *Institute for Latino Studies* 6, no. 4 (2011).

Sartorius, Norman. "Stigma and Mental Health." *The Lancet* 370, no. 9590 (2007): 810–11.

Schabert, Jasmin, Jessica L. Browne, Kylie Mosely, and Jane Speight. "Social Stigma in Diabetes: A Framework to Understand a Growing Problem for an Increasing Epidemic." *Patient* 6, no. 1 (2013).

Serretti, Alessandro, and Laura Mandelli. "Antidepressants and Body Weight: A Comprehensive Review and Meta-Analysis." *Journal of Clinical Psychiatry* 71, no. 10 (2010): 125–72.

Shakher, Jayadave, and Anthony H. Barnett. "Diabetes, Obesity and Cardiovascular Disease—Therapeutic Implications." In *Obesity and Diabetes*, edited by Tony Barnett, Sudhesh Kumar, 151–84. Hoboken, NJ: John Wiley and Sons, 2009.

Shidhaye, Rahul and Michelle Kermode. "Stigma and Discrimination as a Barrier to Mental Health Service Utilization in India." *International Health* 5, no. 1 (2013).

Singer, Merrill. *Introduction to Syndemics: A Critical Systems Approach to Public and Community Health*. San Francisco: Jossey-Bass, 2009.

———. "Aids and the Health Crisis of the US Urban Poor: The Perspective of Critical Medical Anthropology." *Social Science and Medicine* 39, no. 7 (1994): 931–48.

Singer, Merrill, Ann Herring, Judith Littleton, and Melanie Rock. "Syndemics in Global Health." In *A Companion to Medical Anthropology in the 21st Century* edited by Merrill Singer and Pamela Erickson, 159–80. New York: Blackwell Publishing, 2015.

Spring, Bonnie, Kristin Schneider, Malaina Smith, Darla Kendzor, Bradley Appelhans, Donald Hedeker, and Sherry Pagoto. "Abuse Potential of Carbohydrates for Overweight Carbohydrate Cravers." *Psychopharmacology* 197, no. 4 (2008): 637–47.

Stevens-Watkins, Danelle, Brea Perry, Erin Pullen, and Jennifer Jewell. "Examining the Associations of Racism, Sexism, and Stressful Life Events on Psychological

Distress among African-American Women." *Cultural Diversity and Ethnic Minority Psychology* 20, no. 4 (2014): 561–69.
Stuart, Heather. "Violence and Mental Illness: An Overview." *World Psychiatry* 2, no. 2 (2003): 121–24.
Stuart, Heather and Julio Arboleda-Flórez. "A Public Health Perspective on the Stigmatization of Mental Illnesses." *Public Health Reviews* 34, no. 2 (2012): 1–18.
Sutton, Robbie M., Karen M. Douglas, and Leigh M. McClellan. "Benevolent Sexism, Perceived Health Risks, and the Inclination to Restrict Pregnant Women's Freedoms." *Sex Roles* 65, no. 788 (2011): 596–605.
Swan, Suzanne, and David L. Snow. "The Development of a Theory of Women's Use of Violence in Intimate Relationships." *Violence Against Women* 12, no. 11 (2006): 1026–45.
Takeuchi, David T., Margarita Alegría, James S. Jackson, and David R. Williams. "Editorial: Immigration and Mental Health: Diverse Findings in Asian, Black, and Latino Populations." *American Journal of Public Health* 91, no. 1 (2007): 11–12.
Teixeira, M. Elizabeth, and Geraldine M. Budd. "Obesity Stigma: A Newly Recognized Barrier to Comprehensive and Effective Type 2 Diabetes Management." *Journal of the American Academy of Nurse Practitioners* 22, no. 10 (2010): 527–33.
Thomas, Lorrin. *Puerto Rican Citizen: History and Political Identity in Twentieth-Century New York City*. Chicago: University of Chicago Press, 2010.
Ulijaszek, Stanley J., Hayley Lofink. "Obesity in Biocultural Perspective." *Annual Reviews of Anthropology* 35 (2006): 337–60.
Umberson, Debra, Kristin Anderson, Jennifer Glick, and Adam Shapiro. "Domestic Violence, Personal Control, and Gender." *Journal of Marriage and Family* 60, no. 2 (1998): 442–52.
Van Dorn, Richard, Jan Volavka, and Norman Johnson. "Mental Disorder and Violence: Is There a Relationship Beyond Substance Use?" *Social Psychiatry and Psychiatric Epidemiology* 47, no. 3 (2012): 487–503.
Varea, Vincente, Javier Martín de Carpi, Conchita Puig, José Angel Alda, Eva Camacho, Aida Ormazabal, Rafael Artuch, and Lilianne Gómez. "Malabsorption of Carbohydrates and Depression in Children and Adolescents." *Journal of Pediatric Gastroenterology & Nutrition* 40, no. 5 (2005): 561–65.
Vartanian, Lenny R. and Joshua M. Smyth. "Primum Non Nocere: Obesity Stigma and Public Health." *Bioethical Inquiry* 10, no. 1 (2013): 49–57.
Wagner, Birgit, Grit Klinizke, Elmar Brähler, and Anette Kersting. "Extreme Obesity Is Associated with Suicidal Behavior and Suicide Attempts in Adults: Results of a Population-Based Representative Sample." *Depression and Anxiety* 30 (2013): 975–81.
Wang, Y. Claire, Klim McPherson, Steven L. Gortmaker, and Martin Brown. "Health and Economic Burden of the Projected Obesity Trends in the USA and the UK." *The Lancet* 378 (2011): 815–25.
Wang, Youfa, and May A. Beydoun. "The Obesity Epidemic in the United States—Gender, Age, Socioeconomic, Race/Ethnic, and Geographic Characteristics: A Systematic Review and Meta-Regression Analysis." *Epidemiologic Review* 29, no. 1 (2007): 622–28.

Wansink, Brian. "From Mindless Eating to Mindlessly Eating Better." *Physiology & Behavior* 100 (2010): 454–63.

Weaver, Lesley Jo, Emily Mendenhall. "Applying Syndemics and Chronicity: Interpretations from Studies of Poverty, Depression, and Diabetes." *Medical Anthropology: Cross-Cultural Studies in Health and Illness* 33, no. 2 (2014): 92–108.

Whitaker, Robert. "Predicting Preschooler Obesity at Birth: The Role of Maternal Obesity in Early Pregnancy." *Pediatrics* 114, no. 1 (2004): e29–e36.

Whitmore, Catherine. "Type 2 Diabetes and Obesity in Adults." *British Journal of Nursing* 19, no. 14 (2010): 880–86.

Williams, David R., Rahwa Haile, Hector M. González, Harold Neighbors, Raymond Baser, and James S. Jackson. "The Mental Health of Black Caribbean Immigrants: Results from the National Survey of American Life." *American Journal of Public Health* 97, no. 1 (2007): 52–59.

World Health Organization. "Breaking the Cycle Between Mental Ill-Health and Poverty." (2007). http://www.who.int/mental_health/policy/development/1_Breakingviciouscycle_Infosheet.pdf.

Wurtman, Richard J., and Judith J. Wurtman. "Brain Serotonin, Carbohydrate-Craving, Obesity and Depression." *Obesity Research* 3, Suppl 4 (1995): 477S–80S.

Wutich, Amber, Alissa Roth, Alexandra Brewis, and Christopher Boone. "Stigmatized Neighborhoods, Social Bonding, and Health." *Medical Anthropology Quarterly* 28, no. 4 (2014): 556–77.

Yancey, Antronette K., Brian L. Cole, Rochelle Brown, Jerome D. Williams, Amy Hillier, Randolph S. Kline, Marice Ashe, Sonya A. Grier, Desiree Backman, and William McCarthy. "A Cross-Sectional Prevalence Study of Ethnically Targeted and General Audience Outdoor Obesity-Related Advertising." *The Milbank Quarterly* 87, no. 1 (2009): 155–84.

Yost III, William H. "Jonesing for a Taste of Competition: Why an Antiquated Maritime Law Needs Reform." *Roger Williams University Law Review* 1, no. 18 (2013): 52–77.

Zhu, D., I. J. Norman, and A. E. While. "The Relationship Between Health Professionals' Weight Status and Attitudes Toward Weight Management: A Systematic Review." *Obesity Review* 12, no. 5 (2011): 324–37.

Chapter Four

Obesity, Depression, and Weight-Related Stigma Syndemics

Sarah Trainer, Alexandra Brewis, Amber Wutich, and Seung Yong Han

Obesity, especially extreme/severe obesity, has a well-established bidirectional relationship with depression (Brewis 2014; Chapman et al. 2005; Lawson et al. 2010; Luppino et al. 2012; Pratt and Brody 2014b). Causally, weight gain seems to intensify depression, especially for people already considered clinically obese—most obviously through social mechanisms such as increased felt stigma and discrimination (Braziel and Lebesco 2001; Brewis 2014; Rogge 2004). Conversely, depression can lead to weight gain through behavioral changes in appetite and activity patterns, as well as through the obesogenic (obesity-promoting) effects of some biomedical treatments (including certain anti-depressant medications such as the SSRIs) (e.g., Corrigan et al. 2009; Crayton 2012; Haines et al., 2006; Lewis et al., 2011; Major et al., 2014; Neumark-Sztainer et al., 2012; Salvy et al., 2011; Schvey et al., 2011; Vartanian and Novak, 2011; Vartanian and Shaprow, 2008; Wott and Carels, 2010). This relationship is referred to in some research (e.g., Crayton 2012) as a "mutually destructive two-way street," but the connections may extend beyond co-occurrence and amplification of felt symptoms. Alterations in the levels of key hormones such as leptin are implicated in both weight and mood disorders (Carter 2013; Jequier 2002; Lawson et al. 2012). Exposure to a range of stressors, especially at certain key points in development, has also been demonstrated to increase risk (Pike 2005; Gluckman et al. 2007).

In this chapter, we propose a stigma-linked syndemic consisting of social, behavioral, and biological pathways of interaction between obesity and depression. The authors outline a theoretical framework to explain the processes by which felt weight-related stigma can act to create and strengthen a still little-theorized syndemic relationship between obesity and depression (see Lerman 2015 for an exception). To further explicate this relationship, first we briefly outline existing evidence linking obesity and depression, and identify how felt stigma is independently linked to both. We provide a model of theorized stigma mechanisms by which weight gain may lead to depression and back to weight gain. The authors then explore these proposed relationships using three quite different types of anthropological evidence from three very different populations, by drawing on traditional ethnographic in-person interviews with severely obese individuals seeking bariatric surgery, textual data from online diary-style blogs written by overweight or obese (self-identified) people discussing struggles with weight, and responses from a pilot survey among a group of young health trainees of varying sizes. All of these quite different sets of data illuminate interesting perspectives on the ways in which the depression-obesity relationship may be understood.

A key goal is to begin to articulate a more sophisticated anthropological understanding of how stigma connects obesity to depression syndemically, and to provide examples of approaches that can be applied to examine how people perceive and react to these relationships, how they fail to perceive and thus fail to react, or whether they feel able to do so, given structural constraints, as discussed by Lerman elsewhere in this volume. The question of how relevant social actors (including both patients and health care professionals) themselves recognize (or not) such a complex syndemic is important and worthy of further exploration. Such recognition is key to addressing the suffering associated with this proposed obesity-depression syndemic. Importantly, here, the general cultural milieu of the United States does not tend to appreciate the connections and instead tends to focus on obesity as a separate, personally preventable through lifestyle change, etc., physical condition (Boero 2012; Brewis 2011; Rothblum and Solovay 2009; Trainer et al. 2015b).

OBESITY, DEPRESSION, STIGMA, AND SUFFERING: CURRENT EVIDENCE

Obesity

In the United States today, roughly 1 in 50 adults qualifies as severely obese, usually based on a body mass index (BMI) $\geq$40 (Andreyeva et al., 2004; Flegal et al., 2010). Scholars and public commentators have rightly questioned biomedical frameworks that assume a designation of overweight or obese always implies pathology and disease, particularly in instances where classifications of overweight and obese are based on BMI categories $\leq$35, since these are notoriously inaccurate at the individual level (Casper and Moore

2009; Saguy, A. 2013; Trainer et al. 2015b; WHO 2015). Nevertheless, research also overwhelmingly indicates that extreme obesity (regardless of measurement) severely impacts reported health and wellbeing, with serious implications for quality and length of life (Andreyeva et al. 2004; Ballantyne 2003; Burgmer et al. 2014; Karlsson et al. 2007; Thonney et al. 2010).

Obesity and Stigma

"Fatness" is stigmatized in all sectors of U.S. society today, and this stigma negatively impacts almost every aspect of people's lives, including quality of education received, quality of personal relationships, career opportunities, and health care quality and access (Brewis 2011; Puhl and Heuer 2010, 2009). Reported "felt weight-related stigma," or people's anticipation and perceived experiences of being morally judged, excluded, avoided, rejected, or mistreated because of their current or former obesity status (Brewis 2014; Puhl and Heuer 2010, 2009), thus has serious implications in terms of quality of life in and of itself. Severe obesity is particularly stigmatized, both in terms of "misfitting" in physical space (e.g., seats, clothing) and also in terms of encountering constant demoralizing judgments of laziness, sloppiness, and so on (Braziel and Lebesco 2001; Brewis et al. 2016; Rogge 2004). As a result, individuals living with extremely high body weight also experience high levels of stigma, discrimination, social distress, and internalized stress. It is therefore difficult to tease apart the complicated and intertwined issues around health and suffering that make up the daily experiences of people living with severe obesity living in the United States currently, where the pathology surrounding weight is highlighted and the pathology stemming from weight-based discrimination and stigma is all-too frequently overlooked (Braziel and Lebesco 2001; Brewis et al. 2016; Greenhalgh and Carney 2014; Lupton 2013; McCullough and Hardin 2013; Owen 2015; Rothblum and Solovay 2009).

Depression and Stigma

Depression is extremely prevalent in the United States today. Between 2009 and 2012, for example, one study sponsored by the CDC found that more than 7 percent of the U.S. population over twelve years of age had experienced moderate to severe depressive symptoms in the previous two weeks alone (Pratt and Brody 2014a). The quality of life of those who suffer from depression often deteriorates over time, as people with depression tend to be less physically active and less social, to have a negative perception of their current health, to feel more somatic pain, and to have more trouble maintaining a productive career path (Wells et al. 1989). Surveys conducted in 2007 and 2009 for the Behavioral Risk Factor Surveillance System (BRFSS) found that most people surveyed felt that treatment for mental illness is effective, but significantly fewer believed that those with mental illness are treated with kindness and care by others (CDC 2012). Reasons for this include systematically negative portrayals and perceptions of mental illness in public and private institutions, as well as via mass media and legal frameworks, which result in stigmatization and restricted opportunities (Corrigan et al. 2004). On the other hand, the same report from BRFSS found that people living in states with a better social environment for people with mental illness, created by institutional safety nets such as accessible mental health services, were more likely to agree that people are generally caring and sympathetic to those with mental illness than were people states without these resources (CDC 2012). This finding suggests that perceived acceptance of those with mental illness may be influenced by the availability of and per capita spending on mental health services at a local level.

Social support is key to improving the social milieu for those who with mental illness. Recent efforts to combat stigma associated with mental illness, such as the "What a Difference a Friend Makes" campaign, have shown some positive effects (CDC 2012; Corrigan 2012). Considering that both internally produced self-stigma and externally produced felt-stigma prevent many with mental illness from seeking treatment (Givens et al. 2007) and also amplify stress and depressive symptoms, effective interventions to reduce social stigma toward mental illness may contribute to improved mental health.

Obesity and Depression

Depression is associated with chronic diseases, including asthma, arthritis, cardiovascular diseases, cancer, diabetes, and obesity (Chapman et al. 2005; Talbot and Nouwen 2000). However, while other chronic diseases have relatively clear causal relationships—in which depression is an outcome of the other disease—the causal relationship between obesity and depression is bi-directional. Between 2005 and 2010, Pratt and Brody (2014b) found that 34.6 percent of Americans older than 20 years of age were obese and of these, about 7.2 percent of them had reported (the actual numbers were probably greater) moderate to severe depressive symptoms within the past two weeks at the time they were measured (Pratt and Brody 2014b). Conversely, the same research also indicates that approximately 43 percent of American adults with depression are obese. Other studies find even tighter correlates. A Gallup Poll (Mendes 2010) found consistently higher rates of stress, worry, anger, sadness, and diagnosed depression among Americans who were either obese or underweight (based on BMI), compared to overweight or normal-weight individuals. These numbers indicate how prevalent depression is among obese people and vice versa, although the disparities in the numbers reported hint at the complicated nature of the relationship. Furthermore, the numbers do not clearly reveal the nature of the speculated causal relationship. One study (Chou and Yu 2013), for example, noted that atypical depression was more tightly linked with obesity than either classic depression or absence of depression, but the explanations for why this might be have not been clearly established.

Previous attempts to untangle this complex causal relationship yielded mixed results, with most epidemiological studies finding an association but not necessarily pinpointing a causal relationship between obesity and depression (de Wit et al. 2010; Strine et al. 2008). This lack of clarity is due to the reliance of most studies on cross-sectional rather than longitudinal data in collection and analysis. However, the lack of clarity may also be due to the fact that any speculated relationship between depression and obesity may take different forms, depending on cultural context and individual background. For example, a previous meta-analysis (Atlantis and Baker 2008) found that the association between depression and obesity was significant only for women, not for men, although whether this difference reflects gendered disparities in health or simply in reporting is also not clear. Other studies (Carpenter et al. 2000; Dixon et al. 2003) have found significant associations between obesity and depression, regardless of gender, but often with more pronounced trends for young women. Moreover, although a significant association between depression and obesity could not be found in other epidemiological studies using data collected in several non-Western countries (Heo et al. 2006; Ma and Xiao 2010; Simon et al. 2008; Zhao et al. 2009), which might indicate this association is stronger in Western contexts—or again, cultural discrepancies in how obesity and mental health are experienced and reported (Lock and Kaufert 2001; Nichter 1981). When only studies using longitudinal data from the United States were considered in a meta-analysis by Luppino and colleagues (2010), a bi-directional relationship between obesity and depression did emerge.

Theorizing a Weight-Related Stigma, Obesity, and Depression Syndemic

Syndemics typically develop under conditions of profound social inequality, characterized by layers of structural, interpersonal, and symbolic violence (Singer 2009). Certainly, all of these factors, as well as the experience of felt stigma and lack of social support, are observed to elevate both obesity risk and the risk for associated diseases such as depression (Brewis, 2011; Chen et al. 2007; Fettich and Chen 2012; Friedman et al. 2008, 2005; Hatzenbuehler and Link 2014; Hatzenbuehler et al. 2013; Link and Phelan 1995; Mendenhall 2012; Myers and Rosen 1999). Indeed, more ethnographic work done within anthropology and sociology suggests that felt stigma (stemming from obesity, for example) may be a proxy for poorer mental health, given its often-sustained impact on daily wellbeing (Braziel and Lebesco 2001; Brewis et al. 2016; Greenhalgh and Carney 2014; Lupton 2013; McCullough and Hardin 2013; Owen 2015; Rothblum and Solovay 2009).

A syndemic framework, with its emphasis on the social, economic, political, and environmental contexts in which biological physicality is embedded, as well as on the ways in which multiple disease interactions can exacerbate human suffering, becomes extraordinarily helpful in this context, for it aids in tracing out these nested experiences of suffering, disease, and distress (e.g., Lerman 2015; Ostrach and Singer 2012; Singer 2009; Weaver and Hadley 2011; Weaver and Mendenhall 2014). In her 2014 review article on stigma and obesity, Brewis examined the diverse mechanisms that relate weight-related stigma to weight gain, including in contexts of structural uncertainty, insecurity, discrimination and poverty, and inter-personal social exclusion. Brewis argued that all of these exacerbate and amplify one another. In the United States today, obesity has become increasingly an outcome of poverty, food insecurity (especially in key early development phases), and blocked access to education and career opportunities (Tanumihardjo et al. 2007). Adverse environments of this kind also increase risk for depression (Marmot 2012; Nicholson et al. 2008). Thus, increased risk for obesity and depression may develop together, in parallel, in this rather simplistic model.

However, a syndemic perspective, together with our research into obesity stigma (Brewis 2014, 2011; Brewis et al. 2011; Trainer et al. 2015a, 2015b), demands a deeper exploration of the obesity-depression relationship. Over a lifetime, for example, an individual with obesity in the United States is subject to an array of both every day and acute episodes of structural and interpersonal stigma (Braziel and Lebesco 2001; Brewis et al. 2016; Greenhalgh and Carney 2014; Lupton 2013; McCullough and Hardin 2013; Owen 2015; Rothblum and Solovay 2009). Participants detail structural stigmas and indignities that include being forced to ask for seatbelt extenders on airplanes, being unable to fit into booths at restaurants, having difficulty navigating narrow aisles in coffee shops, stores, and classrooms, being unable to fit into the passenger seat of a crowded car, and so on. Interpersonal stigma may include being passed over for promotions at work, coping with casual assumptions of laziness and sloppiness from strangers and acquaintances, and having trouble finding and maintaining romantic relationships. This barrage of social suffering and everyday violence also increases stress and the risk for depression (Brewis 2014; Fettich and Chen 2012). Thus, we see obesity amplifying psychological distress, which is even more true if an individual's felt stigma becomes self stigma: he or she internalizes the constant messages that obesity is not only ugly but also immoral (Dixon et al. 2003; Roberto et al. 2012) and comes to believe and apply such messages to him or herself.

At the same time, however, depression can increase risk for obesity through mechanisms related to stigma. The behavioral pathways here are fairly well understood, particularly as depression and stigma both de-motivate people from adopting regular exercise and also trigger comfort eating and binging (Corrigan et al. 2009; Haines et al., 2006; Lewis et al., 2011; Major et al., 2014; Neumark-Sztainer et al., 2012; Salvy et al., 2011; Schvey et al., 2011; Vartanian and Novak, 2011; Vartanian and Shaprow, 2008; Wott and Carels, 2010).

The biological pathways between obesity and depression are much less clearly explicated at this point. Existing research does indicate that there are some potentially significant connections between obesity, depression, and leptin levels, for example. Leptin, a fat-derived circulating hormone, helps to control (among other functions) food intake (by signaling satiety to the brain), energy expenditure, fat distribution, and insulin sensitivity. Research indicates that leptin may also have antidepressant effects (Lawson et al. 2012). One study (Lawson et al. 2012) showed that low leptin levels were associated with depression in women across the weight and body fat spectrum, although levels tended to be high in women classified as obese. Redistribution of adipose tissue toward greater visceral fat is associated with actual leptin resistance (Carter et al. 2013), however. Thus, another study (Milaneschi et al. 2012) found a significant association in men between high leptin levels and an increased onset of depression when abdominal obesity was also a factor and suggest that visceral fat levels—and the metabolic consequences of visceral fat in particular—may explain these biological co-occurrences.

The glucocorticoids play a complex role in the development and/or exacerbation of a host of physical conditions, since high circulating levels of stress hormones such as cortisol disregulate many of the body's routine functions (e.g., Pike 2005). Metabolic functioning is certainly affected, which influences weight both directly and indirectly (via sleep disturbance, for instance). Cortisol is also significant in the development of depression, both by disturbing daily patterns such as diurnal rhythms and by contributing to genetic variants that increase the risk for depression (Herbert 2013). The glucocorticoids' affects begin prenatally epigenetic evidence suggests possibly even before (Gluckman et al. 2007) and may continue into adulthood and beyond, with profound implications in terms of obesity, depression, and a host of other chronic diseases (Herbert 2013; Pike 2005). Further complicating the picture is the fact that felt maternal stress (including psychosocial stress from experienced stigma) increases the risk of pre-term birth, which in turn increases the risk for chronic disease later on in the child's life (Gluckman 2007; Pike 2007) but so too do maternal depression and maternal obesity, especially when poverty is also a factor (Li et al. 2008). There is even interesting new evidence on the microbiome, gut health, and increased risk for both obesity and depression (Claesson et al. 2012; Dash et al. 2015; Wallace et al. 2011).

Given this complex overlaying of risk upon risk upon risk, the obesity-depression connections beg to be explored using a syndemic framework. As Mendenhall (2012) states in her exploration of the connections between social and psychological suffering among Mexican immigrant women in Chicago, "A syndemics framework describes situations in which adverse social conditions, such as poverty and oppressive social relationships, stress a population, weaken its natural defenses, and expose it to a cluster of interacting diseases" (p. 13).

That being said, a significant component of current obesity stigma in the United States comes from medical and academic works that pathologize larger bodies. Debates over the AMA classification of "obesity" as a disease in and of itself, the language used around obesity and its "comorbidities," and similar issues reveal very legitimate concerns voiced by social scientists (e.g., Casper and Moore 2009; Greenhalgh and Carney 2014; Saguy, A. 2013; Trainer et al. 2015) and by individuals who themselves identify as "fat." Fundamental to these concerns is the fact that research focusing on obesity, suffering, and disease can and has been used to further pathologize and medicalize obesity (Rothblum and Solovay 2009). In that regard, a focus on the more holistic notion of social problems underlying disease clustering, and a nuanced exploration of the syndemic interactions between diseases necessarily takes us beyond simplistic ideas about "comorbidities," as well as a moralizing and myopic focus on individual behavior.

This brings us back to an important question: Do the relevant actors (i.e., those who struggle with obesity and/or depression, and those trained in the health professions) within these syndemics perceive these connections? The authors use three very different studies to interrogate this point, all drawn from this current program of research focused on the lived experience of obesity and related weight-loss struggles in the United States. The first study is a classic ethnography, the second a less conventional web-based project, and the third specifically tests, via a survey, perceptions of syndemic connections in a group of students trained in global health. Together these triangulate an ethnographic perspective on awareness of a contemporary obesity-stigma-depression syndemic in the United States.

BACKGROUND AND CONTEXT OF CURRENT PROJECTS

Bariatric Surgery Patients

The first project described in this paper is based on a multi-year, longitudinal ethnography: a clinic-based study tracking the experiences of bariatric patients as they prepare for and recover from bariatric surgery (most frequently Roux-en-Y gastric bypass and less frequently vertical sleeve gastrectomy) within a large medical system based in the American Southwest and Midwest. This mixed-methods study focused on people's experiences before and after surgery. Detailed repeated interviews, contextualized with long-term participant observation across multiple venues within the hospital and clinic settings, were conducted with participants at the medical system's Southwest location during the period 2014–2016. Participants, who were at different points in the surgery trajectory (preparing for surgery all the way to five years post-surgery), all had a history of extreme obesity, which is what qualified them (along with co-morbidities) for the surgery. A survey was also sent out to all patients who had undergone bariatric surgery within the previous five years at both the medical system's Southwest and Midwest locations. The authors have identified several important themes, all linked in different ways by patients with the size of their physical bodies.

In 2012, roughly 180,000 individuals opted to undergo bariatric surgery (ASMBS 2014a; Mechanick et al. 2013). Clinical data demonstrates bariatric surgery prompts massive and rapid weight loss in the short-term and has substantial benefits for the remission of diabetes, improved lipids, and lowered blood pressure (Adams et al., 2012; Batsis et al., 2008a, 2008b; Belle et al., 2007; Courcoulas et al., 2013; Magro et al., 2008; O'Brien et al., 2013; Odom et al., 2010; Sjöström et al., 2014, 2007, 2004, 1999). It also is associated with improvements in clinical depression (Burgmer et al. 2014) on the one hand and reported rates of weight-related social suffering on the other (Andersen et al. 2010; Ballantyne 2003; Kolotkin et al. 2008; Thonney et al. 2010).

Weight-Loss Bloggers

The context of the second study, in contrast to the bariatric ethnography, is well outside the walls of the traditional clinic space. In this project, we focused on conducting a systematic qualitative study using blogs centered on struggles with weight, body image, and/or weight loss.

At a time when Internet use has saturated many aspects of people's lives (Dumova and Fiordo 2012; Pitts 2004; Reed 2005; Wilkinson and Thelwall 2011), people not only spend more hours online but increasingly craft important social personas and public-private narratives via online venues (Karlsson

2007; de Laat 2008; Monaghan 2005; Pitts 2004; Reed 2005). In our recent internet-based ethnography project, they were particularly concerned with the blogosphere, and the fact that blogs serve as pivotal platforms for ongoing discussions about weight, weight loss, body norms, beauty, and identity (Dicken et al. 2011; Harding and Kirby 2009; de Laat 2008; Leggatt-Cook and Chamberlain 2011; Lopez 2009; Nardi et al. 2004; Pitts 2004; Rausch 2006). The aim of this research was to systematically sample individually-authored, public-access blogs that discuss weight loss and are produced by individuals living in the United States (see Trainer et al. 2016 for a more detailed description of methodologies). Out of the final sample of 234 blogs, 196 were authored by bloggers who identified as either currently overweight/obese or who had been overweight/obese in the past.

RESULTS AND DISCUSSION

Ethnographies of Suffering and Weight

It is notable that in two such different projects as the bariatric ethnography and the blog-based exploration, a common and powerful theme immediately emerged around obesity-linked suffering. The suffering could assume many forms; indeed, it is important to note here that many of the male bloggers and bariatric patients focused exclusively on physical suffering and health issues. Here, however, we focus on psychological suffering and reported depression, trends that emerged much more clearly in the women's narratives from both projects, but did also appear in some men's narratives.[1]

Some of the clearest narratives provided rich examples of intense external stress and trauma, grappling with feelings of depression and stress as a result, and turning to food as a coping mechanism. This pattern showed up repeatedly in the bloggers' stories about themselves and their struggles with weight. One woman, for example, talked about how weight crept up on her in college as a result of unhealthy eating habits, and then later, in the wake of tragic life events, eating, food, and weight became something more. In her after-the-fact recounting, this blogger wove weight struggles into her larger life struggles, including traumas specific to her life and her relationships (including a sick child) as well as community- and city-wide traumas (i.e., Hurricane Katrina). Other bloggers, by contrast, very explicitly made connections between daily experiences of weight-related stigma on the one hand and feelings of shame, guilt, and depression over their weight on the other. Some bloggers—particularly those who currently espoused a Health at Every Size Approach to body acceptance and weight—also made complex connections between previous cycles of dieting their identified "fat" selves toward socially mandated thinness, failing at dieting, self-blame and punishment, and mental distress. Thus, bloggers often identified very different causal pathways between mental distress, stressful environments, specific coping behaviors, and weight—but many of them did draw connections between these.

Bariatric patients told similar stories of overlapping circles of suffering. In a conversation with Russ (a 50-something year old man), held several months before his gastric bypass surgery, he talked at length about the fact that a psychiatrist within the bariatric program had put him on an anti-depressant at the same time that he enrolled in the required pre-surgery "behavioral change" education classes. Although still extremely obese, he reported that he had lost more weight since beginning medication and classes than at any time previously in his adult life. He said that he'd known for decades that he had depression but his job required such high security clearances that he feared going on medication that he would then have to report; instead, he "ate away the pain." Since beginning medication, the urge to use food to medicate had disappeared. Indeed, at the time of the first interview, Russ remarked that he was "only 75 percent certain" he was going to get surgery after all, given the recent sea change in his approach to food.

Valerie and Allison, women who elected to undergo gastric bypass surgery within the program, did not cite clinical depression in quite the same way as Russ but eating to cope with trauma certainly threaded its way through their narratives. Valerie, for example, explicitly made the connection between early childhood sexual abuse and her subsequent turn to food, both because eating was a comfort and also because the resulting fat felt protective. Allison spent her first sixteen years in a highly abusive and chaotic household ruled by her parents' drug habits. She, too, turned to food for comfort and stability. Many of the female bloggers included in the blog-based ethnography related similar stories.

On the one hand, it is important (in light of our concern with careless pathologization of larger bodies) to note that the food-as-a-coping-mechanism technique did in fact "work," from a certain perspective. Russ, Valerie, and Allison, for example, had all overcome significant obstacles and gone on to be highly successful in their chosen fields. On the other hand, the self-blame for unhealthy eating and "out of control" habits was intense and in itself often triggered stress, self-shaming, and self-reports of feeling depressed. Valerie commented that the fat that had once felt protective now felt like a prison from which she could not escape. Moreover, although Russ, Valerie, and Allison had successfully pursued a variety of careers, they also all reported that their success was *in spite* of their weight (a theme strongly echoed by other bariatric patients as well). Russ pointed out that he had to work doubly hard to overcome initial negative impressions of him by superiors and coworkers that equated his physical size with laziness, lack of control, and sloppiness. This produced yet another daily burden with which people struggled.

Valerie's comment about feeling trapped in her body was echoed by other individuals, whose narratives focused less on early psychological trauma increasing their risk for weight gain and more on the current, everyday psychological trauma of being "trapped" in an obese body in a country where weight-based discrimination is the last "safe" prejudice and active fat stigmatizing occurs constantly everywhere. In this scenario, therefore, individuals made direct connections between having a "fat body" and feeling depressed because of it. Alice, for example, a 30-something year old woman also hoping to have gastric bypass surgery, ended her first interview by saying, "I'm basically miserable all the time, I'm miserable about my weight, I'm miserable being fat, I don't like going anywhere because of it." Despite her career accomplishments and her loving and accepting friends, Alice felt her unhappiness over her weight was ruling her life. Similar sentiments were reflected by some bloggers. Many discussed "trading" happiness and health for the momentary pleasure a sweet treat, a stop at a fast food store, etc. The suffering and self-blame stand out in the narratives of both bloggers and bariatric patients. From a theoretical standpoint, it is striking how clearly potential pathways between fraught emotional states (including some instances of diagnosed depression but also, more commonly, to the wear and tear of chronic psychosocial stress and its accompanying elevated chronic cortisol levels) and obese physical states are created and then feed of each other.

A Survey-Based Study of University Global Health Students

The prior sections of this chapter dealt, in different ways, with an ethnographic approach to identifying how those struggling with weight issues perceive the connections between obesity (and to a lesser extent, overweight), weight-related stigma, depression, and suffering. In this respect, our focus was on the experience of being an individual in the United States today, facing some or all of these issues, tracing out the connections between depression and obesity as those most at risk see them (or don't see them). The authors remained curious, however, about professional perspectives on these same issues, and thought it would be interesting to explore the ways in which individuals who have had training in public health and healthcare perceive these same connections between obesity, depression, stigma, and suffering. These are the people, after all, who are charged with helping to address weight issues either in the clinic or through public health efforts.

In this third study, we conducted a network analysis to test how future and current health professionals perceived possible linkages between obesity, stigma, and poverty. Poverty is included here because it is a key feature of most syndemics (Lerman 2015; Mendenhall 2012; Ostrach and Singer 2012; Singer 2009). The authors used surveys with sixty former students from our university department's Global Health track to collect the network data. The surveys were done 3 to 36 months after courses were completed and most of the respondents are now pursuing or already employed in health care fields. The aim was to identify the extent to which people with basic training in global health perceive the strength and directionality of inter-connections between obesity, stigma, and poverty. A further consideration here is that, as instructors in this track, we know that these inter-connections are stressed in class. Because we have taught these classes, however, we know that students come to the classes with very strong opinions about conditions such as obesity and depression, opinions that are heavily influenced by a larger social environment that interprets obesity through a simplistic, stigmatizing lens (Brewis et al. 2015).

A previous study performed in Ireland (Brogan and Hevey 2009) showed that people could express highly consensual and complex models of the etiology of obesity using a survey approach, and we leaned heavily on this previous study's design in the configuration of their research. To our knowledge, this is the first time this approach has been applied to identifying syndemic relationships specifically. Each respondent provided an assessment of the strength of causal relationships between each item and all others. The authors included a number of other conditions in the study, such as diabetes and food insecurity, but here only report the basic model. Using UCI-Net (a tool for social network analysis), we developed a single model from the sixty individual matrices for the four key items: obesity, depression, stigma, and poverty. A basic graphic model of the direction and strength of individual perceived ties between the items is shown in figure 4.1, using data that we collected for this study. The resulting network model demonstrated a high level of consensus among the respondents.

Using responses on perceived strength of a causal relationship, we calculated tie strength (expressed as a percentage) among the four conditions. As discussed in preceding sections, there are reasonable empirical and theoretical reasons to treat these four factors as complex, bidirectional causative and iterative (syndemic) relationships among them all. However, respondents did not perceive all these connections. Using > 65 percent as the threshold to determine strongly perceived causality (i.e., indicating greater consensus than would be indicated by a 50 percent cutoff), respondents saw obesity as a strong cause of both depression and stigma. However, they did not perceive those relationships to be bi-directional, meaning no strong causal relationship was expressed for depression leading to obesity or stigma amplifying obesity.

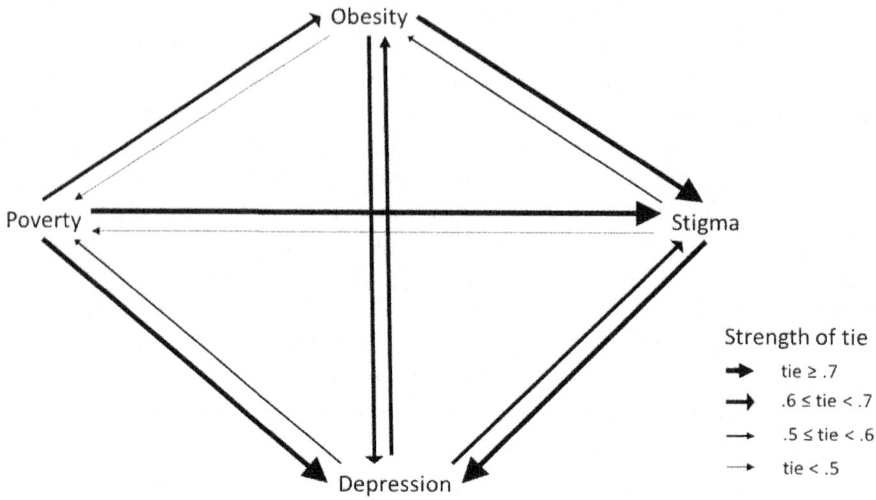

Figure 4.1. Basic network model showing perceived causal relationships among the theorized syndemic conditions. Arrows show the strength of the perceived causal relationship between each item. Analysis was conducted in UCINet.

They did, however, perceive strong bidirectional causal relationships between depression and stigma. While stigma and depression were both perceived to be strongly caused by poverty, respondents did not explicate a strong causative relationship in the other direction. Also no strong tie existed, in either direction, between poverty and obesity, according to respondents. Overall, then, these health professionals were able to articulate some of the connections we hoped to see but they did not appear to be highly aware of a more detailed overarching syndemic model.

CONCLUSIONS

The authors considered two questions at the beginning of this research: (1) Does the stigma-obesity-depression relationship fit a syndemic model? And, (2) To what extent do various social actors embedded within this syndemic perceive it?

Based on this discussion thus far, then, we identify a solid theoretical foundation for an exploration of the syndemic connections between obesity and depression-certainly, through experiences of felt stigma but also seemingly though potential exposures, especially earlier in life, to a range of stressors that affect underlying biology and health. There is good evidence to suggest these relationships are robust, sustained, interwoven with each other and an array of other vulnerabilities, and have significant and important effects on individual and population-level health.

By unpacking the relationship ethnographically, both in interviews with bariatric surgery patients and via the blogs of people documenting their personal struggles with weight, we find that people acknowledge some of syndemic connections between these stigma-linked conditions, as they occur in their own lives, but rhetoric around blame and shame-particularly when internalized-sometimes obscures the linkages. Moralizing messages about an individual's responsibility for maintaining a thin body and a positive outlook in the face of everyday challenges predominate in the United States today and the laser-like focus on individual behavior undermines more nuanced understandings. It makes sense in this regard that the survey responses showed even less knowledge of the syndemic connections and feedback loops. Given dominant biomedical and social explanations of and perspectives on obesity in the United States today (Brewis 2014, 2011), it is not surprising that many people are more comfortable speaking about health, mobility, and physical conditions that predispose them to obesity or that increase risk for it. Nevertheless, within the ethnographic samples in this chapter—the bloggers focused on weight and weight loss and people opting to undergo bariatric surgery—psychological health and ill-health did come up regularly and personal stories of suffering, both externally produced and internalized-were common.

NOTE

1. Significantly, research across multiple lines of inquiry does indicate the on the one hand, American women have felt the impact of weight-related stress more acutely than have their male counterparts (e.g., Bordo; Nichter 2000), and that systemic, gender-based inequalities can put them at greater risk, not only for depression (Belle and Doucet 2003), but also for the amplifying, interwoven effects of a syndemic such as diabetes and depression (e.g., Mendenhall 2012) or even HIV infection and progression (e.g., Ostrach and Singer 2012). Nevertheless, in this research, the number of women in both ethnographic projects vastly outnumbered men and although this disproportionate representation is, itself, striking, it makes firm conclusions difficult. Moreover, it is difficult to ascertain whether female bariatric patients and female bloggers struggled more with depression or were simply more willing to discuss such struggles.

REFERENCES

Adams, T. D., L. E. Davidson, S. E. Litwin, R. L. Kolotkin, M. J. LaMonte, R. C. Pendleton, M. B. Strong, R. Vinik, N. A. Wanner, P. N. Hopkins, R. E. Gress, J. M.

Walker, T. V. Cloward, R. T. Nuttall, A. Hammoud, J. L. Greenwood, R. D. Crosby, R. McKinlay, S. C. Simper, and S. C. Hunt. "Health Benefits of Gastric Bypass Surgery After 6 Years." *Journal of the American Medical Association* 308 (2012): 1122–1131.

American Society for Metabolic and Bariatric Surgery. "Estimate of Bariatric Surgery Numbers." Accessed August 2016. Available at https://asmbs.org/resources/estimate-of-bariatric-surgery-numbers

Andersen, J. R., A. Aasprang, P. Bergsholm, N. Sletteskog, V. Våge, and G. K. Natvig. "Anxiety and Depression in Association with Morbid Obesity: Changes with Improved Physical Health After Duodenal Switch." *Health and Quality of Life Outcome* 8 (2010): 52.

Andreyeva, T., R. Sturm, and J. S. Ringel. "Moderate and Severe Obesity Have Large Differences in Health Care Costs." *Obesity Research* 12 (2004): 1936–1943.

Atlantis, E., and M. Baker. "Obesity Effects on Depression: Systematic Review of Epidemiological Studies." *International Journal of Obesity* 32 (2008): 881–891.

Ballantyne, G. H. "Measuring Outcomes Following Bariatric Surgery: Weight Loss Parameters, Improvement in Co-Morbid Conditions, Change in Quality of Life and Patient Satisfaction." *Obesity Surgery* 13 (2003): 954–964.

Batsis, J. A., A. Romero-Corral, M. L. Collazo-Clavell, M. G. Sarr, V. K. Somers, and F. Lopez Jimenez. "Effect of Bariatric Surgery on the Metabolic Syndrome: A Population-Based, Long-Term Controlled Study." *Mayo Clinic Proceedings* 83 (2008): 897–906.

Batsis, J. A., M. G. Sarr, M. L. Collazo-Clavell, R. J. Thomas, A. Romero-Corral, V. K. Somers, and F. Lopez Jimenez. "Cardiovascular Risk After Bariatric Surgery for Obesity." *American Journal of Cardiology* 102 (2008): 930–937.

Belle, S. H., P. D. Berk, A. P. Courcoulas, D. R. Flum, C. W. Miles, J. E. Mitchell, W. J. Pories, B. Wolfe, and S. Z. Yanovski. "Safety and Efficacy of Bariatric Surgery: Longitudinal Assessment of Bariatric Surgery." *Surgery for Obesity and Related Diseases* 3 (2007): 116–126.

Belle, D., and J. Doucet. "Poverty, Inequality, and Discrimination as Sources of Depression Among U.S. Women." *Psychology of Women Quarterly* 27 (2003): 101–113.

Boero, N. C. *Killer Fat: Media, Medicine, and Morals in the American "Obesity Epidemic."* New Brunswick, NJ: Rutgers University Press, 2012.

Bordo, S. *Unbearable Weight: Feminism, Western Culture, and the Body*. Berkeley, CA: University of California Press, 1993.

Braziel, J. E., and K. Lebesco (eds.). *Bodies Out of Bounds*. Berkeley, CA: University of California Press, 2001.

Brewis A. *Obesity: Cultural and Biocultural Perspectives*. New Brunswick, NJ: Rutgers University Press, 2011.

Brewis, A. "Stigma as a Social Driver of Obesity." *Social Science and Medicine* 118 (2014): 152–158.

Brewis, A., D. Hruschka, and A. Wutich. "Vulnerability to Fat-Stigma in Women's Everyday Relationships." *Social Science and Medicine* 73 (2011): 491–497.

Brewis, A., S. Trainer, S. Y. Han, and A. Wutich. "Publically Misfitting: Living with Extreme Weight and the Everyday Production and Reinforcement of Felt Stigma."

Medical Anthropology Quarterly. Published online before print 7 June 2016. DOI: 10.1111/maq.12309

Brewis, A., A. Wutich, and D. Williams. "Teaching Obesity: Stigma, Structure, and Self." In *Teaching Food and Culture*. C. L. Swift and R. Wilk, eds. (35–48). San Francisco, CA: Left Coast Press, 2015.

Brogan, A. and D. Hevey. "The Structure of the Causal Attribution Belief Network of Patients with Obesity." *British Journal of Health Psychology* (2009): 35–48.

Burgmer, R., T. Legenbauer, A. Muller, M. de Zwaan, C. Fischer, and S. Herpertz. "Psychological Outcomes 4 Years after Restrictive Bariatric Surgery." *Obesity Surgery* 24 (2014): 1670–1678.

Carpenter, K. M., D. S. Hasin, D. B. Allison, and M. S. Faith. "Relationships Between Obesity and DSM-IV Major Depressive Disorder, Suicide Ideation, and Suicide Attempts: Results from a General Population Study." *American Journal of Public Health* 90 (2000): 251–57.

Carter, S., A. Caron, D. Richard, and F. Picard. "Role of Leptin Resistance in the Development of Obesity in Older Patients." *Clinical Interventions in Aging* 8 (2013): 829–844.

Casper, M. J., and L. J. Moore. *Missing Bodies: The Politics of Visibility*. New York: New York University Press, 2009.

Centers for Disease Control and Prevention (CDC). *Attitudes Toward Mental Illness: Results from the Behavioral Risk Factor Surveillance System*. Substance Abuse & Mental Health Services Administration, National Association of County Behavioral Health & Developmental Disability Directors, National Institute of Mental Health, The Carter Center Mental Health Program, 2012.

Chapman, D. P., G. S. Perry, and T. W. Strine. "The Vital Link Between Chronic Disease and Depressive Disorders." *Preventing Chronic Disease* 2 (2005): 1–10.

Chen, E. Y., L. E. Bocchieri-Ricciardi, D. Munoz, S. Fischer, S. Katterman, M. Roehrig, M. Dymek-Valentine, J. C. Alverdy, and D. Le Grange. "Depressed Mood in Class III Obesity Predicted by Weight-Related Stigma." *Obesity Surgery* 17 (2007): 669–671.

Chou, K. L., and K. M. Yu. "Atypical Depressive Symptoms and Obesity in a National Sample of Older Adults with Major Depressive Disorder." *Depression and Anxiety* 30 (2013): 574–579.

Claesson, M. J., I. B. Jeffery, S. Conde, S. E. Power, E. M. O'Connor, S. Cusack, H. M. B. Harris, M. Coakley, B. Lakshminaravanan, O. O'Sullivan, G. F. Fitzgerald, J. Deane, M. O'Conner, N. Harnedy, K. O'Conner, D. O'Mahony, D. van Sinderen, M. Wallace, L. Brennan, C. Stanton, J. R. Marchesi, A. P. Fitzgerald, F. Shanahan, C. Hill, R. P. Ross, and P. W. O'Toole. "Gut Microbiota Composition Correlates with Diet and Health in the Elderly." *Nature* 488 (2012): 178–184.

Corrigan, P. W. "Where is the Evidence Supporting Public Service Announcements to Eliminate Mental Illness Stigma?" *Psychiatric Services* 63 (2014): 79–82.

Corrigan, P. W., J. E. Larson, and N. Rusch. "Self-Stigma and the Why Try Effect: Impact on Life Goals and Evidence-Based Practices." *World Psychiatry* 8 (2009): 75–81.

Corrigan, P. W., F. E. Markowitz, and A. C. Watson. "Structural Levels of Mental Illness Stigma and Discrimination." *Schizophrenia Bulletin* 30 (2004): 481–491.

Courcoulas, A. P., N. J. Christian, S. H. Belle, P. D. Berk, D. R. Flum, L. Gracia, M. Horlick, M. A. Kalarchian, W. C. King, J. E. Mitchell, E. J. Patterson, J. R. Pender, A. Pomp, W. J. Pories, R. C. Thirlby, S. Z. Yanovski, and B. M. Wolfe. "Weight Change and Health Outcomes at 3 Years After Bariatric Surgery Among Individuals with Severe Obesity." *Journal of the American Medical Association* 310 (2013): 2416–2425.

Crayton, J. W. "How to Manage Depression in Overweight or Obese Patients." *Current Psychiatry* 11 (2012).

Dash, S., G. Clarke, M. Berk, and F. N. Jacka. "The Gut Microbiome and Diet in Psychiatry: Focus on Depression." *Current Opinion in Psychiatry* 28 (2015): 1–6.

Dicken, M., S. L. Thomas, B. King, S. Lewis, and K. Holland. "The Role of the Fatosphere in Fat Adults' Responses to Obesity Stigma: A Model of Empowerment Without a Focus on Weight Loss." *Qualitative Health Research* 21 (2011): 1679–1691.

Dixon, J. B., M. E. Dixon, and P. E. O'Brien. "Depression in Association with Severe Obesity: Changes with Weight Loss." *Archives of Internal Medicine* 163 (2003): 2058–2065.

Dumova, T., and R. Fiordo (eds.). *Blogging in the Global Society: Cultural, Political and Geographical Aspects.* Hershey, PA: Information Science Reference, IGI Global, 2012.

Fettich, K. C., and E. Y. Chen. "Coping with Obesity Stigma Affects Depressed Mood in African American and White Candidates for Bariatric Surgery." *Obesity* 20 (2012): 1118–1121.

Flegal, K. M., M. D. Carroll, B. K. Kit, and C. L. Ogden. "Prevalence of Obesity and Trends in the Distribution of Body Mass Index Among US Adults, 1999–2010." *Journal of the American Medical Association* 307 (2012): 491–497.

Friedman, K. E., J. A. Ashmore, and K. L. Applegate. "Recent Experiences of Weight-based Stigmatization in a Weight Loss Surgery Population: Psychological and Behavioral Correlates." *Obesity* 16 (2008): S69–S74.

Friedman, K. E., S. K. Reichmann, P. R. Costanzo, A. Zelli, J. A. Ashmore, and G. J. Musante. "Weight Stigmatization and Ideological Beliefs: Relation to Psychological Functioning in Obese Adults." *Obesity Research* 13 (2005): 907–916.

Givens, J. L., I. R. Katz, S. Bellamy, and W. C. Holmes. "Stigma and the Acceptability of Depression Treatments Among African Americans and Whites." *Journal of General Internal Medicine* 22 (2007): 1292–1297.

Gluckman, P. D., M. A. Hanson, and A. S. Beedle. "Early Life Events and Their Consequences for Later Disease: A Life History and Evolutionary Perspective." *American Journal of Human Biology* 19 (2007): 1–19.

Greenhalgh, S., and M. Carney. "Bad Biocitizens? Latinos and the U.S. 'Obesity Epidemic.'" *Human Organization* 73 (2014): 267–276.

Haines, J., D. Neumark-Sztainer, M. E. Eisenberg, and P. J. Hannan. "Weight Teasing and Disordered Eating Behaviors in Adolescents: Longitudinal Findings from Project EAT (Eating Among Teens)." *Pediatrics* 117 (2006): E209–E215.

Harding, K., and M. Kirby. *Lessons from the Fat-O-Sphere: Quit Dieting and Declare a Truce with your Body*. New York: Penguin Group, 2009.

Hatzenbuehler, M. L., and B. G. Link. "Introduction to the Special Issue on Structural Stigma and Health." *Social Science and Medicine* 103 (2014): 1–6.

Hatzenbuehler, M. L., J. C. Phelan, and B. G. Link. "Stigma as a Fundamental Cause of Population Health Inequalities." *American Journal of Public Health* 103 (2013): 813–821.

Heo, M., A. Pietrobelli, K. R. Fontaine, J. A. Sirey, and M. S. Faith. "Depressive Mood and Obesity in US Adults: Comparison and Moderation by Sex, Age, and Race." *International Journal of Obesity* 30 (2006): 513–519.

Herbert, J. "Cortisol and Depression: Three Questions for Psychiatry." *Psychological Medicine* 43 (2013): 449–469.

Jequier, E. "Leptin Signaling, Adiposity, and Energy Balance." *Annals of the New York Academy of Sciences* 967 (2002): 379–388.

Karlsson, L. "Desperately Seeking Sameness: The Processes and Pleasures of Identification in Women's Diary Blog Reading." *Feminist Media Studies* 7 (2007): 137–153.

Karlsson, J., C. Taft, A. Ryden, L. Sjöström, and M. Sullivan. "Ten-Year Trends in Health-Related Quality of Life After Surgical and Conventional Treatment for Severe Obesity: The SOS Intervention Study." *International Journal of Obesity* 31 (2007): 1248–61.

Kolotkin, R. L., R. D. Crosby, R. E. Gress, S. C. Hunt, S. G. Engel, and T. D. Adams. "Health and Health-Related Quality of Life: Differences Between Men and Women Who Seek Gastric Bypass Surgery." *Surgery for Obesity and Related Diseases* 4 (2008): 651–658.

de Laat, P. "Online Diaries: Reflections on Trust, Privacy, and Exhibitionism." *Ethics and Information Technology* 10 (2008): 57–69.

Lawson, E. A., K. K. Miller, J. I. Blum, E. Meenaghan, M. Misra, K. T. Eddy, D. B. Herzog, and A. Klibanski. "Leptin Levels Are Associated with Decreased Depressive Symptoms in Women Across the Weight Spectrum, Independent of Body Fat." *Clinical Endocrinology* 76 (2012): 520–525.

Leggatt-Cook, C., and K. Chamberlain. "Blogging for Weight Loss: Personal Accountability, Writing Selves, and the Weight-Loss Blogosphere." *Sociology of Health and Illness* 34 (2011): 963–977.

Lerman, S. "'Un Pueblo Tan Dulce': Diabetes, Depression, and Obesity Syndemics in Puerto Rico." MA thesis, University of Connecticut, 2015.

Lewis, S., S. L. Thomas, R. W. Blood, D. J. Castle, J. Hyde, and P. A. Komesaroff. "How Do Obese Individuals Perceive and Respond to the Different Types of Obesity Stigma That They Encounter in Their Daily Lives? A Qualitative Study." *Social Science & Medicine* 73 (2011): 1349–1356.

Li, D., L. Liu, and R. Odouli. "Presence of Depressive Symptoms During Early Pregnancy and the Risk of Preterm Delivery: A Prospective Cohort Study." *Human Reproduction* 24 (2008): 146–153.

Link, B. G., and J. Phelan. "Social Conditions as Fundamental Causes of Disease." *Journal of Health and Social Behavior* (1995): 80–94.

Lock, M., and P. Kaufert. "Menopause, Local Biologies, and Cultures of Aging." *American Journal of Human Biology* 13 (2001): 494–504.

Lopez, L. "The Radical Act of 'Mommy Blogging': Redefining Motherhood Through the Blogosphere." *New Media & Society* 11 (2009): 729–747.

Luppino, F. S., L. M. de Wit, P. F. Bouvy, T. Stijnen, P. Cuijpers, B. W. J. H. Penninx, and F. G. Zitman. "Overweight, Obesity, and Depression: A Systematic Review and Meta-Analysis of Longitudinal Studies." *Archives of General Psychiatry* 67 (2010): 220–229.

Lupton, D. *Fat.* New York: Routledge, 2013.

Ma, Jun, and Lan Xiao. "Obesity and Depression in US Women: Results from the 2005–2006 National Health and Nutritional Examination Survey." *Obesity* 18 (2010): 347–353.

Magro, D. O., B. Geloneze, R. Delfini, B. C. Pareja, F. Callejas, and J. C. Pareja. "Long-Term Weight Regain After Gastric Bypass: A 5-Year Prospective Study." *Obesity Surgery* 18 (2008): 648–651.

Major, B., J. M. Hunger, D. P. Bunyan, and C. T. Miller. "The Ironic Effects of Weight Stigma." *Journal of Experimental Social Psychology* 51 (2014): 74–80.

Marmot, M. "Taking Action on Social Determinants to Improve Mental Health in Urban Settings." Keynote Address: The Social Determinants of Urban Mental Health: Paving the Way Forward. UCL Institute of Health Equity, 2012.

McCullough, M. B., and J. A. Hardin (eds.). *Reconstructing Obesity: The Meaning of Measures and the Measure of Meanings.* New York: Berghahn Books, 2013.

Mechanick, J. I., A. Youdim, D. B. Jones, W. T Garvey, D. L. Hurley, M. M. McMahon, L. J. Heinberg, R. Kuchner, T. D. Adams, S. Shikora, J. B. Dixon, and S. Brethauer. "Clinical Practice Guidelines for the Perioperative Nutritional, Metabolic, and Nonsurgical Support of the Bariatric Surgery Patient-2013 Update: Cosponsored by American Association of Clinical Endocrinologists, The Obesity Society, and American Society for Metabolic & Bariatric Surgery." *Surgery for Obesity and Related Diseases* 9 (2013): 159–191.

Mendenhall, E. *Syndemic Suffering: Social Distress, Depression, and Diabetes among Mexican Immigrant Women*. San Francisco, CA: Left Coast Press, 2012.

Mendes, Elizabeth. "Obesity Linked to Lower Emotional Wellbeing." Accessed August 2015. Available at http://www.gallup.com/poll/143045/obesity-linked-lower-emotional-wellbeing.aspx.

Milaneschi, Y., E. M. Simonsick, N. Vogelzangs, E. S. Strotmeyer, K. Yaffe, T. B. Harris, M. I. Tolea, L. Ferrucci, and B. W. Penninx. "Leptin, Abdominal Obesity and Onset of Depression in Older Men and Women." *The Journal of Clinical Psychiatry* 73 (2012): 1205–1211.

Monaghan, L. F. "Big Handsome Men, Bears, and Others: Virtual Constructions of 'Fat Male Embodiment.'" *Body & Society* 11 (2005): 81–111.

Myers, A. and J. C. Rosen. "Obesity Stigmatization and Coping: Relation to Mental Health Symptoms, Body Image, and Self-Esteem." *International Journal of Obesity* 23 (1999): 221–230.

Nardi, B. A., D. J. Schiano, M. Gumbrecht, and L. Swartz. "'Why We Blog.'" *Communications of the ACM* 47 (2004): 41–46.

Neumark-Sztainer, D., M. Wall, M. Story, and A. R. Standish. "Dieting and Unhealthy Weight Control Behaviors During Adolescence: Associations with 10-Year Changes in Body Mass Index." *Journal of Adolescent Health* 50 (2012): 80–86.

Nicholson, A., H. Pikhart, A. Pajak, S. Malyutina, R. Kubinova, A. Peasey, R. Topor-Madry, Y. Nikitin, M. Bobak, and M. Marmot. "Socio-Economic Status Over the Life-Course and Depressive Symptoms in Men and Women in Eastern Europe." *Journal of Affective Disorders* 105 (2008): 125–136.

Nichter, M. *Fat Talk: What Girls and their Parents Say about Dieting*. Boston, MA: Harvard University Press, 2000.

Nichter, M. "Idioms of Distress: Alternatives in the Expression of Psychosocial Distress: A Case Study from South India." *Culture, Medicine and Psychiatry* 5 (1981): 379–408.

O'Brien, P. E., L. MacDonald, M. Anderson, L. Brennan, and W. A. Brown. "Long-Term Outcomes After Bariatric Surgery: Fifteen-Year Follow-Up of Adjustable Gastric Banding and a Systematic Review of the Bariatric Surgical Literature." *Annals Surgery* 257 (2013): 87–94.

Odom, J., K. C. Zalesin, T. L. Washington, W. W. Miller, B. Hakmeh, D. L. Zaremba, M. Altattan, M. Balasubramaniam, D. S. Gibbs, K. R. Krause, D. L. Chengelis, B. A. Franklin, and P. A. McCullough. "Behavioral Predictors of Weight Regain after Bariatric Surgery." *Obesity Surgery* 20 (2010): 349–356.

Ostrach, B., and M. Singer. "At Special Risk: Biopolitical Vulnerability and HIV Syndemics Among Women." *Health Sociology Review* 21 (2012): 258–271.

Owen, L. "Monstrous Freedom: Charting Fat Ambivalence." *Fat Studies* 4 (2015): 1–13.

Pike, I. L. "Maternal Stress and Fetal Responses: Evolutionary Perspectives on Preterm Delivery." *American Journal of Human Biology* 17 (2005): 55–65.

Pitts, V. "Illness and Internet Empowerment: Writing and Reading Breast Cancer in Cyberspace." *Health* 8 (2004): 33–59.

Pratt, L. A., and D. J. Brody. "Depression in the US Household Population, 2009–2012." *NCHS Data Brief, no 172*. National Center for Health Statistics (2014): 1–8.

Pratt, L. A., and D. J. Brody. "Depression and Obesity in the US Adult Household Population, 2005–2010." *NCHS Data Brief, no 167*. National Center for Health Statistics (2014): 1–8.

Puhl, R. M., and C. A. Heuer. "Obesity Stigma: Important Considerations for Public Health." *American Journal of Public Health* 100 (2010): 1019–1028.

Puhl, R. M., and C. A. Heuer. "The Stigma of Obesity: A Review and Update." *Obesity* 17 (2009): 941–964.

Rausch, P. "Cyberdieting: Blogs as Adjuncts to Women's Weight Loss Efforts." MA thesis, University of Florida, 2006.

Reed, A. "'My Blog Is Me': Texts and Persons in UK Online Journal Culture (and Anthropology)." *Ethnos* 70 (2005): 220–42.

Rogge, M. M. "Obesity, Stigma, and Civilized Oppression." *Advances in Nursing Science* 27 (2004): 301–315.

Roberto, C. A., R. Sysko, J. Bush, R. Pearl, R. M. Puhl, N. A. Schvey, and J. F. Dovidio. 2012. "Clinical Correlates of the Weight Bias Internalization Scale in a Sample of Obese Adolescents Seeking Bariatric Surgery." *Obesity* 20 (2012): 533–9.

Rothblum, E. D., and S. Solovay (eds.). *The Fat Studies Reader*. New York: New York University, 2009.

Saguy, A. *What's Wrong with Fat?* Oxford, UK: Oxford University Press, 2013.

Salvy, S. J., J. C. Bowker, L. A. Nitecki, M. A. Kluczynski, L. J. Germeroth, and J. N. Roemmich. "Impact of Simulated Ostracism on Overweight and Normal-Weight Youths' Motivation to Eat and Food Intake." *Appetite* 56 (2011): 39–45.

Schvey, N. A., R. M. Puhl, and K. D. Brownell. "The Impact of Weight Stigma on Caloric Consumption." *Obesity* 19 (2011): 1957–1962.

Simon, G. E., E. J. Ludman, J. A. Linde, B. H. Operskalski, L. Ichikawa, P. Rohde, E. A. Finch, and R. W. Jeffery. "Association Between Obesity and Depression in Middle-aged Women." *General Hospital Psychiatry* 30 (2008): 32–39.

Singer, M. *Introduction to Syndemics: A Systems Approach to Public and Community Health.* San Francisco, CA: Jossey-Bass, John Wiley & Sons, 2009.

Sjöström, C. D., L. Lissner, H. Wedel, and L. Sjöström. "Reduction in Incidence of Diabetes, Hypertension and Lipid Disturbances After Intentional Weight Loss Induced by Bariatric Surgery: The SOS Intervention Study." *Obesity Research* 7 (1999): 477–484.

Sjöström, L., A. K. Lindroos, M. Peltonen, J. Torgerson, C. Bouchard, B. Carlsson, S. Dahlgren, B. Larsson, K. Narbro, C. D. Sjöström, M. Sullivan, and H. Wedel. "Lifestyle, Diabetes, and Cardiovascular Risk Factors 10 years After Bariatric Surgery." *New England Journal of Medicine* 351 (2004): 2683–2693.

Sjöström, L., K. Narbro, D. Sjöström, K. Karason, B. Larsson, H. Wedel, T. Lystig, M. Sullivan, C. Bouchard, B. Carlsson, C. Bengtsson, S. Dahlgren, A. Gummesson, P. Jacobson, J. Karlsson, A. K. Lindroos, H. Lönroth, I. Näslund, T. Olbers, K. Stenlöf, J. Torgerson, G. Ågren, L. M. S. Carlsson, and the Swedish Obese Subjects Study. "Effects of Bariatric Surgery on Mortality in Swedish Obese Subjects." *New England Journal of Medicine* 357 (2007): 741–752.

Sjöström, L., M. Peltonen, P. Jacobson, S. Ahlin, J. Andersson-Assarsson, Å. Anveden, C. Bouchard, B. Carlsson, K. Karason, H. Lönroth, I. Näslund, E. Sjöström, M. Taube, H. Wedel, P. A. Svensson, K. Sjöholm, and L. M. S. Carlsson. "Association of Bariatric Surgery with Long-term Remission of Type 2 Diabetes and with Microvascular and Macrovascular Complications." *Journal of the American Medical Association* 311 (2014): 2297–2304.

Talbot, F., and A. Nouwen. 2000. "A Review of the Relationship Between Depression and Diabetes in Adults." *Diabetes Care* 23(10): 1556–1562.

Tanumihardjo, S. A., C. Anderson, M. Kaufer-Horwitz, L. Bode, N. J. Emenaker, A. M. Hagg, J. A. Satia, H. J. Silver, and D. D. Stadler. "Poverty, Obesity, and Malnutrition: An International Perspective Recognizing the Paradox." *Journal of the American Dietetic Association* 107 (2007): 1966–1972.

Thonney B., Z. Pataky, S. Badel, E. Bobbioni-Harsch, and A. Golay. "The Relationship Between Weight Loss and Psychosocial Functioning Among Bariatric Surgery Patients." *American Journal of Surgery* 199 (2010): 183–188.

Trainer, S., A. Brewis, D. Hruschka, and D. Williams. "Translating Obesity: Navigating the Front Lines of the 'War on Fat.'" *American Journal of Human Biology* 27 (2015): 61–68.

Trainer, S., A. Brewis, D. Williams, and J. Rosales Chavez, and D. Williams. "Obese, Fat, or 'Just Big'? Young Adult Deployment of and Reactions to Weight Terms." *Human Organization* 74 (2015): 266–275.

Trainer, S., A. Brewis, A. Wutich, L. Kurtz, and M. Niesluchowski. "The Fat Self in Virtual Communities: Success and Failure in Weight-Loss Blogging." *Current Anthropology* 57 (2016): 523–528.

Vartanian, L. R., and S. A. Novak. "Internalized Societal Attitudes Moderate the Impact of Weight Stigma on Avoidance of Exercise." *Obesity* 19 (2011): 757–762.

Vartanian L. R. and J. G. Shaprow. "Effects of Weight Stigma on Exercise Motivation and Behavior: A Preliminary Investigation Among College-Aged Females." *Journal of Health Psychology* 13 (2008): 131–138.

Wallace, T. C., F. Guarner, K. Madsen, M. D. Cabana, G. Gibson, E. Hentges, and M. E. Sanders. "Human Gut Microbiota and Its Relationship to Health and Disease." *Nutrition Reviews* 69 (2011): 392–403.

Weaver, L. J., and C. Hadley. "Social Pathways in the Co-morbidity Between Type 2 Diabetes and Mental Health Concerns in a Pilot Study of Urban Middle and Upper-Class Indian Women." *Ethos* 29 (2011): 211–225.

Weaver, L. J., and E. Mendenhall. "Applying Syndemics and Chronicity: Interpretations from Studies of Poverty, Depression, and Diabetes." *Medical Anthropology: Cross-Cultural Studies in Health and Illness* 33 (2014): 92–108.

Wells, K. B., A. Stewart, R. D. Hays, M. A. Burnam, W. Rogers, M. Daniels, S. Berry, S. Greenfield, and J. Ware. "The Functioning and Well-being of Depressed Patients." *Journal of the American Medical Association* 262 (1989): 914–919.

Wilkinson, D., and M. Thelwall. "Researching Personal Information on the Public Web: Methods and Ethics." *Social Science Computer Review* 29 (2011): 387–401.

de Wit, L., F. Luppino, A. van Straten, B. Penninx, F. Zitman, and P. Cuijpers. "Depression and Obesity: A Meta-Analysis of Community-Based Studies." *Psychiatry research* 178 (2010): 230–235.

World Health Organization (WHO). "BMI Classification." Accessed August 2016. http://apps.who.int/bmi/index.jsp?introPage=intro_3.html.

Wott, C. B., and R. A. Carels. "Overt Weight Stigma, Psychological Distress and Weight Loss Treatment Outcomes." *Journal of Health Psychology* 15 (2010): 608–614.

Zhao, G., E. S. Ford, S. Dhingra, C. Li, T. W. Strine, and A. H. Mokdad. "Depression and Anxiety among US Adults: Associations with Body Mass Index." *International Journal of Obesity* 33 (2009): 257–266.

Chapter Five

The PHAMILIS Stigma Syndemic Among Homeless Women

Ruthanne Marcus and Merrill Singer

The public perception of homelessness is fraught with negative images and stereotypes that can be said to constitute a total stigma environment for people who are without homes. Living under these conditions has identifiable consequences for the health and well-being of people who are homeless, including, as described in this chapter, suffering from a distinctive stigma syndemic that increases the health burden of those deemed to fit the constructed social category of being homeless.

Despite endurance of adverse portrayal and discrimination as an identifiable category of people, in fact, people who are homeless are not a fixed or undifferentiated population nor is homelessness a stable unchanging condition. Rather, the face of homelessness has been transformed since the images of the Bowery and Skid Row were etched in the public's imagination during the early twentieth century, a gallery of images that depicted homeless, drunk men gathering aimlessly on urban street corners (Hopper 2003; Rossi 1989; Wagner 1993). In the 1960s, homeless people in the United States, predominantly older white men, were living in inexpensive single-room occupancy (SRO) hotels, mission shelters, or temporarily in jails. In the 1950s and 1960s only 3 percent of the homeless population were women (Bassuk 1993). Furthermore, in the 1960s, mental health reforms closed many psychiatric facilities and forced mentally ill persons onto the street, leaving them to sleep in the cold, in doorways, on park benches or culverts, under bridges, or in other outdoor or nonpermanent locations (Rossi 1989). In the 1970s, economic stagnation, rising inflation, decline in real wages, the significant loss of manufacturing jobs, and high unemployment levels led to a rise in the number of homeless people (Glasser and Bridgman 1999). As Skid Rows vanished in many large cities, the homeless population also declined, as many pensioners moved to subsidized housing for the elderly. The composition of the homeless population changed significantly in the 1980s when the gentrification of urban areas created a lack of affordable housing and an increase in companies with unattainable high-tech jobs requiring specialized education forced people onto the streets and other nonpermanent locations (Burt 1992; Hopper 1988; Rossi 1989). Also during this decade, state and federal welfare programs were reduced, real estate prices rose, lower-paid service-industry jobs and part-time work increased, affordable housing decreased, and the departure of manufacturing industry reduced available well paid employment (Burt 1992). Due to the convergence of all these factors, at this time there was a large increase in the number of visibly homeless men and women on the streets making them much harder for polite society to ignore (Burt 1992; Rossi 1989). During the period 1985–1990, unlike in earlier decades, the proportion of homeless women came to equal the number of homeless men (Lehmann et al. 2007).

Welfare reform during the 1980s and 1990s further altered this population as younger women, mothers and their children were forced to seek residence on the streets, in shelters, subway stations, bus stations, and other public places (Glasser and Bridgman 1999; Rossi 1989). These changes notwithstanding, homeless people remain subject to daily categorization as undesirable, disreputable, damaged, and blameworthy for their failure to live up to social expectations about personal success, acceptable residence, and proper self-display.

Women who are living without shelter represent a growing proportion of the homeless population in the United States (Homelessness 2013). Of the approximately 3.5 million people who are homeless; one-third are women (U.S. Department of Housing and Urban Development 2011). Homeless women suffer from an array of health and social problems and these are exacerbated by multiple layers of social stigma that adhere to substance abuse, physical, emotional and sexual abuse, social loss, residential instability, and perpetual poverty. It is this population and their experience with the effects of stigma and structural violence that is the focus of this chapter.

Understanding this population entails untangling a number of complexities. The first of these has to do with a multitude of intertwined influences that line the pathway to homelessness, including predisposing, exacerbating, and intervening factors that shape the lived-experience of homeless women. Although presented here heuristically as discrete factors they are overlapping and co-existing variables. Predisposing factors, such as poverty and living in unstable families (single motherhood, divorce, estranged relationships) lead to homelessness, whereas exacerbating factors, such as abuse, trauma, mental illness, and substance abuse, worsen the lives of people who are homeless. Certain intervening factors, such as incarceration, disability, early pregnancy, and custody battles, further complicate their homeless situation. And at every level these factors are driven by and entwined with stigma.

In this chapter we analyze this complexity using Critical Medical Anthropology (CMA) theory (Baer et al. 2003; Singer 2004). From this perspective, the stigmatization of homelessness in society is the result of built-in structural inequities in housing, education, employment, law enforcement, access to health care and needed resources, and achievement of valued social statuses, all of which comprise a sweeping pattern of discriminations against the poor and ethnic and other minorities. Therefore, homelessness in the United States is linked directly to the ideologies and processes of capitalism and to power and to the ways these are rationalized in society in a context of massive and growing inequalities. Thus, we argue here that the homeless are stigmatized because they are said to make no valuable contribution to society/economy (Belcher and DeForge 2012). Rather, they are portrayed as social failures and a drag on those deemed to be respectable and worthy citizens. The contribution of such treatment to the misery of the homeless and to the creation of a blamable object is a specter that haunts dominant ideology about the poorest members of society (Singer and Page 2013). Having such a population provides both a negative role model to help discipline the rest of society and a scapegoat to blame for the problems of modern life.

In short, people who are homeless are heavily stigmatized for five reasons (Jones et al. 1984): (1) they are the bottom rung of the broader stigmatized strata of the poor, a group seen as responsible for its own failure in society; (2) they are forced to spend considerable time on the streets or in public places and are, therefore, visible to others (including those in positions of authority), and they are often viewed as disruptive; (3) being without regular shelter, they have difficulties cleaning themselves or their clothes and can be considered aesthetically unappealing and unhygienic (and hence a health threat); (4) they may have mental illness or substance use disorders (Link et al. 1997, 1995; Phelan et al. 1997); and (5) because the homeless serve as among the most easily targeted blamable populations upon which to assign culpability for structurally caused problems of contemporary society. Many homeless people as a result may struggle to hide their stigmatized identities (Quinn and Earnshaw 2011), such as being someone with a mental illness or having HIV infection, as a way to reduce their experience of ridicule. Recognizing the range of stigmatizing conditions affecting people who are homeless helps reveal the multiple layers of oppression and marginalization they face.

Homelessness stigma directly affects the personal experience of a shared social suffering that is impacted by mental illness (Corrigan 2005; Rüsch et al. 2005), substance abuse (Ahern et al. 2007; Earnshaw et al. 2013), physical and sexual abuse (Coffey et al. 1996; Overstreet and Quinn 2013), and poor physical health (Bassuk et al. 1998; Benbow et al. 2011; Gelberg and Arangua 2006; Hwang et al. 2011; Rabiner and Weiner 2012). These intertwined and multifactorial structural and personal conditions create a stigma-driven syndemic unique to people who are homeless.

The mosaic of health, behavioral, and social problems of homeless women are interactive and this intersection of factors worsens their overall health status. In this light, we describe what they call the *PHAMILIS stigma syndemic* (acronym spelled out below) they observed among homeless women, as a set of multilayered denigrated conditions comprised of the relationships that exist between physical and mental health problems, substance abuse, and physical, emotional and sexual abuse, significantly compounded by the effects of social loss, residential instability, and perpetual poverty. The authors developed the argument presented in this chapter based on life history analyses using data collected in a field study of homeless women ($n = 30$) living in a shelter in rural Connecticut in 2010–2011.[1] The shelter is located in a town of just over 4,000 people in northeastern Connecticut, near the Massachusetts and Rhode Island borders.

Small towns are rarely explored as locations to study homelessness (most often considered an urban issue) yet this setting provided a unique opportunity to study homeless women and their life experiences. The *Entré* shelter is an emergency facility with 60 beds for families and single men and women with a 60-day stay limit. The facility provides referrals to housing, employment, mental health, and substance use services. The purpose of this chapter is to describe women's experiences with, and propose the model for, the homeless stigma syndemic that emerged from their analysis.

A SYNDEMIC CALLED PHAMILIS

A syndemic approach offers a theoretical framework that emerged from CMA. This model helps in understanding the complexities of homelessness and provides a window of insight on its causation and challenges. In a syndemic, there is a synergistic interaction of two or more co-existing or sequential diseases or other health conditions (e.g., mental illness) that contributes to an excess burden of ill health in a social group or population (Singer and Clair 2003). The clustering of diseases in a population, and hence the conditions that foster the potential for disease interaction, are facilitated by structural factors like physical and structural violence, including poverty, discrimination, abuse, and social trauma. Women, in particular, are subject to interacting conditions that are exacerbated by social structural factors affecting their lives (Meyer et al. 2011; Ostrach and Singer 2012). These intertwined factors constitute the syndemic here labeled PHAMILIS (read as families)—Physical Health problems, Abuse (physical, sexual, emotional), Mental Illness, Loss, Instability, and Substance abuse (alcohol, tobacco, and other drugs). These domains typify and, within the context of broader structural factors, help explain the lived experience and the making of homelessness at the individual level. Structural factors that create the social conditions that foster homelessness include social policies and practices that produce cyclical economic downturns and loss or lack of access to jobs, as well as restrictions on housing opportunities, the policing of the poor, and related enactments of power and social control in support of an architecture of inequality (Lyon-Callo 2004; Susser 1996). Syndemics rely on two interrelated interactions: first, at least two health conditions interacting adversely with one another in a given social or structural context, which in the case of PHAMILIS involves a set of physical health conditions, physical and sexual abuse, mental illness, and substance abuse in settings of homelessness; second, the creation and aggravation of these health conditions by a set of social conditions, which in PHAMILIS include various stigmatized forms of social loss and instability, and poverty. These multiple interactions in their varying combinations, in turn, result in both a heightened disease burden and contribute to the occurrence and reoccurrence of homelessness.

PHAMILIS AND THE EXPERIENCE OF STIGMA

The constructs that comprise the PHAMILIS syndemic reflect multilayered stigmatized conditions affecting homelessness (Earnshaw and Chaudoir 2009). The women interviewed for this study, for example, expressed feelings of being unjustly treated by society, shelter staff and other residents, and most importantly by their families. Primarily because of the stigma associated with being homeless, women tried to hide their situation. They spoke about the profound shame and embarrassment they felt from being at the shelter.

The shelter is in a small town and the location of the shelter is well known to the townspeople. "Mary," (a pseudonym, as are all participant names) one of the interviewed women, had worked in town for many years before coming to the shelter, so she knew many local residents. She had relocated to a state in the Western United States and after many years got divorced, lost her primary source of income, and subsequently returned to the area. She discussed her reluctance to go into her former workplace or even to walk around the neighborhood for fear of running into someone she knew when she previously lived in the area. Mary was quite concerned that people would know that she was homeless and would judge her negatively.

This fear and perceived stigma also affected children staying at the shelter. Sometimes to hide their homelessness they would walk down the street to get on the school bus rather than get on near the shelter. Children also got off the bus down the street so other students on the bus did not see where they were staying. Some women also hid their location and said that they do not tell people where they live. As Mary put it: "and no one knows I'm in a homeless shelter. I mean on Facebook I just crack jokes like it's every day." This need to conceal their housing status illustrates their shame and desire to keep their situation a secret. It also provides insight into how their everyday lives affect how they conceptualize homelessness. For example, "Laura" described her views on being considered homeless and who was aware of where she was staying:

> I don't tell people. My friends don't know. Her [daughter's] father doesn't know. Only about three people know. Only 'cuz if you find out I'm not going to lie. No they don't know but if they know and they find out that doesn't make me a bad person cause I'm homeless . . . I mean I could tell everybody and if they treated me different then I don't need to talk to you anyway cause if one slight difference change in me then you're not friends with me because of me, you're friends with me because of what I have or what I had . . . Being homeless doesn't make you a bad person . . . what you do when you become homeless defines who you are.

The complex factors contributing to the PHAMILIS stigma syndemic are impacted by circumstances that predispose women to homelessness, exacerbate their life situation, and intervene in their developmental trajectory. The interrelatedness of poverty, physical health problems, abuse (psychological, sexual, physical, substance abuse), mental illness, loss, and instability are the central domains identified in the lives of homeless women as depicted in figure 5.1 and described below, using data that we collected for this study.

Physical Health

The first component of the PHAMILIS stigma syndemic is Physical Health. This involves a bidirectional interaction as poor physical health affects homelessness and conversely homelessness can affect physical health. The physical health problems reported by homeless women in this study include heart disease, diabetes, seizures, chronic obstructive pulmonary disease (e.g., emphysema and chronic bronchitis), asthma, arthritis, musculoskeletal problems, or dental problems among other acute and chronic health conditions (Gelberg and Linn 1989; Gelberg et al. 1990; Hwang 2001). Many of these

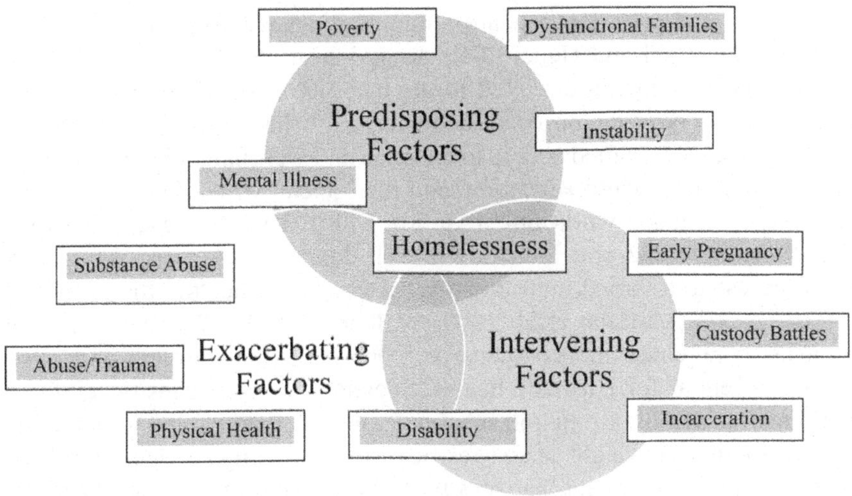

Figure 5.1. PHAMILIS Syndemic Model of Homeless Women

are stigmatizing conditions that affect how society relates to, discriminates against, and stereotypes homeless women.

Habitual self-medicating illicit drug use also increases the likelihood of infection with HIV, Hepatitis C Virus (HCV), as well as sexually transmitted infections (STIs) due to both high risk sexual behaviors (e.g., multiple partners, low condom use, sexual violence) and the mixing of sex and drug use (Khantzian 1985; Loeliger et al. 2016; Ostrach and Singer 2012). Women in the lead author's study mentioned poor health as restricting or limiting their ability to work or making them disabled and unable to obtain employment, resulting in their inability to afford stable housing. Some participants had worked or were currently working in low paying service positions with few, if any, health benefits, which delayed or restricted their accessing health care. Moreover, most felt that working class jobs contributed to their chronic health conditions, such as back (e.g., disc degeneration or osteoarthritis) or heart (e.g., hypertension) problems exacerbated by stress (Cohen et al. 2007; Yudkin et al. 2000). One woman described in detail being epileptic, which she felt was a result of serious physical abuse in childhood including head trauma. Another felt that as a child she was singled out among her siblings and abused by her father because she had Type I diabetes. Almost all the women smoked cigarettes and thus were at greater risk for lung disease and various cancers, including those of the head and neck.

Several of the women in this research were morbidly obese, a dynamic risk factor for physical health problems (e.g., diabetes, osteoarthritis, cardiovascular disease, and poor dental health), mental illness (discussed below), and weight stigma (Puhl and Heuer 2010; Rogge et al. 2004). Overweight and obesity in poor women are related to the inability to obtain good nutrition, complicated by poverty, no or inadequate health insurance, limited health care over time, constrained access to exercise and well-paid jobs, inappropriate and incomplete health education, and the societal view of poor women's bodies as "a devalued work tool" (Aguirre 2000). The relationship between being overweight and poor nutrition is well described (Aguirre 2000) with limited access to a varied, nutritionally balanced, and healthy diet, affected by food deserts (Morland et al. 2002; Walker et al. 2010) and the lack of resources to purchase more expensive foods containing protein and other nutrients essential for adequate health. Societal views on obesity reinforce discrimination against women in schools, in the job market, and in obtaining housing. Their overweight status restricts their mobility, creates problems in providing child care, and narrows their life chances in what has been described as a society in which obese persons are the "last acceptable targets of discrimination" (Puhl and Brownell 2001:788).

Poverty and homelessness exacerbate the physical health consequences of obesity by adding stress and depression which result in elevated cortisol levels and subsequent higher rates of chronic health conditions, such as memory loss, diabetes, and a weakened immune system (Gragnoli 2012). Other biological pathways contributing to the PHAMILIS syndemic, such as the effects of cultural consonance on elevated blood pressure levels as described by Dressler and colleagues (Dressler et al. 2005), have been reported. Similar syndemics affecting homeless women, for example diabetes and depression, have been described (Mendenhall 2012) as well as other syndemic interactions between diabetes, obesity, poverty, and mental illness (Lerman 2015).

Obesity-related chronic medical conditions such as cardiovascular disease, diabetes, and the co-occurring medical effects of poor dental health are exemplary of the PHAMILIS syndemic. Obese individuals tend to make infrequent visits to the dentist, and most often when they have a problem and not for prophylaxis. These patients have trouble accessing dental care and many dentists are reluctant to provide necessary care due to ergonomic access problems in the treatment area. Issues related to obesity also contribute to inadequate dental hygiene including poor diet (e.g., sugary snacks and soft drinks), uncontrolled heartburn (i.e., gastro-esophageal reflux), and frequent vomiting (Stillwell Accessed January 23, 2016).

As discussed at length by Raskin in the companion book that will follow this volume, oral health disparities are also created by inequities in dental health insurance, unequal access to dental care, lack of education, drug or alcohol use, and poor nutrition, and compounded by various forms of stigma.

Lack of dental care can begin in childhood if children are unable to attain access to dentists and preventive treatment, and they ultimately develop dental caries, missing teeth, and oral malformations at an early age (Carrion et al. 2011; Castañeda et al. 2010; Horton and Barker 2010). Into adulthood, suffering stigma and discrimination in work and other critical life settings can be affected by bad teeth (Horton and Barker 2010). An individual's teeth and mouth are visible to others and can become the basis for criticism, rejection, unfairness, and consequent loss of self-esteem. Limited or absent dental health care due to inequities in dental insurance among the poor adversely impact oral health (Edelstein 2002).

Mary described her experience with a two-class system in dental health care where people with Medicaid receive inferior treatment:

> I had to go to a dentist who had tattoos all over his arm, who looked like a biker who basically ripped my tooth out, which—I thought for sure I was gonna get dry socket—which has not completely healed yet. That's been a month now. That's my experience with how they treat people on Medicaid. Maybe it's me being paranoid, but that's my experience. . . . No, I've had a tooth pulled and a fake one put in but I was treated with dignity [when she used private insurance]. This was like this guy came in, rip, and just went on his way to the next one.

Mental Illness

A second health component of the PHAMILIS syndemic is mental illness which affects women's relationships, their ability to attain and maintain employment, and their daily functioning (Corrigan 2005; Rüsch et al. 2005). More than two thirds of homeless mothers have a mental illness, including post-traumatic stress disorder (PTSD), substance abuse and depression (Bassuk et al. 1998; Desmond 2006; Gelberg and Linn 1989).

Not all the women in this research disclosed suffering from a mental illness; however, of the 30 women interviewed, 22 (73 percent) mentioned some type of mental health issue. Several women had a depressive illness, the most frequently discussed condition, which affected their daily lives with consequences such as hospitalization or suicide attempts. "Sue," a woman in her late fifties with grown children, discussed her recent bout with depression:

> Ya know whatever they [hospital staff] said I just, I couldn't think. I couldn't hold a thought, very scattered, very anxious, very depressed. And then I went to an outpatient service—[name of program] at the hospital for it was either 3 or 4 weeks I'm not sure. I found out a lot of stuff just talking that I didn't . . . realize. And by the time I got out of there my diagnosis was major depression, anxiety disorder. I was oh I'm not going to be able to think of the word now,

> agoraphobic. Prior to that when I was at home. I couldn't leave, I couldn't, I couldn't even go out on the back porch. I could not leave the house. . . . I was really starting to go under but I didn't, I didn't know that.

Some of the women were being treated for depression, others had lived with the illness for many years, and others were coping with it in their own way. Those who had struggled for longer periods of time often were more nonchalant, discussing their mood and feelings in an unemotional manner. "Margaret" discussed how depression had affected her life in the following way:

> Psychiatric issues—mostly depression because of the situation. Not bein' with my kids. Not bein' able to support them or myself but I mean it was the right decision. I know that as much as it hurts them not bein' here with me, I know that it's better for them mentally 'cuz it's hard enough of a change goin' without mom to have too many changes. . . . It started in May and every time I think I'm strivin' and doin' better and gettin' on the beaten path to get back on my feet, something else happens and I hit a roadblock and I just sink right back into the depression. It just like starts all over again. It's not where I wanted to be—not where I pictured myself bein' at 39. . . . Nobody asks for depression. Nobody asks for most problems or health problems that come into their life. I could see if I was a druggy or something, but I mean I'm just like everybody else. Get up in the morning, go to work, get your kids off to the bus, go to work, come home, make supper, get your kids to bed, do your cleaning and go to bed that night and get up and do it all over the next mornin'.

The second most common mental illness was anxiety. Generalized anxiety is difficult to separate from situational anxiety created by being homeless which worsened the women's health problems and promoted ill health, especially stress-related diseases (e.g., hypertension, heart disease) or diet-related problems (e.g., overweight and obesity, nutritional deficiencies). The women who spoke about their anxiety discussed it as a life-long factor that they faced, seldom identifying their current feelings as anxiety.

Drug Abuse

Mental illness is closely linked with drug abuse, which includes all mood/mind altering drugs and alcohol and tobacco. The women who discussed drug use in their lives were often coping with depression, anxiety, personality disorders, and low self-esteem. Personal drug use in early years or by family members negatively impacted their ability to maintain a stable life and to deal with life stressors of jobs, housing, or relationships. Too often people self-treat their mental illness by using drugs such as alcohol, tobacco, or illegal drugs that temporarily alleviate some of their pain and suffering (Khantzian

1985). Drug use has been identified as a key component of syndemic interactions with significant adverse health outcomes (Singer 2014; Stall et al. 2003; Van Tieu and Koblin 2009).

Drug or alcohol use by the women themselves or a family member was quite prevalent with almost half ($n = 14$; 47 percent) mentioning ever using drugs either in adolescence or adulthood. Involvement in drug use may have social or economic motivators as relationships are sometimes built upon shared participation in drug consumption. Additionally, buying and selling drugs, or exchanging drugs for sex, food, housing, or other commodities, may be a means of economic survival. Substance use was a central theme in the life stories told by many of the women and some were in recovery. Some attributed their substance use to childhood exposure through their parents.

Several women described being given drugs by husbands or partners. This method of control or demonstrating power had a direct impact on women's feelings of self-esteem and independence, and further affected their mental and physical health. "Rose," for example, spoke about her abusive relationship and the toll alcohol and other drugs had taken on her life: "[My husband] was very abusive, you know, alcohol, drugs, the same thing over and over, alcohol and drugs, that's my whole life, alcohol and drugs, that's all I've seen." She described how this exposure had led her to continued drug use which haunted her most of her life.

> like I said, I wasn't much of a drinker. I was after the pills, actually, you know . . . I've tooken a lot. I've tooken like barbiturates, and I've tooken speed, and I've tooken—I've took Percocet, but I don't like those pills no more. If I'm hurting, I would take a Tylenol, you know, just no more. You would just not think I would be wild, but I was. I was just wild. That's all I knew, that's the violence, everything, and never got in trouble and never got caught with the law.

Some of the women had childhoods that were plagued by alcoholic parents or their own alcohol use as described by Rose:

> That's a cycle with my past, you know. He [her father] used to give us beer in a Dixie cup. We'd go out and get snow and put snow in it. At first, I didn't like it, and then afterwards, I started liking the beer. I was about six, seven years old. It was a problem. It started very young. It's like everywhere I turn, my family has always had an issue with drinking.

Abuse

Abuse is another stigmatized condition within the PHAMILIS syndemic. As noted, this broad domain includes psychological or emotional abuse, sexual abuse, and physical abuse. Most instances of abuse are hidden from view and rarely discussed due to the feared severe consequences of disclosing it. Experience of abuse has damaging lifelong effects and contributes substantially to women's risk of homelessness (Baker et al. 2010; Browne 1993; Hamilton et al. 2011; Ponce et al. 2014). The number of women who reported they had experienced a form of abuse in their lives was startling. Of the women interviewed, 13 (43 percent) had been physically abused, either as a child or as an adult. Most of these women were abused by their father or step-father during childhood or by a partner in adulthood. Eight mentioned sex abuse by their father, step-father, or other relatives. At least one-third of the women had been emotionally abused by someone, including their mother, father, or a partner, who frequently suffered from drug use disorders. Emotional or psychological abuse occurred when a parent or partner damaged the woman's self-esteem by controlling her, insulting her, or otherwise demoralizing her. This psychological distress left the woman unable to fully care for herself or her children, make her own decisions without the fear of criticism, or function independently. The detrimental effects of this form of abuse left scars on the women as painful as physical abuse.

Witnessing violence in their homes and community was also damaging to their psyche (Romero-Daza et al. 2005). Women reported a significant level of sexual abuse by a family member or family "friend." This violation of their bodies carried over into intimate relationships with partners and made them vulnerable to homelessness and further abuse (Bassuk et al. 2001; Davies-Netzley et al. 1996; Goodman et al. 1997; Green et al. 2012; Stein et al. 2002). They desperately sought attention and belonging that had been lacking in their younger years and too often their adult relationships were fraught with additional abuse. Intimate partner violence (IPV) was common and some of the women had spent time at domestic violence shelters prior to arriving at the *Entré* shelter. Suffering personal abuse had become a routine, if dreaded, part of their lives and each episode increased their susceptibility to further abuse, commonly resulting in mental health problems (Singer 2006). Stigma associated with IPV is multifactorial. Women involved in abusive relationships are stigmatized by society (cultural stigma), they often blame themselves for their abuse (internalized stigma), and they fear rejection if others find out about the abuse (anticipated stigma) (Overstreet and Quinn 2013).

Several of the women had been involved in relationships with men who physically abused them, while others were violated emotionally, or sexually. "Alice" described her abusive relationship with her husband and how it affected her children, the stability in their lives, her homeless situation, and her use of drugs:

> I've actually been considered homeless since June of 2009. I went to a transitional domestic violence program in [another town nearby] and moved up here.

> My abuser broke into my apartment and I had to move up here away from that city. He knows [where I am now] but he's moved on. He was just real mad. He is no longer, but he's no longer in my life anymore and I just came [here] for a fresh start, got a job at the school system. My sons were happy . . . but it's kind of a hard situation. . . . It didn't work, and I stuck it out for a year and a half after he was born and I just couldn't do it no more. I was on drugs and—I don't wanna say double pain—but just an excuse to get high.

Social and Structural Conditions

Beyond the interaction of diseases or behavioral conditions, syndemics unfold under harsh social, structural, and ecological conditions. The adverse social conditions described below predisposed women to homelessness and worsened their physical and mental health, in particular poverty and dysfunctional families began in childhood and were primary factors influencing their life trajectories. Further loss and instability intervened in their complex lives and caused additional pain and suffering.

Poverty

Poverty was the overarching predisposing stigmatizing construct that affected the homeless women from early childhood throughout their lives. Although not all the women who were interviewed came from poor natal families, they generally came to find themselves in situations where they were unable to utilize their resources and provide for themselves or their family. Poverty creates a risk environment in which people must cope with discrimination and multiple health disparities (Marmot 2005; Rhodes et al. 2005) and health consequences (Everson et al. 2002). Poor women face unequal access to health care, marginalized treatment by health-care providers, class discrimination, gendered inequalities, competing priorities, denial of health problems, and the inability to leverage social capital and economic resources to provide adequate health care for their families. Most of the women interviewed did not discuss being poor or growing up in poverty, yet their current situation being at the shelter illustrated this indisputable fact. They were relying on financial support, often from the government, for their health insurance, food, and housing subsidies, among other assistance, but this source is not accessible without admonishment, social hurdles, and changing ground rules. Their natal family's financial support was generally non-existent or sporadic, and women could not depend on them economically. This was primarily because their families were also impoverished, living on the edge, sometimes family members were alcoholics or drug users themselves, or due to the fact that their relationships with their families were strained or had been severed.

Lack of steady income whether from a job or an entitlement program made the women's daily existence chaotic and challenging, affecting their ability to find a place to live and pay their bills. Being poor affected all aspects of their lives. For example, having a car was a luxury. Those who owned their own car were either dealing with car repair bills, broken brake lines, or feeling they were taken advantage of by the other shelter residents who wanted to hitch a ride to a local store. At the shelter, people with cars were generous about transporting other residents to appointments, shopping, or jobs; all for a price. If someone was going to a store they would bring back snacks, Mountain Dew, and cigarettes for others who paid them. Vehicle ownership was a status symbol since so few shelter residents had a car. It represented freedom to leave the shelter during the day or in the evening to go see friends or family; to visit children living in another city. Having a vehicle expanded options when looking for housing or employment or to attend medical appointments. Some of the women mentioned living in their car prior to arriving at the shelter.

Dysfunctional Childhood Relationships

All family relationships are complex but these women described stories of complicated emotions of love and hate that were at times difficult to fathom. Love, or lack of it, was woven into all of the women's life stories. Their relatives often consisted of parents who were alcoholics, working several jobs to make ends meet, or they were divorced. Their siblings may have had different fathers and the women were raised by various relatives. Many had been hurt or rejected by their family. A few had been emancipated as teenagers because of their tumultuous relationships with their parents, usually their mother. This lack of familial support and nurturing may have contributed to subsequent dysfunctional relationships with boyfriends and husbands that involved early parenthood, substance use, and domestic violence. "Mary Beth," a young woman in her twenties who had come to the shelter from "down South" with her husband, his son, and their baby daughter, exemplifies this complex situation:

> but my mom, she disowned me when I was younger, and then my sister was taken from her by her dad. Then she just raised my [other] sister. I was in a foster home until I was of legal age of [state] law statute. They emancipated me at 15. I was basically kicked out on the curb and I was like homeless and then my mom let me come live with her and her husband at the time, but he didn't like me so he threw me out. I think that's kind of why I ran into [father of her first child] and then I got pregnant so young, because I was 17.

Physical, sexual, or emotional abuse from family or partners revolved around issues of power. Many of the women felt put-down, bullied, or belittled by parents or partners. Often the women were involved in power struggles with their mother. Sue's relationship with her mother illustrates this pattern:

> I was told all the time I was growing up when I would try to explain something that [I] had done wrong and I would say "I thought" "Don't think, I'll think for you. I'll tell ya." It's like, ya know that gets to you, too.

Carrie discussed power struggles with partners. She had an embattled relationship with her mother and then she dealt with multiple relationships with men that further broke her spirit. Here she explained how she was treated by one boyfriend. She had a son with him at a young age and then her boyfriend used his ultimate power to report her to the Connecticut Department of Children and Families [DCF] and he and his mother obtained custody of the boy.

> So about three months after I had my son, me and him were living at his mother's house. And I just decided enough was enough ya know every time I told him something it would go in one ear and out the other. His opinion was always on top of mine. Holier than thou attitude. Wouldn't listen to anything I would have to say. Basically I was just there. I wasn't even . . . ya know what I mean? . . . He was in charge of everything. Even if I yelled at him he wouldn't even . . . ya know got to the point where I would be yelling at him and he still wouldn't be listening. Like yeah whatever. Wouldn't even comment back to anything I said. He made me feel like this big.

Loss

Loss was an overarching theme identified in this research, and a central condition of the PHAMILIS stigma syndemic. Not routinely identified as a stigmatizing condition, homeless women who experienced loss in their lives were often alone, isolated, and viewed negatively by society. The women described loss of their childhood, loss of possessions when they lost their home, loss of a partner, or loss of custody of their children. They suffered from emotional loss, material loss, and loss of love, freedom, privacy, and self-esteem; all of these affected their feelings about themselves, their ability to organize their lives, and their inner resources to cope and bound back from missteps and misfortune. Some loss was financial occurring with eviction, relocation, or relationships. Emotional loss occurred when the women were robbed of their childhood or their innocence when they had alcoholic or incarcerated parents, dysfunctional families, or experienced sexual abuse. Too often their relationships ended abruptly or painfully resulting in loss of romantic love. These homeless women were coping with the structural violence resulting from the loss of freedom or privacy that involved power relations encountered while living in a shelter or dealing with social service systems or government entities. These string of losses added to the social suffering of homelessness.

Instability/Relocation

Another interwoven social construct affecting the PHAMILIS stigma syndemic was instability, a common predisposing factor leading to homelessness. The homeless women described "doubling-up" with family and friends or being thrown out of their homes, being evicted, displaced, or frequently relocating in childhood and as adults. Moving to different locations or shuffled from home to home either due to divorce, rejection by family members, or poverty created a chaotic living situation. Some of the women had been foster children and were then left on their own after "aging out" of the system at the age of 18.

The women's chaotic lives were further upended by numerous residential moves during childhood, relocation to different areas, and being shuffled between various extended family members. This pattern continued in their adult life as they moved from town to town and in and out of shelters or other housing to find stability. Instability can be defined in multiple ways and it may or may not adversely affect an individual's life if there are adequate resources and social support. Without these, however, disruptions may take a toll on well-being. Instability may involve relocation and it can arise from physically moving from place to place or from mental illness or substance abuse that makes it difficult to maintain relationships, jobs or housing. "Audrey," for example, made light of the mobility she experienced during her childhood. When asked where she grew up, she explained:

> I was born in Maine. I stayed there for a while. I think we moved here when I was like six to eight, and we lived in [nearby city] for a long time. We lived there for like six years. Now there's five of us children. My oldest sister was born in Maine. My next sister was born in Maryland. My brother was born in New York. I was born back in Maine, and then my little brother was born in [another city in] Maine. I have gypsies for parents.

Others had to leave their prior location due to abuse, divorce, or eviction and had nowhere to go but a shelter. Their social networks were disrupted by moving but this was very often a positive change since their past social ties were frequently detrimental, filled with rejection, negative influences, or marred by abuse. The women described their previous locations and social networks as contributing to undesirable behaviors that caused problems for them. They believed they needed to establish true social support systems and begin a more positive lifestyle. Alice's relief about moving to a new area exemplifies this perspective:

> Being up here, I could be anybody and no one has to know my past. It's like a different life up here . . . It feels real good. Once I get in the apartment I'll feel a whole lot better. I feel like I can breathe again.

Intervening Social Issues

While poverty, loss, and dysfunctional relationships are chronic conditions affecting the lives of homeless women, certain other social issues intervened in their lives sporadically and influenced their pathway to homelessness. These issues upset their ability to maintain a stable, positive life. Moreover, most intervening factors were socially marginalizing and reflected social discrimination. The women believed that some of these factors were beyond their control (e.g., loss of a child through DCF, incarceration of a family member) and others were life decisions or unplanned events that altered their course (e.g., early parenthood). These actions affected future decisions such as finishing high school or continuing onto college, and pursuing careers in a field of their choice. DCF involvement and the ridicule of being considered a "bad mother" severely impacted the women's self-esteem and feelings of self-worth. With the label of "convict" or "criminal," women personally involved in the criminal justice system or with men in the system, dealt with criticism and discrimination in job and housing searches.

Early parenthood has numerous complications and consequences as it can abruptly end or delay high school graduation, destroy relationships with parents, and create challenges with employment and careers. Caring for a baby and oneself as a teenager is difficult financially and emotionally. Alice, who at 38 years old had a 19 year-old son at the shelter with her, is an example of this situation:

> Yeah, I finished high school. I got married at 17. I had my son. I finished high school at 17—I'm sorry, 19. I graduated June the year he was born and I got married at 17 'cuz I got pregnant and I had a bad miscarriage and went downhill from there. I should never have gotten married. If I could go back I wouldn't change my kid, but I wish I could go back. Oh, my God. I would go to college, and I want better for my kids.

Often the fathers of the babies born to the women when they were teenagers were no longer involved in their lives. Most of the women had several relationships with men after their early pregnancy. Not all of these were positive. When asked if she finished high school, for example, Diane explained, "No, I dropped out. I went and got my GED . . . when I was pregnant. It's like every time I get my life together, it's like, I make one stupid decision. It's usually involving men, definitely involving men."

One of the major risks or worries experienced by the women was fear of losing custody of their children to DCF. "Tessa," for example, was very concerned that she would be vulnerable to losing her child if DCF found out she had moved locations and was staying at a homeless shelter.

Some of the women had lost custody of their children and were fighting with the court and/or family to regain guardianship. These women felt they had been unjustly blamed or accused for their behavior, which resulted in loss of custody (e.g., neglecting their child, using drugs or alcohol). All of the women who described their involvement with children's services felt that they had a right to regain custody or to receive adequate visitation rights to their child.

Another issue that interfered with acquiring a stable life was involvement in the criminal justice system. None of the women mentioned doing time in jail or prison except as adolescents when they were involved in the juvenile justice system. Several of the women in the study were involved with men who were serving prison or jail time frequently as a result of substance use involvement which resulted in arrest, either for possession of illegal drugs, theft to support a drug habit, selling drugs, or driving under the influence. Often these men were the fathers of their children, adding additional stress, instability, and loss to their lives. "Marilyn," for example, dealt with an abusive relationship and then her partner was sent to prison.

> And then my kids' father was very abusive. Broken ribs, cracked jaws, I tried to poison him. [I: Were you married?] Noooooooooo. I wouldn't marry him. Noooo. He's asked me. Twice. But then he went to jail and I pawned the rings. What the hell am I going to do with rings? They don't mean anything to me. No. I don't think I ever wanted to marry him . . . But I've seen him [in jail] because I want money from him, so I do what I have to do to get what I have to get. [I: How long has he been incarcerated?] Three years now. Three years. Four years. Something like that. Probably not [getting out] for another—he got sentenced 20 years, it's pending after 11. He allegedly sexually assaulted his older daughter from his previous relationship. Don't know if that's true. I'm not sure that even happened. Part of me that says that oh man I've spent almost 14—I've been with this man almost half of my life, no way he woulda done that. Then part of me says well, there must've been something. He was sentenced. Then part of me is like well, they put people in jail for 20, 30 years to turn out to be innocent. It happens.

DISCUSSION AND CONCLUSIONS

The authors' research with homeless women revealed that their lives are intertwined with interconnected themes of loss, sexual abuse, violence, dysfunctional and/or broken natal families, mental health issues, drug abuse, DCF intervention, incarceration, and for most a history of living in poverty and its associated insults and insecurities. All of these predisposing, exacerbating, and intervening factors in concert create complex lives that have led to homelessness and poor health. Furthermore, these factors are shrouded in layers of stigma, which serve as powerful drivers of the life pathways followed by these women, and which result in pathways of adverse interaction between disease and other health factors. First, there is the social context in which decisions are made, events occur, and health/mental health is created. Of particular importance in this regard is structural violence (Farmer 2004; Lyon-Callo 2001) which is evidenced by power differentials in the women's personal lives, within the shelter, in encounters with the social service and criminal justice systems, and with the dominant society generally. Structural violence is at the heart of stigma and is notable because it is built into the structure of social arrangements and is hence less overtly visible than actual physical violence. Lyon-Callo (2001) specifically addresses this unequal power distribution as it affects homeless women and contributes to their experience of structural violence arguing: "Domination through processes of class exploitation, racial injustice, unequal educational opportunities, and gendered inequality are . . . all fairly easy to document components of homelessness" (Lyon-Callo 2001:295).

Second, unequal social relationships are enforced by stigmatization. The result of these "conjunctures of vulnerability" (Ribera and Hausmann-Muela 2011) commonly is enduring damage to the subordinate individual's self-esteem, especially as this pattern is reinforced by other built-in components of the overarching structure of social inequality. A consequence of living in this kind of emotional risk environment for homeless woman is a heightened sense of need for support and of social acceptance and belonging. As a result, they continued to make problematic decisions over their life course, a pattern that can only be understood within the contexts of stigma and structural violence.

Finally, other intervening factors, such as early pregnancy or incarceration, that contributed to an unstable life also were shaped by social structures of inequality and constitute additional outcome of structural violence. If the women became pregnant as teenagers, they often were not welcomed to stay in their natal homes, due to stigma and discrimination, rejection, disappointment, or the inability to afford another mouth to feed. In part, this pattern reflects the cultural pattern of blaming the individual for socially disapproved events and behaviors, which in this case is highly gendered as boys are not as commonly forced from their natal homes for fathering a child out of wedlock. These women entered into early adulthood with the responsibility of caring for a baby, often as a single parent, and trying to find a place to live and to make ends meet. They sometimes sought security and stability by rushing into subsequent relationships that were adverse and sometimes abusive. The men they became involved with at times had criminal histories due to drug charges or other infractions that limited options for housing. Moreover, incarceration, in itself, is disruptive to family life. Yet patterns of incarceration illustrate that involvement in the criminal justice system reveals that social class is a significant determinant of who gets "punitively policed, prosecuted, and sentenced" (Pettit and Western 2004).

In sum, by proposing the PHAMILIS syndemic model this chapter captures the complexity and interaction of the multitude of stigmatizing factors experienced directly by homeless women but emanating from various levels of the prevailing social structure that contours their lives. The myriad health problems of homeless women are syndemically entwined and mutually enhancing, and driven overall by stigma. Thus, trauma in childhood and adulthood can provide the psychological motivation for drug abuse and a lifestyle that is prone to increased sexual and other risky behaviors that can lead to HIV or other sexually transmitted infections. It is the ongoing interaction of these factors that defines the struggles of homeless women and shapes their experience and understanding of being homeless or living in a homeless shelter. Recognizing the syndemic nature of these factors, we argue, provides a basis for intervention development that recognizes and actually addresses the full set and multifaceted enmeshed nature of the factors causing and maintaining homelessness. Responding to syndemics, particularly stigma-driven syndemics, requires multi-component, intersectorial intervention models. As Mendenhall (2012:113) stresses, "In a country in which great wealth often overshadows and perpetuates great inequalities, the lack of attention to comprehensive, integrated health care for the poor is unacceptable." Beyond health care, lack of attention to the housing care needs of the poor, as well as neglect of the synergistic relationship between poor health and poor housing, is no less acceptable.

NOTE

1. The study was designed to use qualitative research methods to create an ethnographic account of the ideas, beliefs, and concerns homeless women have about their lives from childhood to the present (Bates et al. 2007; Needle et al. 2003; Trotter et al. 2001). The lead author conducted one in-depth interview each with 30 women staying at the *Entré* Emergency Shelter (pseudonym) to learn about their life histories and to identify cultural domains shared by the women. Data collection occurred with a convenience sample of women staying at the shelter with a partner or alone,

including those who had children and those who didn't, and women staying at the shelter with their children. Only women over the age of 18 years were included. For the purpose of giving "voice" to the women, each was assigned a pseudonym for attributing their quotes—these are used here. Data analysis consisted of qualitative ethnographic descriptions of the semi-structured interviews. The authors conducted analysis using a modified grounded theory technique (Bernard 2002; Corbin 2008) focusing on patterns and themes that arose from the textual data, as well as from pre-established codes that were identified as constructs from a review of the literature (Bernard 2002). The research was approved by the Institutional Review Board at the University of Connecticut.

REFERENCES

Aguirre, Patricia. "Socioanthropological Aspects of Obesity in Poverty." In *Obesity and Poverty: A New Public Health Challenge.* M. Peña and J. Bacallao, eds. Washington, DC: Pan American Health Organization, 2000.

Ahern, Jennifer, Jennifer Stuber, and Sandro Galea. "Stigma, Discrimination and the Health of Illicit Drug Users." *Drug and Alcohol Dependence* 88, nos. 2–3 (2007): 188–96.

Baer, Hans A., Merrill Singer, and Ida Susser. *Medical Anthropology and the World System*. Westport: Praeger, 2003.

Baker, Charlene K., et al. "Domestic Violence, Housing Instability, and Homelessness: A Review of Housing Policies and Program Practices for Meeting the Needs of Survivors." *Aggression and Violent Behavior* 15, no. 6 (2010):430–439.

Bassuk, Ellen L. "Homeless Women—Economic and Social Issues: Introduction." *American Journal of Orthopsychiatry* 63, no. 3 (1993):337–339.

Bassuk, Ellen L., John C. Buckner, Jennifer N. Perloff, and Shari S. Bassuk. "Prevalence of Mental Health and Substance Use Disorders Among Homeless and Low-Income Housed Mothers." *American Journal of Psychiatry* 155, no. 11 (1998):1561–1564.

Bassuk, Ellen L., Jennifer N. Perloff, and Ree Dawson. "Multiply Homeless Families: The Insidious Impact of Violence." *Housing Policy Debate* 12, no. 2 (2001): 299–320.

Bates, Christopher, Merrill Singer, and Robert T Trotter. "Part I: Background on the CARE Act, RARE, and the Care System Assessment Demonstration Project—The RARE Model of Rapid HIV Risk Assessment." *Journal of Health Care for the Poor and Underserved* 18, no. 3 supplement (2007):16–34.

Belcher, John R., and Bruce R. DeForge. "Social Stigma and Homelessness: The Limits of Social Change." *Journal of Human Behavior in the Social Environment* 22, no. 8 (2012):929–946.

Benbow, S., C. Forchuk, and S. L. Ray. "Mothers with Mental Illness Experiencing Homelessness: A Critical Analysis." *Journal of Psychiatric and Mental Health Nursing* 18, no. 8 (2011):687–695.

Bernard, H. Russell. *Research Methods in Anthropology: Qualitative and Quantitative Approaches*. Walnut Creek: AltaMira Press, 2002.

Browne, Angela. "Family Violence and Homelessness: The Relevance of Trauma Histories in the Lives of Homeless Women." *American Journal of Orthopsychiatry* 63, no. 3 (1993):370–384.

Burt, Martha R. *Over the Edge: The Growth of Homelessness in the 1980s*. New York: Russell Sage Foundation, 1992.

Carrion, Iraida V., Heida Castañeda, Dinorah Martinez-Tyson, and Nolan Kline. "Barriers Impeding Access to Primary Oral Health Care Among Farmworker Families in Central Florida." *Social Work in Health Care* 50, no. 10 (2011):828–844.

Castañeda, Heide, Iraida V. Carrion, Nolan Kline, and Dinorah Martinez-Tyson. "False Hope: Effects of Social Class and Health Policy on Oral Health Inequalities for Migrant Farmworker Families." *Social Science & Medicine* 71, no. 11 (2010):2028–2037.

Coffey, Patricia, Harold Leitenberg, Kris Henning, Tonia Turner, and Robert T. Bennett. "Mediators of the Long-Term Impact of Child Sexual Abuse: Perceived Stigma, Betrayal, Powerlessness, and Self-Blame." *Child Abuse & Neglect* 20, no. 5 (1996):447–455.

Cohen, S., D. Janicki-Deverts, and G. E. Miller. "Psychological Stress and Disease." *Journal of the American Medical Association* 298, no. 14 (2007):1685–1687.

Corbin, Juliet M. *Basics of Qualitative Research: Techniques and Procedures for Developing Grounded Theory*. Los Angeles, CA: Sage Publishing, Inc., 2008.

Corrigan, Patrick W. *On the Stigma of Mental Illness: Practical Strategies for Research and Social Change*. Washington, DC: American Psychological Association, 2005.

Davies-Netzley, Sally, Michael S. Hurlburt, and Richard L. Hough. "Childhood Abuse as a Precursor to Homelessness for Homeless Women with Severe Mental Illness." *Violence and Victims* 11, no. 2 (1996):129–142.

Desmond, Meredith. "ACOG Recommendations for Improving Care of Homeless Women." *American Family Physician* 73, no. 9 (2006):1655.

Dressler, William W., Mauro C. Baileiro, Rosane P. Ribeiro, and José Ernesto Dos Santos. "Cultural Consonance and Arterial Blood Pressure in Urban Brazil." *Social Science & Medicine* 61, no. 3 (2005):527–540.

Earnshaw, Valerie A., and Stephenie R. Chaudoir. "From Conceptualizing to Measuring HIV Stigma: A Review of HIV Stigma Mechanism Measures." *AIDS and Behavior* 13 (2009):1160–1177.

Earnshaw, Valerie, Laramie Smith, and Michael Copenhaver. "Drug Addiction Stigma in the Context of Methadone Maintenance Therapy: An Investigation into Understudied Sources of Stigma." *International Journal of Mental Health and Addiction* 11, no. 1 (2013):110–122.

Edelstein, Burton L. "Disparities in Oral Health and Access to Care: Findings of National Surveys." *Ambulatory Pediatrics* 2, no. 2 (2002):141–147.

Everson, Susan A., Siobhan C. Maty, John W. Lynch, and George A. Kaplan. "Epidemiologic Evidence for the Relation Between Socioeconomic Status and

Depression, Obesity, and Diabetes." *Journal of Psychosomatic Research* 53, no. 4 (2002):891–895.

Farmer, Paul. "An Anthropology of Structural Violence." *Current Anthropology* 45, no. 3 (2004):305–325.

Gelberg, Lillian, and Lisa Arangua. "Homeless People." In *Social Injustice and Public Health*. B. S. Levy and V. W. Sidel, eds. New York: Oxford University Press, 2006.

Gelberg, Lillian, and Lawrence S. Linn. "Assessing the Physical Health of Homeless Adults." *Journal of the American Medical Association* 262, no. 14 (1989):1973–1979.

Gelberg, Lillian, Lawrence S. Linn, Richard P. Usatine, et al. "Health, Homelessness, and Poverty: A Study of Clinic Users." *Archives of Internal Medicine* 150 (1990): 2325–2330.

Glasser, Irene and Rae Bridgman. *Braving the Street: The Anthropology of Homelessness*. New York: Berghahn Books, 1999.

Goodman, Lisa A., Mary Ann Dutton, and Maxine Harris. "The Relationship Between Violence Dimensions and Symptom Severity Among Homeless, Mentally Ill Women." *Journal of Traumatic Stress* 10, no. 1 (1997):51–70.

Gragnoli, Claudia. "Depression and Type 2 Diabetes: Cortisol Pathway Implication and Investigation Needs." *Journal of Cellular Physiology* 227, no. 6 (2012): 2318–2322.

Green Harold D., Jr., et al. "Association of Childhood Abuse with Homeless Women's Social Networks." *Child Abuse & Neglect* 36, no. 1 (2012):21–31.

Hamilton, A. B., I. Poza, and D. L. Washington. "'Homelessness and Trauma Go Hand-in-Hand': Pathways to Homelessness among Women Veterans." *Women's Health Issues* 21, no. 4 (2011):S203-S209.

Hopper, Kim. "More Than Passing Strange: Homelessness and Mental Illness in New York City." *American Ethnologist* 15, no. 1 (1988):155–167.

———. *Reckoning with Homelessness*. Ithaca: Cornell University Press, 2003.

Horton, Sarah and Judith C. Barker. "Stigmatized Biologies: Examining the Cumulative Effects of Oral Health Disparities for Mexican American Farmworker Children." *Medical Anthropology Quarterly* 24, no. 2 (2010):199–219.

Hwang, Stephen W. "Homelessness and Health." *Canadian Medical Association Journal* 164, no. 2 (2001):229–233.

Hwang, Stephen, et al. The Health and Housing in Transition Study: A Longitudinal Study of the Health of Homeless and Vulnerably Housed Adults in Three Canadian Cities. *International Journal of Public Health* 56, no. 6 (2011): 609–623.

Jones, Edward E, Robert A. Scott, and Hazel Markus. *Social Stigma: The Psychology of Marked Relationships*. New York: W. H. Freeman and Company, 1984.

Khantzian, Edward. "The Self-Medication Hypothesis of Addictive Disorders: Focus on Heroin and Cocaine Dependence." *American Journal of Psychiatry* 142, no. 11 (1985):1259–1264.

Lerman, Shir. "Un Pueblo Tan Dulce": Diabetes, Depression, and Obesity Syndemics in Puerto Rico." MA thesis, University of Connecticut, 2015.

Link, Bruce G., Sharon Scwartz, Robert Moore, Jo Phelan, Elmer Struening, Ann Stueve, and Mary Ellen Colten. "Public Knowledge, Attitudes, and Beliefs About

Homeless People: Evidence for Compassion Fatigue?" *American Journal of Community Psychology* 23, no. 4 (1995):533–555.

Link, Bruce G., Elmer L. Struening, Michael Rahav, Jo C. Phelan, and Larry Nuttbrock. "On Stigma and Its Consequences: Evidence from a Longitudinal Study of Men with Dual Diagnoses of Mental Illness and Substance Abuse." *Journal of Health and Social Behavior* 38, no. 2 (1997):177–190.

Loeliger, Kelsey B., Ruthanne Marcus, Jeffrey A. Wickersham, and Frederick Altice. "The Syndemic of HIV, HIV-Related Risk and Multiple Co-Morbidities Among Women Who Use Drugs in Malaysia: Important Targets for Intervention." *Addictive Behaviors* 53 (2016):31–39.

Lyon-Callo, Vincent. "Homelessness, Employment, and Structural Violence." In *The New Poverty Studies: The Ethnography of Power, Politics, and Impoverished People in the United States*. J. Goode and J. Maskovsky, eds., 293–318. New York: New York University Press, 2001.

———. *Inequality, Poverty, and Neoliberal Governance: Activist Ethnography in the Homeless Sheltering Industry*. Peterborough, Ontario: Broadview Press, 2004.

Marmot, Michael. "Social Determinants of Health Inequalities." *The Lancet* 365, no. 9464 (2005):1099–1104.

Mendenhall, Emily. *Syndemic Suffering: Social Distress, Depression, and Diabetes Among Mexican Immigrant Women*. Walnut Creek, CA: Left Coast Press, 2012.

Meyer, Jaimie P., Sandra A. Springer, and Frederick L. Altice. "Substance Abuse, Violence, and HIV in Women: A Literature Review of the Syndemic." *Journal of Women's Health* 20, no. 7 (2011):991–1006.

Morland, Kimberly, Steve Wing, and Ana Diez Roux. "The Contextual Effect of the Local Food Environment on Residents' Diets: The Atherosclerosis Risk in Communities Study." *American Journal of Public Health* 92, no. 11 (2002):1761–1768.

National Alliance to End Homelessness. *The State of Homelessness in America 2013*. Washington, DC. 2013

Needle, Richard H., Robert T. Trotter II, Merrill Singer, and Louis Herns Marcelin. "Rapid Assessment of the HIV/AIDS Crisis in Racial and Ethnic Minority Communities: An Approach for Timely Community Interventions." *American Journal of Public Health* 93, no. 6 (2003):970–979.

Ostrach, Bayla, and Merrill Singer. "At Special Risk: Biopolitical Vulnerability and HIV/STI Syndemics Among Women." *Health Sociology Review* 21, no. 3 (2012):258–271.

Overstreet, Nicole M., and Diane M. Quinn. "The Intimate Partner Violence Stigmatization Model and Barriers to Help-Seeking." *Basic and Applied Social Psychology* 35, no. 1 (2013):109–122.

Pettit, Becky, and Bruce Western. "Mass Imprisonment and the Life Course: Race and Class Inequality in U.S. Incarceration." *American Sociological Review* 69, no. 2 (2004):151–169.

Phelan, Jo, Bruce G. Link, Robert E. Moore, and Ann Stueve. "The Stigma of Homelessness: The Impact of the Label 'Homeless' on Attitudes Toward Poor Persons." *Social Psychology Quarterly* 60, no. 4 (1997):323–337.

Ponce, Allison N, Martha Staeheli Lawless, and Michael Rowe. "Homelessness, Behavioral Health Disorders and Intimate Partner Violence: Barriers to Services for Women." *Community Mental Health Journal* 50, no. 7 (2014):831–840.

Puhl, Rebecca M. and Kelly D. Brownell. "Bias, Discrimination, and Obesity." *Obesity Research* 9, no. 12 (2001):788–805.

Puhl, Rebecca M. and Chelsea A. Heuer. "Obesity Stigma: Important Considerations for Public Health." *American Journal of Public Health* 100, no. 6 (2010):1019–1028.

Quinn, Diane M., and Valerie A. Earnshaw. "Understanding Concealable Stigmatized Identities: The Role of Identity in Psychological, Physical, and Behavioral Outcomes." *Social Issues and Policy Review* 5, no. 1 (2011):160–190.

Rabiner, M. and A. Weiner. "Health Care for Homeless and Unstably Housed: Overcoming Barriers." *Mount Sinai Journal of Medicine* 79, no. 5 (2012):586–592.

Rhodes, Tim, Merrill Singer, Philippe Bourgois, Samuel R. Friedman, and Steffanie A. Strathdee. "The Social Structural Production of HIV Risk Among Injecting Drug Users." *Social Science and Medicine* 61 (2005):1026–1044.

Ribera, Joan Muela and Susanna Hausmann-Muela. "The Straw That Breaks the Camel's Back Redirecting Health-Seeking Behavior Studies on Malaria and Vulnerability." *Medical Anthropology Quarterly* 25, no. 1 (2011):103–121.

Rogge, Mary Madeline, Marti Greenwald, and Amelia Golden. "Obesity, Stigma, and Civilized Oppression." *Advances in Nursing Science* 27, no. 4 (2004): 301–315.

Romero-Daza, Nancy, Margaret Weeks, and Merrill Singer. "Conceptualizing the Impact of Indirect Violence on HIV Risk Among Women Involved in Street-Level Prostitution." *Aggression and Violent Behavior* 10, no. 2 (2005):153–170.

Rossi, Peter. *Without Shelter: Homelessness in the 1980s*. New York: A Twentieth Century Fund Paper, 1989.

Rüsch, Nicolas, Matthias C. Angermeyer, and Patrick W. Corrigan. "Mental Illness Stigma: Concepts, Consequences, and Initiatives to Reduce Stigma." *European Psychiatry* 20, no. 8 (2005):529–539.

Singer, Merrill. "Critical Medical Anthropology." In *Encyclopedia of Medical Anthropology: Health and Illness in the World's Cultures*. Melvin Ember and Carol R. Ember, eds., 23–30. New York: Springer Science, 2004.

———. *The Face of Social Suffering: The Life History of a Street Drug Addict*. Long Grove, IL: Waveland Press, 2006.

———. "The Infectious Disease Syndemics of Crack Cocaine." *Journal of Equity in Health* 3, no. 1 (2014):32–44.

Singer, Merrill, and Scott Clair. "Syndemics and Public Health: Reconceptualizing Disease in Bio-Social Context." *Medical Anthropology Quarterly* 17, no. 4 (2003):423–441.

Singer Merrill, and J. Bryan Page. *The Social Value of Drug Addicts: The Uses of the Useless*. Walnut Creek, CA: Left Coast Press, 2013.

Stall, Ron, Thomas C. Mills, John Williamson, and Joseph A. Catania. "Association of Co-Occurring Psychosocial Health Problems and Increased Vulnerability to HIV/AIDS Among Urban Men Who Have Sex With Men." *American Journal of Public Health* 93, no. 6 (2003):939–942.

Stein, Judith A., Michelle Burden Leslie, and Adeline Nyamathi. "Relative Contributions of Parent Substance Use and Childhood Maltreatment to Chronic Homelessness, Depression, and Substance Abuse Problems Among Homeless Women: Mediating Roles of Self-Esteem and Abuse in Adulthood." *Child Abuse & Neglect* 26, no. 10 (2002):1011–1027.

Stillwell, K David. "Obesity Complicates Dental Health—Be Proactive!" Obesity Action Coalition, 2016. Accessed January 23, 2016. http://www.obesityaction.org/educational-resources/resource-articles-2/obesity-related-diseases/obesity-compli cates-dental-health.

Susser, Ida. "The Construction of Poverty and Homelessness in US Cities." *Annual Review of Anthropology* 25 (1996):411–435.

Trotter, Robert T., Richard H. Needle, Eric Goosby, and Merrill Charles Singer. "A Methodological Model for Rapid Assessment, Response, and Evaluation: The RARE Program in Public Health." *Field Methods* 13, no. 2 (2001):137–159.

U.S. Department of Housing and Urban Development, Office of Community Planning and Development. The 2010 Annual Homeless Assessment Report to Congress. 2011.

Van Tieu, Hong and Beryl Koblin. "HIV, Alcohol, and Noninjection Drug Use." *Current Opinion in HIV & AIDS* 4 (2009):314–318.

Wagner, David. *Checkerboard Square: Culture and Resistance in a Homeless Community*. Boulder: Westview Press, 1993.

Walker, Renee E., Christopher R. Keane, and Jessica G. Burke. "Disparities and Access to Healthy Food in the United States: A Review of Food Deserts Literature." *Health & Place* 16, no. 5 (2010):876–884.

Yudkin, John S., Meena Kumari, S.E. Humphries, and Vidya Mohamed-Ali. "Inflammation, Obesity, Stress and Coronary Heart Disease: Is Interleukin-6 the Link?" *Atherosclerosis* 148, no. 2 (2000):209–214.

Chapter Six

Dangerous Bodies, Unpredictable Minds

HIV/AIDS, Mental Disorders, and Stigma Syndemics in Western Kenya

Elizabeth J. Pfeiffer, Harrison M. K. Maithya, Mary A. Ott, and Kara Wools-Kaloustian

Disease interactions between HIV/AIDS and mental health disorders are well documented in high-income countries, with research demonstrating that the additive effects of suffering from both conditions work synergistically to produce adverse health outcomes, such as increasing viral loads and lowering CD4+ T cell counts and immune function, thus leaving patients vulnerable to opportunistic infections and accelerating the progression to AIDS (Boarts et al. 2006). While the relationships between these epidemics have been less well examined in sub-Saharan Africa, recent studies in Kenya report not only high rates of both HIV/AIDS (Murray et al. 2012) and common mental disorders across the general population (Steel et al. 2014), but also suggest a strong association between the two (Ng'ang'a 2011).

> People with HIV start drinking so they can forget [they are living with HIV/AIDS] . . . so they may not be stressed and feel like [they] are in a normal situation [again]. Because . . . you are sick and you know that you are the cause of that sickness and that you have even infected your own wife. What would you do? You start drinking. The moment your wife discovers that she is also sick, what will she do? She will come to have a mental disorder. That is what makes someone become addicted to alcohol. And that is why you can see that at least 1/3 of the population—they are insane. (Anonymous Participant)

These blunt comments were shared by a casual laborer during an impromptu group discussion centering on the shared perception that, in the recent past, there had been a noticeable increase in the use of potent, yet cheap and illegal forms of alcohol, such as *chang'aa*,[1] among residents living in a small trading center in western Kenya. While several explanations were offered,[2] those present for this conversation agreed with the sentiments put forth by the man quoted above. Indeed, when asked to describe the biggest challenges facing community members, almost every person interviewed mentioned the growing number of individuals described as "idle" and "useless drunkards." In turn, such residents were regularly characterized as "reckless" and accused of carelessly, sometimes purposefully, perpetuating the spread of HIV. As the man cited above effectively demonstrates, the ongoing social, moral, and emotional stressors and individualized blame evoked by HIV infections were construed not only as major contributors to the increased prevalence of mental disorders, but also imagined to have caused "insanity" among a substantial proportion (33 percent) of the population in this marginalized highway community (Das and Poole 2004). It was social stressors, forces and conditions that were perceived to link and drive the mutually enhancing epidemics of HIV/AIDS and mental disorders (namely depression and chronic alcoholism) in ways that not only (re)produced deleterious biological consequences for some, but simultaneously perpetuated the stigma associated with HIV/AIDS in this part of the world. As this example exemplifies, to adequately understand and address health problems in Kenyan communities, it is necessary to critically explore the complicated ways that social, psychological, and physiological conditions converge and become syndemic (Mendenhall et al. 2015).

It is worth noting that although the past decade has witnessed dramatic improvements in understandings of HIV/AIDS and a drastic increase in HIV counseling, testing, and antiretroviral therapies (ART), mental health care services have not been included as part of this "scale up" in many communities of the Global South (Kleinman 2009). Similarly, while some data point to the idea that the stigmas associated with mental illness may be even greater than those associated with HIV/AIDS in Kenya (Jenkins et al. 2013), the latter epidemic has received considerably more scholarly and public health attention. This neglect likely reflects some of the challenges of integrating even basic mental health services in African countries (see Jenkins et al. 2013), as well as an unintended consequence of the prioritization of HIV/AIDS global health programing, funding, and policy development that has overshadowed other health issues and concerns (Prince and Marsland 2014). Furthermore, literatures centering on the deleterious health effects of stigma are often developed in distinct domains, with one body of work, for example, focusing on AIDS-related stigma, and yet another on mental illness stigma (Hatzenbuehler, Phelan, and Link 2013). Very little research has questioned the ways that these domains may actually intersect with one another.

Despite initial hopes that more equal access to ART would eliminate processes of AIDS-related stigma (Castro and Farmer 2005), studies continually suggest that treatment alone is insufficient (Wyrod 2011). To better understand how and why this stigma persists, work is needed to describe the syndemic of HIV/AIDS and mental health disorders, while keeping in mind the broader social, political, cultural, economic, scientific, and historic contexts fueling it in communities of the Global South. Furthermore, there is a paucity of ethnographic research that investigates the subjective, lived experiences and interpretations of the effects of this syndemic and its associated stigmas in sub-Saharan Africa. Drawing on syndemics theory, which focuses attention on disease/disease interaction in social context, and literatures on social stigma, as well as empirical data gathered during ethnographic research in a highway trading center located in Rift Valley Province, Kenya, the current study contributes to these gaps through a critical exploration of the interactions between HIV/AIDS and mental health disorders, with a particular focus on how the intertwining social stigmas associated with both conditions, drive the synergy. We contend that a focus on the perspectives and beliefs of those experiencing, interpreting, and/or resisting processes of stigma in situ (Kleinman et al. 1995) offers a more holistic and detailed understanding of these linked epidemics and can inform current and future global health policies and programs in efforts to improve HIV services and care in this part of the world.

METHODOLOGICAL AND THEORETICAL CONTEXTS

The lead author gathered the data presented in this chapter as part of two larger studies conducted in the same community. The first was an intensive ethnographic project centered on the intertwining linguistic, social, and structural drivers of AIDS-related stigma during a period of increased HIV testing and services (Pfeiffer 2014). The second was a qualitative study exploring the social and structural barriers to HIV testing and linkage to HIV treatment and care among men. With permissions from Institutional Review Boards in the United States and Kenya, the research was conducted over a total of 14 months (May–August 2010, October 2011–April 2012, July–September 2012, October–November 2014). The studies incorporated a wide range of methods, including daily participant observation in diverse settings (e.g., clinics, bars, homes) and at various events throughout the community (e.g., burials, engagement parties) and semi-structured interviews. Data were further collected and triangulated using life-history interviews, informal conversations with key consultants, gathering/reading newspaper articles, and through the systematic collection of conversational journals (Watkins, Swidler, and Biruk 2011). The first author and research assistants conducted the interviews in English or Kiswahili, depending on the participant's preference, and most were audio recorded,[3] transcribed, and translated into English.

The first author analyzed the data by using an iterative thematic coding approach that is common in ethnographic research (Ryan and Bernard 2003). Both the notion that HIV/AIDS-related stigma had transformed alongside the scale up of HIV services and the perception that those living with HIV/AIDS were increasingly suffering from psychological problems were persistent themes that emerged across the data through the wide range of methodologies employed. To understand these themes, this chapter draws on theories of syndemics and stigma. Syndemics theory postulates that diseases are not independent; they work together in complex ways to exacerbate harmful health consequences, especially among populations living in conditions characterized by poverty, stress, malnutrition, social inequalities, and structural violence (Singer 2009). We further draw on theories that conceptualize stigma as a complex social process that is dependent upon social, economic, and political power (Link and Phelan 2001), and as part of an ongoing struggle over the maintenance and legitimization of myriad forms of inequalities, including those associated with gender, sexuality, class, and race/ethnicity (Parker and Aggleton 2003). We aim to demonstrate the ways that social and structural processes of stigma served as pathways linking unequal social relations and the (re)production of suffering and negative biological outcomes associated with this syndemic, especially among already marginalized members living in the community (Singer and Clair 2003).

ETHNOGRAPHIC CONTEXT

The fieldwork took place in a community located in Uasin Gishu District in the Midwestern part of Rift Valley Province. In contrast to other areas of Kenya, this portion of the western highlands hosts an especially favorable climate with fertile land suitable for sustaining a productive farming/agricultural base (Kamungi 2009), and the field site consists of rolling landscapes and rural communities united by a small trading center. Strategically located along a major trans-African highway, the physical layout of the trading center, as well as the services and goods available in it, accommodated the various needs/desires of those living in and nearby, as well as the dozens of truck drivers who passed through daily. The trading center housed a District Hospital that served an estimated 200,000 individuals and a population of approximately 11,000 during the study period (private communication). A broad mix of Kenya's 42 ethnic groups is found in this part of Kenya, but the population is mostly Kikuyu[4] or Kalenjin.[5]

This part of the country has experienced chronic ethnic, social, economic, and political turmoil since (at least) the British colonial period, when colonists displaced indigenous populations from their lands, which polarized and sharpened the distinctions between cultural groups and ethnic identities (Ashforth 2009; Kamungi 2009; Lynch 2011). These historic legacies continue to fuel and sustain land-use conflicts and competition over the available resources in Kenya. Postcolonial politicians have yet to resolve such issues, and instead have, at times, drawn upon them to incite violence across ethnic lines, and as a strategy for mobilizing political support and maintaining power and interests. Persisting tensions are epitomized by the episodes of violent conflict that accompanied the Kenyan presidential elections in 1992, 1997, and 2007/2008. The most damaging episode occurred when lawlessness erupted following the perceived rigging of the 2007/2008 presidential elections (Ashforth 2009; Kamungi 2009; Lynch 2011). While the 2007/2008 postelection violence (PEV) and fighting took on varying forms, according to Ashforth (2009), Kalenjins engaged in the ethnic cleansing of Kikuyus caused the majority of deaths, destruction, and displacements. It is perhaps not surprising then that the study area—with high percentages of individuals identifying as Kikuyu or Kalenjin—was at the epicenter of the conflict, where approximately 1,320 homes and numerous farms and businesses were destroyed and over 5,000 residents were displaced (Goodrich et al. 2013). At the time of this research, area residents were still struggling to recover—economically, socially, emotionally, and politically—from the disastrous effects of the PEV, and the community characterized by spiraling inequality, corruption, political and economic insecurity, high rates of unemployment, and an increased reliance on competitive informal and/or illegal economies (e.g., prostitution and the brewing, distribution and sale of illegal forms of alcohol/brews and drugs).

HIV/AIDS AND MENTAL HEALTH DISORDERS: INTERTWINING EPIDEMICS

In Kenya, at the time of this study, an estimated 1.6 million adults were infected with HIV (NASCOP 2009) and women had a prevalence rate that was 40 percent higher than men at 7.6 percent and 5.63 percent, respectively (NASCOP 2014). Despite a recent decline in the national prevalence rate to 5.6 percent (NASCOP 2014), the number of new HIV infections remained high, with 101,560 people infected in 2013 (NASCOP 2014). Data confirm both that individuals living with HIV under good viremic control do not transmit the virus (M. Cohen et al. 2011), and that there is a mortality benefit with early antiretroviral treatment (The Insight START Study Group 2015; PEPFAR 2012; UNAIDS 2014). In 2010, a rigorous home counselling and testing (HCT) campaign was launched in Kenya (CSIS 2009), with teams going door-to-door to offer free and confidential HIV rapid tests to individuals, couples, and families across the county. Those who tested positive were immediately referred to a Comprehensive Care Centre (CCC), where ART are available free of charge. During the research, HCT teams were making their way in and around the trading center, which has hosted a CCC since 2003 that was serving over 1,700 HIV-infected individuals (private communication).

Epidemiological studies estimating the prevalence of mental disorders among the general population in Kenya suggest that they are common, with rates hovering around 10 percent (Jenkins et al. 2012; Steel et al. 2014). Anthropologists studying mental illness in this country have attributed these high levels to structural violence, food insecurity, gender inequality, inadequate healthcare and services, as well as the social stressors associated with living in communities with high burdens of chronic illnesses (Copeland 2011; Mendenhall et al. 2015). Prevalence studies conducted in the context of health care facilities in Kenya reveal especially high rates of mental illness among patients (Jenkins et al. 2012; Aillon et al. 2014). For example, researchers studying alcohol use found that reported rates of hazardous drinking are high among outpatients in both general medicine (68 percent) and HIV (53 percent) clinics (Papas et al. 2011, 2012). Similarly, a cross-sectional study conducted in 10 health facilities found that as many as 42 percent of research participants exhibited depressive symptoms (Ndetei et al. 2009). A significant finding from this latter project was that only 4.1 percent of the study population had a diagnosis of a psychiatric condition. Such high prevalence rates are disconcerting, especially given the extremely limited availability of psychiatric services and other mental health resources, which include only one psychiatrist available for every 500,000 individuals (Jenkins et al. 2010a; Jenkins et al. 2010b). People living with a wide variety of mental, neurological, substance abuse disorders in Kenya rarely have access to the treatment and services they need generally, and particularly in HIV/AIDS-related care (Mayston et al. 2012).

It has been well documented that as HIV attacks an individual's nervous system, it can cause HIV-associated neurocognitive disorders (HAND), which can have a damaging impact on overall brain function (Clifford and Ances 2013). Emerging evidence suggests that in the era of universal access to ART, milder forms of HAND are becoming increasingly prevalent as people are living longer lives with HIV infections (Kaul 2009). Being diagnosed with HIV and the associated side effects of the disease can thus increase a person's vulnerability to a wide range of mental health disorders, including adjustment, mood, anxiety, and substance abuse (Berg, Michelson, and Safren 2007). These two epidemics thereby interact synergistically to produce adverse physiological health outcomes. Yet the mild degree of cognitive symptoms of HIV cannot, in and of itself, account for the high prevalence of mental health disorders in HIV-infected patients.

While the exact pathways between HIV/AIDS and mental health disorders are not yet fully understood (Singer 2014), preliminary evidence suggests that this biological synergism is mediated by myriad human behaviors—such as poor eating habits, unsafe sexual practices, increased smoking/drinking, decreased sleep, non-adherence to ART, delayed entry into and decreased retention in HIV-related care—that accelerate HIV's progression to AIDS (Mayston et al. 2012). Other scholars have proposed that psychological stress may also play an important role in this synergism, noting in particular the toxic biological and behavioral effects on individuals who experience stressful events and chronic stress, in ways that ultimately influence the pathogenesis of physical disease, including the regulation of immune and inflammatory processes that have the potential to influence depression, some cancers, and myriad infectious, autoimmune and coronary artery diseases (S. Cohen, Janicki-Deverts, and Miller 2007). This latter body of work considers not only the behavioral changes that occur as individuals adapt or cope with such stressors, but also the stressor-elicited immunologic and endocrine response systems that are activated and work in concert with the autonomic nervous and other physiological systems to increase the risk of physical and psychiatric disorders that lead to worse AIDS-related outcomes (S. Cohen, Janicki-Deverts, and Miller 2007). This growing body of evidence suggests that the biological and behavioral responses to stress processes triggered after exposure to chronic and socially stigmatizing events (Hatzenbuehler, Phelan, and Link 2013; Lick. Durso, and Johnson 2013) could potentially account for some of the synergy between mental health disorders and HIV disease progression (S. Cohen, Janicki-Deverts, and Miller 2007). In these ways, mental, physical and social health and well-being become intricately related to one another in ways that shape the everyday lives, experiences and perceptions of people. As this chapter demonstrates, life stressors, including those associated with HIV stigma appear to sometimes drive mental disorders, and the stigmas associated with both conditions interact in a mutually enhancing spiral to produce deleterious biological health consequences.

CHANGING PUBLIC PERCEPTIONS: HIV/AIDS-RELATED STIGMA (RE)DEFINED

Participants consistently reported that stigma had not only been reduced in recent years, but that it had changed over time, making remarks such as "stigma is . . . no longer like [it was] before" and "[stigma] is still there, but it isn't . . . like before" (anonymous participant). These shifts were always linked in the minds of locals to improved awareness of the disease and the increased accessibility of ART in the community. As one rural Kalenjin woman framed things,

> Because those last times [before ART] . . . people [living with HIV/AIDS] were totally rejected. But now anyone can live with that person because you cannot even know that the person is sick anymore. So long as the person knows early enough to get [ART], no one can ever know! It is not like those other times . . . because before people did not know what the problem was yet . . . [and] those medicines were not there. You could . . . know that person [was HIV+] because . . . the rashes [appeared]. . . . It could be very bad. But now people can live very well. (*Rural Kalenjin woman*)

As the woman cited above makes explicit, processes of social stigma were perceived to have been reduced due to increased knowledge and the introduction of free ART, which could allow HIV to remain relatively undetectable in a body. This made it nearly impossible to know whom to discriminate or stigmatize. ART were thus construed not only to have simply reduced death, dying, and total social rejection, but also to be useful in their ability to conceal what would otherwise eventually become a visibly stigmatizing condition.

Curious about how locals defined stigma and to determine whether or not it was perceived as a completely imported concept (along with global health HIV programs and services), the lead author and researcher inserted lines of questioning on the topic during interviews with key consultants. General responses are succinctly reflected by one man's remarks: "I can remember stigma [before there was ART]. Anyone who died of AIDS was put in some polythene [plastic] papers to send the message that nobody should come near that body. . . . [The body] was dangerous." A woman echoed this logic and extended it when she juxtaposed the stigma associated with HIV/AIDS before and after the increase of HIV services:

> The stigma we had early for those infected with HIV/AIDS—before the wazungu [white people associated with HIV global health programs] and the ART came—was a big one. People were locked away so they would not infect anyone else. And if people learned that someone had HIV/AIDS and was having sex with others, the community would kill that person to stop [him or her] from spreading the disease. . . . Also, people have always hated those with chronic diseases and mental problems. In the past, no one would allow a person with a mental problem to marry into their families—it was taboo. (*Anonymous participant*)

As this woman makes clear, stigma manifested itself more intensely early in the epidemic. It took the form of physical isolation—even the killing of those harboring the virus but who refused to abstain from sex—as a local strategy adopted to stop the spread of the disease before the introduction of ART. But she goes on to add the notion that community members "have always hated those with chronic diseases and mental problems," thus suggesting that stigma had changed since "the wazungu and ART came." In other words, since the scale up of HIV testing, treatment, and care, stigma and people living with HIV/AIDS had come to be equated with having "mental problems." Thus, as stigma came to manifest itself in new ways, so too did the local knowledge used to draw upon and think about those living with the virus. In response, bodies were no longer overtly physically isolated, but rather were socially differentiated in more subtle ways (e.g., marital taboos).

Indeed, the idea of a person living with HIV getting married was described by the general public as being unacceptable and as one of the greatest challenges facing those who were infected. One man stated this plainly during an interview: "Nowadays, it is not accepted to be married to an HIV+ person because even if you wanted to get married, you must first be tested . . . and if you are found positive—marriage is disqualified—automatic." When the lead researcher went on to explore the possibility of discordant individuals marrying (one person was living with HIV and the partner was not infected), interviewees were appalled by the question. One Kalenjin woman instantly replied that "[being married with a man who was known to be infected with HIV] would be like sticking my head in a pot of boiling water!" Another man was more polite in tempering the way he may have actually felt about the idea: "According to me, it is not good for an HIV positive to marry into my family."

The very question about discordant individuals marrying violated a very basic local logic that marriage was about reproduction, and thus, not a context for condoms, abstinence, and/or any of the safe sex practices promoted by and through HIV prevention programs. A Kalenjin man explained this directly during an interview: "You know, Kalenjins believe that procreation is first in marriage . . . marriage is not . . . actually . . . for companionship. The factor number one is that marriage is for procreation." In many parts of sub-Saharan Africa, being married (with offspring) continues to be one of the most significant markers of a respectable adult person. Reproduction was at the heart of the marital union, and as a consequence, living with HIV/AIDS posed a major threat, especially among those who were not yet married and with children, and thus had not yet achieved the coveted status of respectable adult.

Local understandings of stigma were also shifting to incorporate and draw on already existing logics about people with mental illness. That is, stigma was described as affecting (or potentially affecting) the minds of particular individuals. For example, one man shared that "nowadays . . . it seems . . . if someone finds that they are HIV+, it is like they get psychologically affected." Similarly, a woman shared her perception that locals were experiencing new types of "problems nowadays" because of stigma. She offered the following logic to justify her beliefs: "People with HIV have a lot of problems nowadays. They feel despised . . . and because of that despise, you find that the person now has troubling thoughts. They have stress and [so] they [suffer] even more sickness!"

While many interviewees emphasized the ways that HIV/AIDS "nowadays" affected the minds of individuals, such notions quickly moved the interview content away from a general discussion of "mental disturbances" toward a moral discussion of a person's impairment in social functioning and/or tendency toward (or potential for) social rule violation (see Barrett's [1988] discussion of schizophrenia). The mental disturbances being caused by HIV/AIDS were described as causing such individuals to engage in socially deviant behaviors (e.g., committing suicide, intentionally spreading the disease to others). This relocated the danger from their physical bodies (at least semantically) into their minds and social interactions. One resident said,

> If people have HIV, sometimes they are just going around—living in that other way—without even caring. . . . I have heard many stories of people leaving letters when they die of all the people they have infected—intentionally! It is just that they [those living with HIV] have psychological problems . . . and that does happen here so much. (*Anonymous participant*)

The individual quoted above suggests that HIV caused "psychological problems" and thus made those who were infected to live "without caring." In so doing, the stigma associated with mental illness (rather than the stress/risk of potential social marginalization associated with HIV) gets drawn upon to justify treating HIV-positive individuals differently. Those suffering from mental disorders were thus blamed for the ongoing and intentional spread of the virus.

The increase in HIV testing services seemed to have amplified and intensified the local perception that those living with HIV/AIDS were increasingly suffering from mental illnesses among the general population. For example, at one point, gossip began to circulate about a woman who allegedly tested positive during the HCT program. A Kalenjin woman and key consultant shared details of the gossip she had heard, while also offering her own interpretation of the situation:

> I think she had hysteria. Right after [the HCT testing] she rented a [hotel] room with a Congolese truck driver. . . . After that . . . she went running up and down in the village, grabbing [her private parts] and saying that she isn't satisfied [sexually] by the husband and wants more sex. She was saying, "Somebody help me!" . . . People say that the woman started shouting, "I won't die alone!" And now I have been hearing that she has started to seduce . . . men. . . . People are talking now, "Take care of [be careful around] that wife!" (*Key consultant*)

Whether or not this gossip was true is beyond the scope of this chapter. The point to be made, instead, is that locals desired to share the details of this type of story with one another. Luise White (2000) contends that gossip exposes the shared anxieties and uncertainties associated with everyday life in a community at a given moment in time. The discourse about individuals not wanting to "die alone," was regularly parroted by residents and used to describe bitter individuals living with HIV who malevolently spread the virus to others, and were documented early on during the AIDs epidemic (see Whyte 1997). This gossip both reflected and reinforced the anxiety-producing belief that individuals diagnosed with HIV might potentially have a psychological reaction that could cause harm to others. This cast the HIV infected body as dangerous, in new ways, and in so doing, perpetuated not only the idea that those living with HIV were sexually hyper and deviant, immoral, and malicious, but also the stigma and anxieties associated with this syndemic during a period of increased services. The gossip thus also served to justify the local response to "take care" around or discriminate this particular woman.

This "psychologization" of stigma (see Kleinman 1988, 1599) likely reflects the complex intertwining of local observations, experiences, beliefs, as well as anti-stigma campaigns and interventions. Scholars have already noted that anti-stigma programs, developed by global health experts primarily from abroad were, early on in the epidemic, universalized and transported around the globe as part of prevention packages that some have described as "briefcase concepts" (see Liu 2009). Such programs have historically been rooted in western, social-psychological approaches, which tend to conceptualize stigma as a static "thing" or characteristic that is located within (the mind of) a particular individual (Parker and Aggleton 2003:14). Anthropologists and sociologists have argued that the psychologically grounded, and thus individually focused, anti-stigma education campaigns put the onus on individuals and their "personal choices." In so doing, they unintentionally aggravate processes of stigma by casting blame on particular individuals and/or categories of people, while shifting attention away from the social and structural inequalities sustaining stigma and constraining the "choices" being made (Castro and Farmer 2005:54; Parker and Aggleton 2003; Yang et al. 2007).

SELECTIVE CONCEALMENT

Nearly everyone interviewed—whether living with HIV or not—shared that because HIV continued to evoke notions of sexual immorality and potential physical, mental, and social dangers, an HIV-positive diagnosis should be kept private. As one Kalenjin woman stated,

> I think Kenyans . . . they only think that you get HIV through . . . immorality. There is no other option! So if you are HIV+, you equal immoral. So I think because we have never changed and realized that you can get HIV through other means or ways [other than through immoral sexual acts] . . . I think we still have to have those private parts of our lives. Because that will give you the confidence to continue on with your activities so that you are able to fit in the society. (*Anonymous participant*)

A young Nandi man, Kibet,[6] further exemplifies this point when he justified his plan to never disclose his seropositive status to anyone:

> [Being diagnosed with HIV] is a really hard experience. It is very serious. And it is very, very dangerous. You fear very much that anyone might come to know . . . because they will start announcing to everyone [whispering]: "Someone is sick!" And then the discrimination will start. Slowly people will start to fear you. Slowly people will be avoiding you. And you know for me, it is really dangerous because I am young. I am not married yet. I do not have kids. And I do not yet have a job. (*Kibet*)

For Kibet, the threat of being cut off from various forms of social and interpersonal relationships (e.g., finding a marital/sexual partner) because of an HIV+ diagnosis, evoked a sense of danger, being different, and a potential marker of the beginning signs of the breakdown of the person (Lock and Nguyen 2010, 73).

A pastor of a local congregation continued to maintain the need for privacy in terms of handling one's HIV/AIDS status:

> It is important to keep that one [HIV+ status] a secret . . . because . . . others may embarrass you if they know. As long as you have known that this is the problem that you are in . . . and your spiritual counselor or your doctor . . . has given you the proper guidelines of what to do with this problem that you are in, to me it can be secret. . . . If this is the case, it should be kept secret—for the sake of protecting yourself. . . . Because sometimes in society . . . somebody can lose anger and then they can easily throw words around about you. So . . . being secret is a bit important. (*Pastor*)

As the cleric quoted above suggests, it was important for people living with HIV/AIDS to be vigilant in practicing selective concealment in order to preserve their social reputation yet get the proper care, services, and support they needed. Moving between the contexts of the clinic and larger community therefore required careful negotiations that have been documented by scholars working in southern Africa (Frank and Rödlach 2013). Indeed, it was easier for wealthier individuals to maintain this balancing act because they were able to afford the costly practice of travelling far distances to attend clinics and minimize the chance that someone might see them.

Commonly articulated strategies of hiding a seropositive status from others were to never disclose and to conceal ART usage, both of which allowed those living with the virus to appear symptom-free and thereby able to preserve their social relationships. One man made an intriguing statement about how stigma used to be, before ART. He noted that in the earlier years of the epidemic, polythene had been used to wrap deceased bodies, but "we no longer put bodies in polythene; now people are hiding the drugs—taking them out of the bottles and putting them in polythene." This allowed people to take their ART publicly, while also being able to make claims about other ailments that they were suffering from but were less stigmatizing. Indeed, between the highway and the CCC was a path along a row of bushes that literally contained dozens of empty bottles of antiretrovirals and other medications associated with HIV (e.g., cotrimoxazole).[7] While concealment was an essential practice used to avoid stigmatization and social marginalization, it also reinforced the deleterious effects of HIV. That is, people who tested positive might not link into, adhere to, or remain in care because of their need to conceal.

The availability of ART and the ability to conceal an HIV+ status brought both relief and anxiety to those living at the research site. Locals felt that ART had helped the community because it had drastically reduced the number of deaths. One man stated,

> Those ART are very important because if we could have no drugs, we could have lost many. People are very grateful to [the CCC] because when they came here, we have no deaths anymore. . . . Earlier we were burying people every day, but now those [death] rates have gone down. Now . . . [the death rate] is very low. (*Anonymous participant*)

This relief, however, was not without new types of anxieties among residents, and thus fueled stigmatizing discourses and practices regarding the dangers associated with those living with HIV/AIDS. Specifically, alongside the frequent articulation that it was important to keep an HIV+ status a private matter, came fears about not knowing who was infected with the virus. For example, one man shared a concern that people (women in particular) using ART were more "admirable," and therefore could easily seduce men. From his position, the ability of those to hide an HIV+ status was a major contributor to the perceived high rates of infection among young men in the area. He shared the following remarks.

> There are many [people living with HIV/AIDS] in [this community]. You can just go and look at the person and they may be finished [very sick inside] . . . [but] . . . because she is using medication, when you actually look at her . . . she is admirable. . . . This lady will then just start to seduce the man and he takes her home. And when this man comes to the point [later] that he needs marriage, he cannot find one lady in this area because everybody knew that he slept with an HIV+ woman. (*Anonymous participant*)

On a handful of occasions, people shared the idea that antiretrovirals were becoming a problem for locals, precisely because they allowed people to conceal the disease from others longer, and thus could also secretly and maliciously spread the disease. This, in turn, intensified local gossip and in so doing, fueled local anxieties, stigma, and the need to more ardently practice selective concealment. One participant concluded,

> [In this community] we . . . have those people who say that these drugs have come to bring us [new] problems. The person who is positive knows [he is] positive but when [he] takes these drugs, he looks very much healthy and so he spreads it—knowingly! And if he is a very unkind person, he may go on spreading it . . . quickly! (*Anonymous participant*)

LIVING WITH HIV/AIDS AND NAVIGATING STIGMA IN KENYA

Subjective experiences with stigma among those living with HIV/AIDS were diverse and often contradictory. People rarely described their experiences simply as "Yes, I have felt/been stigmatized" or "No, I have never felt/been stigmatized." Instead, most presented such processes as contingent and shifting. Specifically, sometimes individuals described that they might be rejected in one context (e.g., at church) but accepted in the next (e.g., at the CCC). Stigma was sometimes a problem, and at other moments, it was not. But the possibility of being stigmatized was always described as a potential, which made it feel ominous.

To provide an example, one woman reported that she only rarely experienced stigma because of HIV/AIDS. On most days, she claimed, she could keep HIV/AIDS out of her sense of self, her daily life, and interpersonal relationships (Charmaz 1997). This was not true, however, when she became noticeably ill. During these times, she said, she could not escape her internal feelings of stigma and fears of social abandonment. Whenever she became sick, her usual interpersonal dynamics with others suddenly changed. This, she reasoned out loud, was because people knew that she was living with HIV, which meant that others also knew that any illness could potentially result in her demise. For this woman, the shift in the ways others responded to her verbally in such moments, always made her feel considerably worse. During a semi-structured interview, she recalled the last time she had experienced this type of shift in her relationships with others: "When I look weak, people say 'You are about to die.' The last time this happened, it made me cry so much that I became even sicker and I even ended up having to go to the hospital!" The state of her relations with others (and their stigmatizing comments) had a very real impact upon her physical health and well-being.

Another woman also mentioned that the stigma associated with HIV served as a driver of her self-reported depression. She explained her current circumstances:

> I am depressed. . . . I am okay with the [ART], but the appetite is so much. But I am given no food. I am [no longer] supported because my husband says that I must go to my brothers for support. But the brothers say, "No—you must go to the husband." My father says that the [CCC] gives free food, money, and medicine, so I should be going there. But I do not get money there. . . . My family does not give me support for transportation to get my ARTs and so they don't want to be associated with me anymore . . . they say they don't care if I eat or not, because I am on my way [dying]. . . . Everyone says I am on my way dying.

The woman quoted above was neither being well cared for by those in her kin networks because of her HIV status, nor did she qualify for monetary assistance or food relief at the CCC. Despite having access to ART and basic health care, she felt depressed as she confronted the stressful realities of being cut off from other equally important resources—social, emotional, mental health, financial, and nutritional. At the same time, the notion that people living with HIV/AIDS should ultimately be cared for by a CCC was a convenient way for their families, friends, and community members to withdraw their own support and resources, and thus served as a form of self-preservation in this resource-poor place.

During semi-structured or life-history interviews, many people living with HIV/AIDS reported some incident of having been or having felt stigmatized (see Jacoby 1994)—usually in the form of a verbal attack, sometimes in the form of neglect, and only rarely in the form of overt physical abuse. Verbal attacks and neglect were construed as being at least as dangerous, if not more so than corporeal attacks because they left little, if any, proof for locals to complain about or to use as evidence against a person who stigmatized another. One employee at the CCC made this belief evident:

> Stigma . . . that is still a challenge here in Kenya. It is very difficult to intervene in such cases. Apart from when one has been physically assaulted. Or a child has been thrown out of school. Or someone has been chased out of employment . . . there are laws on that. . . . But stigma may be very hard to intervene because . . . proof is difficult. And those patients don't want to expose their families to such ridicule. So even if [our clients/patients have] a problem in the home, they will not tell you. [We at the clinic] try to encourage them, counsel them.

In general, people working at the CCC felt that there was little they could do to help their clients who were experiencing stigma, outside of offering encouraging words and very basic counseling. This was not only because they lacked the proper resources to do so, but also because their clients were rarely forthcoming about such matters (they felt a shared moral obligation not to shame their family members or themselves by complaining about abuses). Furthermore, it was often difficult to find any evidence to use or justify interventions against stigmatizers.

While only a select few individuals stated that they had never experienced or worried about any form of stigma or discrimination, even though they openly shared their seropositive status with others,[8] everyone interviewed had personally witnessed and/or heard about someone being stigmatized, usually in the form of gossip and/or through the media. Several interviewees shared that they had never experienced any form of stigma or discrimination, but then quickly qualified that this was because they concealed their HIV status as a strategy to avoid such problems. One woman made it clear that she had seen others being abused in various parts of Kenya for being HIV+, which is what she claimed continued to motivate her to keep her own seropositive status private. She stated,

> No one knows that I am HIV+. I have witnessed others of my status being abused with words and physically. I am not special, so I can go through the same thing. Once I was at [another town] where business women were buying potatoes to resell. Now the victim [one living with HIV] wanted her [share] of the potatoes [to sell] but she was told by another, "I cannot talk or share with a skeleton like you!"

In the context of a community marked by extreme poverty and disparities, sometimes stigmatizing and discriminating discourses and practices were used during fierce attempts to disadvantage a competitor and to maintain control over already scarce resources.

During life-history interviews, a handful of people living with HIV/AIDS shared extreme experiences with processes of stigma and discrimination, and in so doing, their lives unveiled some of the pathways through which deleterious biological health consequences are produced and reproduced through harmful social and structural conditions, forces, relations, and inequalities. Specifically, such individuals provided details of the damaging and cumulative effects of life stressors, including those associated with being cut off from important social and kin networks after being diagnosed with HIV. As a result, they reported struggling with the additional burdens of a wide range of self-diagnosed mental disorders. Here we highlight one of these cases to illuminate the physiological and synergizing effects of the intertwining of HIV/AIIDS, mental disorders, stigma, and other stressful events and social forces.

A Kikuyu woman, Wanja, offered her own subjective experiences and perspectives of suffering simultaneously from HIV/AIDS and a mental disorder. Specifically, through a series of life-history interviews, Wanja traced the various trajectories of her life that first resulted in an HIV infection, and eventually to a struggle to overcome chronic alcoholism. Wanja had, at one point, been a married housewife and farmer living in Central Province. Her husband had a well-paying job and together they had four children. When her spouse died unexpectedly from an accident, Wanja's life became considerably more turbulent. She began moving across the country from one job to another. She explained, as a widow with multiple kids, the initial mobility required by her work had eventually been eased when her children went to live with her mother in her rural homestead in Central Province. Wanja did not make very much money but sent what she could to her mother and children.

She described that things became overwhelming after she learned that her mother had poisoned (and killed) the youngest son for becoming too much of "a burden" on the household's already scarce resources. Wanja spoke at great length about grappling with her anger, angst, and internal struggle to forgive her mother. When she landed a job working on the farm of a Kalenjin family, in a rural area in Rift Valley Province, she was grateful and relieved by the great distance that separated her from the mother. It was when she was living just outside the trading center (the field site) that Wanja, in an effort to try to conceive another boy to replace the one who had been lost, became infected with HIV. As she explained,

> [A Kalenjin man had been pursuing me for some time] . . . and people were saying that I was somehow abnormal [for not being in a sexual relationship with a man]. . . . That is when I . . . thought, "Why should I live desperate when there are men?" . . . So . . . we made love! . . . [Later] he told me, "If you are not going to give birth—to give me a kid—I think there is . . . no need of me staying with

> you." . . . I prayed [to] God and thought, "May you give me another boy [to replace the one who had been poisoned]." So I had decided . . . and I got pregnant. . . . I was almost to give birth . . . when I was told by another . . ., "You know what? I never wanted to discourage you, but . . . do you know that you will be a second wife?" I never believed. I thought that that lady was jealous! But then she kept on telling me such things [until eventually I came to meet the first wife, who was also pregnant]. . . . After I gave birth, I told the husband, "Don't think I was interested [in being] . . . married. Me, I was married to a person who gave dowry to my people and I cannot go to another home. So, let us say that we have wasted time with each other." And I told him [that] and I became very strict. I went on with my work. . . .
>
> Around the time when the boy was . . . 5 years [he] started becoming sick. . . . It was always something like pneumonia. . . . [And later] . . . I started becoming sick. . . . I came to the hospital. I was given . . . all sorts of medicine. . . . The medicine was good . . . but nothing changed. . . . [A doctor] told me, "Have you ever had your blood checked?" I said, "No." She said, "Go and be checked in the blood." . . . I was [HIV] positive. . . . So . . . I brought . . . my child [and] he was found [HIV] positive. I told God, "Oh God, although the life will be short, give us happiness."
>
> I came to the [CCC] . . . where I met . . . the father of my child. . . . I met him at the [CCC] . . . sitting in line. [Laughing] Queuing! He . . . call[ed] me [and was saying things such as], "You know . . . I am sorry! . . . I had no mind then." . . . I told him, "So you knew it was this way [you were living with HIV]? And you were that way [HIV+]? . . . You wanted to waste me [infect me with HIV]?" . . . At the next [CCC] visit . . . I met [his first] wife [and that confirmed] . . . where I had got the virus. It is from this man. And . . . that is the time I started becoming weak. . . . From there I started becoming a drunkard. I started drinking. I started taking alcohol. Because I found that I was nothing . . . different. (*Wanja*)

After Wanja began drinking heavily, she recalled a series of spiraling hardships, including losing several jobs, becoming homeless, and being raped numerous times while intoxicated. For Wanja, it was not the HIV diagnosis that triggered her heavy drinking per se, but rather it was a strategy through which she coped after a series of stressful events, including a realization that she had been infected by a man she otherwise believed had wanted to marry her. She felt alone, "different," like "nothing," and blamed herself for having been foolish—as a previously hard-working and responsible woman who did not sleep around or engage in careless or reckless sex—and duped by a man who had only been pretending to care about and want to provide for her and their child. For Wanja, the felt stigma associated with HIV was a driver of her mental disorder. An unemployed widow and single mother, she faced the challenges of the syndemic of HIV, chronic alcoholism, and the harmful social and stigmatizing conditions that accompanied her marginalized social status (a poor woman, widow, person living with HIV, and alcoholic) in relative isolation. At the same time, the ongoing self-blame (of having been infected and for having infected her young son), her living conditions, and the gender-based violence that she endured all worked together to amplify her susceptibility for HIV reinfection, contracting other sexually transmitted infections, and other opportunistic infections known to have deleterious biological consequences in that they accelerate the progression of HIV. At the same time, the combining effects of this syndemic put others in the community at risk for HIV transmission, and in so doing, Wanja experienced further stigmatization as a community resident with a "psychological problem," who was therefore imagined by others to be purposefully and callously spreading the virus.

DISCUSSION / CONCLUSION

Myriad life stressors, including those stemming from the associated social processes of HIV/AIDS-related stigma, put individuals at high risk for mental health disorders. Mental health disorders and their related stigmas, in turn, were associated with worsening HIV disease. This is especially true among individuals who are cut off from the necessary resources provided to them through their social and kin networks. In Kenya, stigma is especially powerful in this regard for two primary reasons. First, in the context of extreme economic marginalization and limited access to resources, family members are sometimes simply unable to provide the support necessary for their loved ones living with chronic illnesses. The second reason is because an adult's sense of normal or "respectable" personhood is linked explicitly to particular social relationships (e.g., marital), and the powerful synergy of both HIV and mental disorders had the potential to interrupt current and the potential for future relationships. In this setting, and as exemplified through the narratives and subjective lived experiences of interviewees presented throughout this chapter, the stressors of stigma associated with HIV/AIDS was a driver of mental health disorders, which are equally stigmatized conditions. In these ways, this stigmatized syndemic constituted a reinforcing spiral.

Personal narratives among the general public and of people living with HIV/AIDS suggest that HIV-related stigma has, in fact, shifted from fear of the physical to fear of the mental. As HIV treatment programs continue to be successful in helping individuals conceal the physical manifestations of HIV in this part of the world, the stigma has been transformed by taking on the logic of fears of mental disorders among those infected. This new manifestation of stigma both caused and reinforced mental disorders at multiple levels, including that of the individual (through feelings of isolation, depression, and alcoholism at the risk of loss of family, home, livelihood); societal (as persons are shunned by their families and communities); and structural (as those suffering from and those in positions to care for individuals facing chronic illnesses are unable to access the proper medical care and the resources necessary to maintain nurturing environments). Individuals learned to cope with these mutually reinforcing stigmas by practicing selective concealment. However, concealment may, in fact, be a further source of stress (Lick, Durso, and Johnson 2013) and reinforce the taboos and prevent the linkage to and retention in care required to curb the HIV epidemic.

As this chapter demonstrates, biological and social lives are mutually constitutive (Lock and Nguyen 2010). If the *2030 Agenda for Sustainable Development* goals to end the epidemics of AIDS, tuberculosis, malaria, hepatitis, and neglected tropical diseases (UN 2015) are to be seriously attempted and attained, it will first have to be acknowledged—and then acted upon in both the biomedical and social science worlds—that "it is impossible to maintain a marked division between the biological body and its social context" (Lock and Nguyen 2010, 2). As scholars, practitioners, and policy makers united by and committed to understanding and ameliorating HIV/AIDS, these biosocial realities must be incorporated and drawn upon in the creation and development of future programs and policies centering on HIV/AIDS. The treatment of these reinforcing conditions will require addressing both HIV and mental health treatment and the driving social stigmas associated with both conditions, together.

NOTES

1. Studies in western Kenya have found that the ethanol content in an average serving of chang'aa was the equivalent to two U.S. standard drinks (Papas et al. 2010).
2. Other explanations included poverty, joblessness, laziness, peer pressure, and as a coping mechanism to reduce high levels of stress, which were attributed not only to HIV/AIDS, but also to unemployment, everyday violence, and the demoralizing effects of the 2007/2008 post-election violence in Kenya.
3. On a handful of occasions, participants were willing to be interviewed but specifically requested that they were not audio recorded. These interviews are documented by extensive field notes.
4. The largest ethnic group in Kenya.
5. A linguistic and political-social category that actually incorporates several different ethnic groups (see Lynch 2011).
6. Kibet and all other names are pseudonyms used to protect the confidentiality of the participants.

7. Most bottles were empty, but some were full. A healthcare worker explained that some people did not like taking ART, often because they did not feel sick. But many had learned that if you did not attend your monthly clinic appointment, someone from the CCC would show up at your house, sending the message to your neighbors that you were living with the virus. As a consequence, a few people would get their ART, throw them into the bushes, and go about their lives without ever using them. The following month they would repeat the ritual.

8. It should also be noted that informants who consistently reported never having experienced any stigma were also employed by the CCC in varying capacities.

REFERENCES

Aillon, Jean-Louis, David M. Ndetei, Lincoln Khasakhala, Washington Njogu Ngari, Hesbon Otieno Achola, Selestine Akinyi, and Simone Ribero. 2014. "Prevalence, Types and Comorbidity of Mental Disorders in a Kenyan Primary Health Centre." *Social Psychiatry Psychiatric Epidemiology* 49(8):1257–68.

Ashforth, Adam. 2009. "Ethnic Violence and the Prospects for Democracy in the Aftermath of the 2007 Kenyan Elections." *Public Culture* 21(1):9–19.

Barrett, Robert J. 1988. "Interpretations of Schizophrenia." *Culture, Medicine and Psychiatry* 12:357–88.

Berg, Carla J., Susan E. Michelson, and Steven A. Safren. 2007. "Behavioral Aspects of HIV Care." *Infectious Disease Clinics of North America* 21(1):181–200.

Boarts, Jessica M., Eve M. Sledjeski, Laura M. Bogart, and Douglas L. Delahanty. 2006. "The Differential Impact of PTSD and Depression on HIV Disease Markers and Adherence to HAART in People Living with HIV." *AIDS and Behavior* 10:253–61.

Castro, Arachu, and Paul Farmer. 2005. "Understanding and Addressing AIDS-Related Stigma." *American Journal of Public Health* 95(1):53–59.

Charmaz, Kathy. 1997. *Good Days, Bad Days*. New Brunswick, NJ: Rutgers University Press.

Clifford, David B., and Beau M. Ances. 2013. "HIV-Associated Neurocognitive Disorders." *The Lancet Infectious Diseases* 13(11): 976–86.

Cohen, Myron S., Ying Q. Chen, Marybeth McCauley, Theresa Gamble, Mina C. Hosseinipour, Nagalingeswaran Kumarasamy, James G. Hakim, et al. 2011. "Prevention of HIV-1 Infection with Early Antiretroviral Therapy." *New England Journal of Medicine* 365(6):493–505.

Cohen, Sheldon, Denise Janicki-Deverts, and Gregory E. Miller. 2007. "Psychological Stress and Disease." *Journal of the American Medical Association* 298(14):1685–87.

Copeland, Toni J. 2011. "Poverty, Nutrition, and a Cultural Model of Managing HIV/AIDS among Women in Nairobi, Kenya." *Annals of Anthropological Practice* 35(1):81–97.

CSIS (Center for Strategic and International Studies). 2009. *AMPATH*. Retrieved from http://smartglobalhealth.org/blog/entry/ampath-an-integrated-model-of-healthcare-in-rift-valley-province-kenya/.

Das, Veena, and Deborah Poole. 2004. *Anthropology in the Margins of the State*. Santa Fe, NM: SAR Press.

Frank, Emily, and Alexander Rödlach. 2013. "To Disclose or Not to Disclose." *Journal of Southern African Studies* 39(1):119–33.

Goodrich, Suzanne, Samson Ndege, Sylvester Kimaiyo, Hosea Some, Juddy Wachira, Paula Braitstein, John E. Sidle, et al. 2013. "Delivery of HIV Care during the 2007 Post-Election Crisis in Kenya." *Conflict and Health* 7:25. Retrieved from https://conflictandhealth.biomedcentral.com/articles/10.1186/1752-1505-7-25.

Hatzenbuehler, Mark L., Jo C. Phelan, and Bruce G. Link. 2013 "Stigma as a Fundamental Cause of Population Health Inequalities." *American Journal of Public Health* 103(5):813–21.

The Insight START Study Group. "2015 Initiation of Antiretroviral Therapy in Early Asymptomati HIV Infection." *The New England Journal of Medicine* 373:795–807.

Jacoby, Ann. 1994. "Felt versus Enacted Stigma." *Social Science and Medicine* 38(2):269–74.

Jenkins, Rachel, David Kiima, Frank Njenga, Marx Okonji, James Kingora, Dammas Kathuku, and Sarah Lock. 2010a. "Integration of Mental Health into Primary Care in Kenya." *World Psychiatry* 9:118–20.

Jenkins, Rachel, David Kiima, Marx Okonji, Frank Njenga, James Kingora, and Sarah Lock. 2010b. "Integration of Mental Health in Primary Care and Community Health Workers in Kenya: Context, Rationale, Coverage and Sustainability." *Mental Health in Family Medicine* 7:37–47.

Jenkins, Rachel, Frank Njenga, Marx Okonji, Pius Kigamwa, Makheti Baraza, James Ayuyo, Nicola Singleton, Sally McManus, and David Kiima. 2012. "Prevalence of Common Mental Disorders in a Rural District of Kenya, and Socio-Demographic Risk Factors." *International Journal of Environmental Research and Public Health* 9:1810–19.

Jenkins, Rachel, Caleb Othieno, Stephen Okeyo, Julyan Aruwa, James Kingora, and Ben Jenkins. 2013. "Health System Challenges to Integration of Mental Health Delivery in Primary Care in Kenya." *BMC Health Services Research* 13:368. Retrieved from http://bmchealthservres.biomedcentral.com/articles/10.1186/1472-6963-13-368.

Kamungi, Prisca Mbura. 2009. "The Politics of Displacement in Multiparty Kenya." *Journal of Contemporary African Studies* 27(3):345–64.

Kaul, Marcus. 2009. "HIV-1 Associated Dementia Update on Pathological Mechanisms and Therapeutic Approaches." *Current Opinion in Neurology* 22(3):315–20.

Kleinman, Arthur. 1988. *The Illness Narratives*. New York: Basic Books.

———. 2009. "Global Mental Health: A Failure of Humanity." *The Lancet* 374:603–604.

Kleinman, Arthur, Wen-Zhi Wang, Shi-Chuo Li, Xue-Ming Cheng, Xiu-Ying Dai, Kun-Tun Li, and Joan Kleinman. 1995. "The Social Course of Epilepsy." *Social Science & Medicine* 40:1319–30.

Lick, David J., Laura E. Durso, and Kerri L. Johnson. 2013. "Minority Stress and Physical Health." *Perspectives on Psychological Science* 8(5):521–48.

Link, Bruce G., and Jo C. Phelan. 2001. "Conceptualizing Stigma." *Annual Review of Sociology* 27:363–85.

Liu, Shao-hua. 2009. "Contested AIDS Stigmatization in Southwest China." *Human Organization* 68(4):395–405.

Lock, Margaret, and Vinh-Kim Nguyen. 2010. *An Anthropology of Biomedicine*. Malden, MA: Wiley-Blackwell.

Lynch, Gabrielle. 2011. *I Say to You*. Chicago: The University of Chicago Press.

Mayston, Rosie, Eugene Kinyanda, Nathaniel Chishinga, Martin Prince, and Vikram Patel. 2012. "Mental Disorder and the Outcome of HIV/AIDS in Low-Income and Middle-Income Countries." *AIDS* 26 Suppl 2:S117–35.

Mendenhall, Emily, Gregory Barnabas Omondi, Edna Bosire, Gitonga Isaiah, Abendnego Musau, David Ndetei, and Victoria Mutiso. 2015. "Stress, Diabetes, and Infection: Syndemic Suffering at an Urban Kenyan Hospital." *Social Science & Medicine* 146:11–20.

Murray, Christopher J. L., Theo Vos, Rafael Lozano. Mohsen Naghavi, Abraham D. Flaxman, Catherine Michaud, Majid Ezzati, et al. 2012. "Disability-Adjusted Life Years (DALYs) for 291 Diseases and Injuries in 21 Regions, 1990–2010: A Systematic Analysis for the Global Burden of Disease Study 2010." *Lancet* 380:2197–2223.

NASCOP (National AIDS and STI Control Programme). 2009. *Kenya AIDS Indicator Survey 2007*. Retrieved from http://stacks.cdc.gov/view/cdc/12122/.

———. 2014. *Kenya HIV Prevention Revolution Road Map*. Nairobi, Kenya: Ministry of Health.

Ndetei, David M., Lincoln I. Khasakhala, Mary W. Kuria, Victoria N. Mutiso, Francisca A. Ongecha-Owuor, and Donald A. Kokonya. 2009. "The Prevalence of Mental Disorders in Adults in Different Level General Medical Facilities in Kenya." *Annals of General Psychiatry* 8:1.

Ng'ang'a, P. 2011. *Prevalence of Anxiety and Depression among HIV/AIDS Patients Attending the Comprehensive Care Centre (CCC), Kenyatta National Hospital (KNH)*. University of Nairobi.

Papas, Rebecca K., Benson N. Gakinya, Joyce B. Baliddawa, Steve Martino, Kendall J. Bryant, Eric M. Meslin, and John E. Sidle. 2012. "Ethical Issues in a Stage 1 Cognitive Behavioral Therapy Feasibility Study and Trial to Reduce Alcohol Use among HIV-Infected Outpatients in Western Kenya." *Journal of Empirical Research on Human Research Ethics* 7(3):29–37.

Papas, Rebecca K., John E. Sidle, Benson N. Gakinya, Joyce B. Baliddawa, Steve Martino, Michael M. Mwaniki, Rogers Songole, et al. 2011. "Treatment Outcomes of a Stage I Cognitive-Behavioral Trial to Reduce Alcohol Use Among Human Immunodeficiency Virus-Infected Out-Patients in Western Kenya." *Addiciton* 106:2156–66.

Papas, Rebecca K., John E. Sidle, Emmanuel S. Wamalwa, Thomse O. Okumu, Kendall L. Bryant, Joseph L Goulet, Stephen A. Maisto, R. Scott Braithwaite, and Amy C. Justice. 2010. "Alcohol Content of Traditional Brew in Western Kenya Using Culturally Relevant Methods." *AIDS Behavior* 14(4):836–44.

Parker, Richard, and Peter Aggleton. 2003. "HIV/AIDS-Related Stigma and Discrimination." *Social Science and Medicine* 57(1):13–24.

PEPFAR (U.S. President's Emergency Plan for AIDS Relief). 2012. *PEPFAR Scientific Advisory Board 3rd Meeting*. Retrieved from http://www.pepfar.gov/documents/organization/200669.pdf.

Pfeiffer, Elizabeth J. 2014. "Viral Stories." PhD diss., Department of Anthropology, Indiana University Bloomington.

Prince, Ruth J., and Rebecca Marsland. 2014. *Making and Unmaking Public Health in Africa: Ethnographic and Historical Perspectives*. Athens, OH: Ohio University Press.

Ryan, Gery W., and H. Russell Bernard. 2003. "Techniques to Identify Themes." *Field Methods* 15:85–109.

Singer, Merrill. 2009. *Introduction to Syndemics: A Critical Systems Approach to Public and Community Health*. San Francisco, CA: Jossey-Bass.

Singer, Merrill. 2014. "Syndemics." In *The Wiley Blackwell Encyclopedia of Health, Illness, Behavior, and Society*, edited by William C. Cockerham, Robert Dingwall, and Stella R. Quah, 2419–23. Malden, MA: Wiley-Blackwell.

Singer, Merrill, and Scott Clair. 2003. "Syndemics and Public Health." *Medical Anthropology Quarterly* 17(4):423–41.

Steel, Zachary, Claire Marnane, Changiz Iranpour, Tien Chey, John W. Jackson, Vikram Patel, and Derrick Silove. 2014. "The Global Prevalence of Common Mental Disorders: A Systematic Review and Meta-Analysis 1980–2013." *International Journal of Epidemiology* 43(2):476–93.

UN (United Nations). 2015. *Transforming Our World: The 2030 Agenda for Sustainable Development*. New York: United Nations. Retrieved from https://sustainabledevelopment.un.org/content/documents/21252030%20Agenda%20for%20Sustainable%20Development%20web.pdf.

UNAIDS (Joint United Nations Programme on HIV/AIDS). 2014. *90–90–90 An Ambitious Treatment Target to Help End the AIDS Epidemic*. Geneva: UNAIDS. Retrieved from http://www.unaids.org/sites/default/files/media_asset/90–90–90_en_0.pdf.

Watkins, Susan Cotts, Ann Swidler, and Crystal Biruk. 2011. "Hearsay Ethnography." In *The Handbook of the Sociology of Health, Illness, and Healing*, edited by Bernice A. Pescosolido, Jack K. Martin, Jane D. McLeod, and Anne Rogers, 431–45. New York: Springer.

White, Luise. 2000. *Speaking with Vampires*. Berkeley: University of California Press.

Whyte, Susan Reynolds. 1997. *Questioning Misfortune*. Cambridge: University of Cambridge Press.

Wyrod, Robert. 2011. "Masculinity and the Persistence of AIDS Stigma." *Cult Health Sex* 13(4):443–56.

Yang, Lawrence Hsin, Arthur Kleinman, Bruce G. Link, Jo C. Phelan, Sing Lee, and Byron Good. 2007. "Culture and Stigma." *Social Science and Medicine* 64:1524–35.

Chapter Seven

Biomedical Moralities

HIV Community Stigma and Risks for HIV/STI Syndemics

Nicholas Emard

Stigma, most famously defined in Erving Goffman's (1963) work on "spoiled identities," has become a multi-faceted, dynamic, and permeable variable in social science research. Social stigma intersects with the damaging layers of structural violence such as racism, classism, and homophobia (Smith et al. 2012). Parker and Aggleton (2003) address stigma as a fluid aspect of societal attitudes, framing it as a constantly changing social process. In the same vein, the HIV/AIDS epidemic has become immensely different, both biomedically and socially. Since the time that HIV/AIDS was popularly portrayed as a "gay cancer" nearly 35 years ago (Shilts 1987), the face of HIV has also changed. People do not walk around with IV poles trailing alongside them, they do not typically bear the lesions of Kaposi's sarcoma, and they do not have to take 15 pills a day. For those who have access to medications to manage it, HIV has become mostly invisible, yet even with this cloak of invisibility stigma has seemingly become ever more evident.

This chapter examines ways that multiple forms of stigma, enacted and perpetuated within HIV communities on HIV-positive bodies, can affect the overall health of community members. I argue that the hegemony of biomedicine perpetuates *biomedical moralities* wherein "good" HIV patients are completely adherent to medications and promote healthy behaviors—ones that perpetuate idealized HIV management. In an attempt to limit potential HIV spread and protect HIV community identity, drug use, unprotected sexual intercourse, and lack of bodily management are stigmatized and deemed immoral (Goffman 1963). Thus, stigma not only manifests among HIV-positive members within their communities but also, and especially, outside of their shared space. The proposal here is that biomedicine and its advancing treatment of HIV thereby reinforce and even engender a structural violence that reproduces HIV stigma, that then becomes embodied *within* HIV communities. Resulting intra-community dynamics increase members' risks for deleterious health consequences through interactions between within-group HIV stigma, substance use, unprotected sexual intercourse, and reduced medication adherence—increasing overall risk for HIV/STI syndemics.

Syndemics theory is a highly effective model used to address the multiple social factors, including stigma that HIV-positive individuals, particularly men who have sex with men (MSM), face. I became interested in applying lessons from existing syndemics literature to the in-group stigma I saw among HIV-positive MSM at his fieldwork site. During data collection, I clearly saw that prospective, ethnographic research on syndemic interactions revealed the lived experiences of people affected by syndemic interactions. This in-group HIV stigma syndemic is the focus of the chapter presented here.

SYNDEMIC SITE—THE COMMUNITY CENTER

Tucked in what looks like a back alley, Fight AIDS Boston (FAB),[1] an HIV community center, is located in an inconspicuous brownstone surrounded by restaurants and apartments. At the front of the building, minimally painted white characters shine through the windows, a faded volunteer sign flaps flimsily in the wind, and a tarnished bike rack adorns the spattered concrete sidewalk. Each unobtrusive aspect enhances a passerby's ability to stroll past the community center without a second glance. Such obscurity may be purposeful.

I inquired about FAB's location early on and was informed by the site supervisor that during the 1990s this "tucked away" aspect was pragmatic, allowing members to sneak in and out unobserved during the early stages of the epidemic. The back entrance looks like most city alleys: black trash-laden pavement, a fire escape that zigzags down the building in intersecting patterns, and greenish dumpsters that sit beside each building. The inconspicuous entrance was an escape for many members to freely move in and out. Once inside the building the layout resembles a rectangle. A prominent honey oak countertop tucked underneath the L-shaped staircase compels guests to greet the desk person. If a visitor is downstairs around noon—lunchtime—they can observe members pack into the boxy space like sardines in a can. And like an open tin can, their bodies spill onto the staircase with eagerness to get some grub.

At the top of the stairs, visitors are forced to pick a direction. Almost automatically, one is compelled to go left—hypnotized by fluorescent signs and sun-drenched table tops—into the art room. This space is multi-purpose, offering members a place to receive a haircut, a station for making jewelry, or in the month of October, a showcase for the best painted pumpkin. The various Minions pumpkins, made in anticipation of the new "Minions" movie, were particularly well crafted artistic renditions. The red brick walls are lined with black shelves with glass fronts that hold a rainbow of colored paper, multiple paint sets, and an array of miscellaneous knick-knacks. If you can manage to get through the art room without being distracted, the cafeteria lies just beyond.

Fieldnotes Excerpt—The Cafeteria

> Walking into the cafeteria is like going back into high school. The clam-yellow walls are papered with current events and happenings of that week, carefully written in bright colors on white paper. Fashioned in checkered patterns, the rectangular tables allow the pale yellow tabletops to visually intersect with the cool grey floor. Five or six yellow and green flimsy plastic chairs adorn each table. When the clock strikes twelve, or a few minutes after, the wooden stairs screech under the members' pounding feet as each person races to get their designated spots in line. Chatting about, they form the usual sequential link and hastily go down the stainless steel counter collecting their food. Most are warm and friendly, yelling "HEY" to the staff members that they know, often cracking jokes as they pass. A persistent kind of warmth remains. Maybe it's the red brick walls that account for exactly half of the room, or the intersecting mint green molding around the windows. Or, perhaps, the history of shared meals and traumatic losses. Whatever it may be, the shared diagnosis connects the community in more ways than one. Togetherness lingers.
>
> An outsider does not immediately feel this overwhelming sense of belonging. Social groups form and each group of friends has their own designated spot in the cafeteria. They sit with each other every day; those are their people. (Fieldnotes, 2015)

I first entered the dining room that day as an appendage of a staff member, sitting at the staff member's table, talking to whomever she talked to, eating what she ate, and trying to blend in. Feeling out the members—their willingness to talk to new people, their openness to share their table, and their scrutiny of his own experiences—was not easy. Certain groups were easier to talk to than others. Most inquired about my volunteer position, while others just sat and ate as he tried to elicit information from them. People at new tables were often welcoming when approached.

Conversation became the hard part. Often, conversations centered on the weather or recent movies to remain on neutral topics. When I felt established at a certain table, I would inquire about aspects of stigma they may have faced. Each person had his or her own response, some more similar than others. Trying to understand the social dynamics of the table provided more insight into stigma than any amount of exiguous conversation that I could provoke. The cafeteria, a liminal space, offered pivotal ethnographic insights into in-group stigma and community social dynamics, informing the theoretical arguments of this chapter.

STIGMA

> I find that the biggest disconnect with people in general, whether you are a professional or not, is communication. If the language isn't understood on both levels, you know, what I anticipate [and] what I think the meaning of stigma is . . . could be very different from you or anyone else. (Grant)

During an interview, Grant discussed the different meanings and language used to describe HIV stigma. He suggests that perceptions of stigma are different for everyone and language is especially important within medical and professional settings. In Goffman's (1963) conception, "an individual who might have been received easily in ordinary social intercourse possesses a trait that can obtrude itself upon attention and turn those of us whom he meets away from him. . . . He possesses a stigma, an undesired differentness from what we had anticipated," he posses a *spoiled identity* (Goffman 1963, 15). In this chapter, Goffman's foundational definition of stigma and his concept of "spoiled identities" are used to expand upon the nuances of stigma as they have long been, and continue to be, associated with HIV/AIDS.

Stigma can be dialogical, experiential (subjective, inter-personal, contextual), internalized, or simply a product of other people's biases. Goffman's definition of stigma most notably refers to "the situation of the individual who is disqualified from full social acceptance" and any "attribute that is deeply discrediting" (1963, 2). From these aspects of stigma, concepts like "enacted stigma," "self-stigma," and "layered stigma" all play a role in how academics measure, evaluate, and write about stigma. Yet, HIV-positive individuals may experience and describe stigma differently, as amorphous or rigid, depending on who you ask. Some participants in my study had a clear definition of stigma, such as: disclosing someone's status, being discriminated against for employment, or having someone refuse to drink from their cup.

Others, like Grant, acknowledged that stigma is different for everyone. Stigma, in the eyes of participants, was recognized as some level of discrimination stemming from either lack of education, prejudice, or fear. They often spoke about stigma in terms of Goffman's concept that is based in a lack of social acceptance, but did not always account for the ways academics categorize and represent social stigma.

Much of public health and psychological research on the experiences of people living with HIV describes "enacted stigma" (Gray 2002; Scambler 2009; Lekas, Siegel, and Leider 2011), or the ways in which HIV-negative people discriminate, judge, or negatively interact with HIV-positive people. This directly describes participants' sense that the stigma they experience may stem from prejudice or fear. Yet little literature to date examines how stigma is enacted between or among individuals *within* HIV communities.

The intersectionality and multilayered nature of stigma and how it is facilitated or used to justify discrimination, can also be based on fixed aspects of one's identity. Kimberle Crenshaw (1991) first used the term "intersectionality" to describe the layering of racism and sexism that perpetuates violence against Black women. Crenshaw and others sought to highlight the gendered and racial dimensions of discrimination in Black and feminist communities (Crenshaw 1991). Intersectionality theory, more broadly, is used to examine how social identities, particularly among minorities, intersect with systems and structures that reinforce oppression and discrimination (Crenshaw 2014). Bowleg mentions how public health research can use intersectionality to talk about social categories. She described it as:

> a theoretical framework that posits that multiple social categories (e.g., race, ethnicity, gender, sexual orientation, socioeconomic status) intersect at the micro level of individual experience to reflect multiple interlocking systems of privilege and oppression at the macro, social-structural level (e.g., racism, sexism, heterosexism). (2012, 1267)

Scambler (2009), like Goffman's definitions, adds that stigma based on attributes—such as race, ethnicity, and sexual preference—may also adversely affect health. While many HIV-positive individuals may feel stigmatized by their serostatus, stigma related to class, sexuality, age, and ethnicity can combine with and compound HIV-related stigma to create multiple intersecting and overlapping stigmas. Such compounding stigmas can impact health and worsen overall disease burden contributing to syndemic interactions (Merrill Singer 2006).

Ritsher and Phelan define internalized stigma as, "when an individual perceives stigma existing in the culture and expects to be treated with devaluation and rejection" (2004, 258). This sets the stage for Steward et al.'s further clarification of forms of stigma related to HIV:

> When stigma is internalized . . . it results in prejudice and may lead to enacted stigma; when it is internalized . . . the consequence is "self-stigma." In the latter

case, people's self-concept is congruent with the stigmatizing responses of others; they accept the discredited status as valid. (2008, 446)

When individuals accept these forms of devaluation and "self-stigma" they appear more likely to engage in behaviors risky for their health. Jefferies et al. note, "the pervasiveness of HIV stigma and its potential to compromise health warrant greater understanding of HIV stigma experienced by young MSM in the United States" (2015, 59). While Jefferies' study included specifically young MSM, a greater understanding of HIV stigma experienced by *and between* MSM generally is needed to elucidate the potential social conditions that can exacerbate biological interactions between known risk factors for HIV stigma and other opportunistic diseases, to produce syndemics.

Much has been written about HIV-positive MSM perceiving stigma from the predominantly heterosexual world around them (Lee, Kochman, and Sikkema 2002; Singer and Clair 2003; Rao et al. 2007; Rintamaki et al. 2006; Van Der Straten et al. 1998) and from HIV-negative members of gay and MSM communities (Courtenay-Quirk et al. 2006; Smith et al. 2012). Smith et al. outlined stigma related to, "discrimination and rejection by HIV-negative gay men, stigma related to aging, changes in physical appearance, race/ethnicity and self-stigma" (2012, 406). In these findings, perceived stigma was associated with "risky" sexual behaviors (such as unprotected anal intercourse, multiple sexual partners, etc.), alcohol consumption, recreational drug use, lack of engagement in health care, and medication non-adherence (Smith et al. 2012; Halkitis et al. 2012). Additionally, HIV-related stigma and discrimination have also been found to have a negative impact on people living with HIV, acting as deterrents to HIV-testing, serostatus disclosure, and linkage and retention in care (Smith et al. 2012).

Overall, current HIV stigma research positions stigmatized or 'spoiled' identities (Goffman 1963) as a form of symbolic violence (Bourdieu 1986): when HIV-positive individuals or communities perceive and perhaps accept (consciously or subconsciously) negative notions of themselves based on cultural and societal evaluations. Bourdieu's concept of "symbolic violence" reflects the ways violence is enacted upon individuals with their own complicity (Bourdieu and Wacquant 1992). Such societal evaluations result in misrecognition of individuals with HIV, ones that depict them as somehow "less than fully human" (Padilla 2009, 155). This is the process by which external forms of structural and symbolic violence, oppression, and discrimination become embodied on the psyches and bodies of HIV-positive people through the internalization of HIV stigma (Lee, Kochman, and Sikkema 2002; Brouard and Wills 2006).

HIV-positive MSM face multiple structural oppressions based on aspects of their identities that put them at increased risk for syndemics. They may be a greater risk for syndemic interactions because of structural violence related to homophobia, interpersonal homophobic violence, associations with substance use, mental health status, unprotected sexual behavior, and workplace discrimination, and so on (Halkitis et al. 2012; Dyer et al. 2012; Stall, Friedman, and Catania 2008; Merrill Singer 2006) The impacts of homophobia, poverty, drug use and racism likely all influence stigma, and subsequent sociobiological interactions, that HIV-positive community members face from outside the community. However, in this proposed syndemic, biomedical hegemony facilitates and exacerbates *intra*-community interactions and perpetuates stigma that is harmful to health—in-group stigma which may be grounded in stereotypes about one's race, how/when one acquired HIV, perceived substance use, or socioeconomic status.

The author conducted intensive ethnographic research to investigate perceptions of stigma within a long-standing, specific HIV community in the greater Boston area,[2] where a campaign focused on reducing HIV stigma was already underway. The author synthesized data from his larger qualitative study to inform the development of the syndemic model proposed in this chapter.[3]

The author encountered some limitations to exploring aspects of structural stigma at FAB, because stigma was a topic that had already been addressed and actively targeted within the community center with "anti-stigma campaigns" featuring shirts, bandanas, and parades before I began my research. This may well have been why some members claimed that there "*was no stigma*"; they were 'tired' of talking about stigma. This often forced me to shift focus to other aspects of the community members' HIV stories, ones that they did not necessarily consider to be immediately related to stigma. Increasingly, I discovered that the stigma at FAB came from aspects of members' identities that were fostered through the biomedical moralities embodied and indoctrinated into community values. The resulting "community ethics" related to HIV care and other bodily and health expectations functioned as veiled discrimination, which is why members did not consider it stigma. Moreover, stigma may have been incorporated as a part of their daily lives as people living with HIV, as Mendenhall's (2012) participants suggest.

No Safe Place from Stigma—Pathways of Syndemic Interaction

This section outlines pathways of interaction between the in-group stigma at FAB and multiple disease or biological factors that compound the deleterious health effects of HIV syndemics. The specific syndemic proposed here consists of stigma enacted by HIV-positive MSM toward other HIV-positive MSM that co-exist within this HIV community, and that deleteriously exacerbates interactions between HIV, risk behaviors for other STIs, reduced medication adherence, and substance use. These pathways of interactions are likely applicable to other similar settings. Exchanges and reinforcement of in-group HIV stigma serve as the structural factors that drive interactions between various overlapping and intersecting biological and behavioral factors. As mentioned, the biological/behavioral factors include substance use, reduced medication adherence, increased susceptibility for other STIs, and increased sexual risk-taking. Any of these factors in combination increase risks for syndemics, and elevate HIV-positive MSMs' overall burden of and risks for known HIV/STI syndemics (Stall et al. 2003; Merrill Singer 2006; Ostrach and Singer 2012; Lyons, Johnson, and Garofalo 2013; O'Leary 2014).

Stigma at Fight AIDS Boston (FAB)

Beginning as a stand-alone agency, FAB prides itself on the ability of its members to unite and guide the organization. The organization was conceived during a Thanksgiving meal in the late 1980s or early 1990s, when AIDS-diagnosed individuals gathered to share food, mourn losses, and offer sentiments of support. This meal, now known as the annual "Celebration of Life" dinner, was just that: a celebration of life with an AIDS diagnosis. Since its founding, the word *member*, instead of "client" or "patient," has been used at FAB, because people who go to the center are members of a community. Thus "long-time member" often implies social obligations to new members ('others') as a part of the informal criterion for community membership (Fieldnotes).

FAB has gone through many changes. "Jeff," an active member, describes the impact of a major financial scandal in the center's history, when an executive director embezzled money. He states, "I was able to see it [the center] implode and rebound because of the whole financial problems that they had [in that era] . . . it was covered in the newspapers. I mean it was SCANDAL! It was a real scandal; and this community doesn't do well with scandals."

After the financial debacle he references, Jeff said the organization gained a new director, however this person was said to lack a 'sense of the community' and subsequently left. Following this vacancy, the center hired as an interim director a long-time AIDS activist from the area who, Jeff says, "brought the center back to its roots." Jeff emphatically claims, "I just decided to latch onto him [the new director]. So I'd get all the dirt first."

However, by expressing, "this community does not do well with scandal" it seems that Jeff wanted me to understand how the previous directors' betrayal and departure (respectively) shook many members' confidence, illustrating how tight-knit and interdependent FAB has been for a long time.

In 2012, the agency was, for financial reasons and after the embezzlement scandal, forced to merge with a larger local multi-service agency that provides individualized treatment programs to primarily homeless people recovering from alcohol and drug addiction. This change in member demographics—from mostly gay men to people recovering from addiction—was jarring for some members. Most were unwilling and unhappy about being affiliated with other organizations that did not share the same core values and history. "Steve," a long-time member, talks about conflicts that emerged within the community:

> The overall mission statement has stayed pretty true, despite all the things that have changed—which includes the demographic of its membership by virtue of the shift of the demographic of the epidemic. So, you may well know that it started out as a local South End gay male group and, then began bringing on members who were bisexual or straight identified . . . but as the demographic of the HIV community in the Boston metropolitan expanded, so did the demographics coming through the door. There was at least one crisis point where the original demographic majority felt they were losing the center's focus, and that the center was expanding too far from its original clientele base. So there was quite a challenging year or so. There was push back and resentment, and people who felt that the organization needs to follow the demographic needs of the epidemic—not of the original group- that put us in conflict with donors. (*Steve*)

Steve's comments suggest that the conflict between original (mostly gay, HIV-positive) members and new (mostly substance-using, HIV-positive, many also MSM) members was intensely strong. Many original donors did not give their support to FAB once they thought the mission of providing support specifically to gay men with HIV was compromised. This local social history accounts for some of the dichotomy that still divides the "community" today. In this way, a socially defined "community" identity can perpetuate stigma—by saying who does and does not belong. Despite the conflict, the community nevertheless offers support for all affected with HIV/AIDS—all members have a place, but often times not all are equally embraced.

Arch, another long-time community member, describes the ways that members separate themselves into cliques while eating lunch in the cafeteria. A retired medical professional in his 60s, Arch comes in and out of FAB with his partner, visiting whenever they come back from vacation, often wearing fluorescent flower-laden shirts from their travels. Noting the same conflicts that arise with the changing of demographics and the ways new members behave within the established community, Arch says the following:

> Up until about six years ago, I think it was more of a larger gay population [at FAB], and it seemed to be more of the somewhat straight-laced gay group. Umm, then when there was a merged [a take-over] . . . the clientele and members then seemed to have made a switch that seem to include a much larger percentage of substance abusers, people who are at a lower economic level, people who may not have good or any housing, and more of a mix of women and men . . . the group that now makes up a larger part than previously tends to be less considerate of people's private spaces; in terms of . . . not being quite while announcements are being made and having to be reminded to do or not do certain . . . issues of conduct. (*Arch*)

While Arch is stating the change in demographics, he is ultimately telling the story of why members create and perpetuate such in-group tensions. He finds that the former population was a "somewhat straight-laced gay group," implying the standard of conduct established by members with more 'cultural capital' are taken more seriously and reinforced. Newer members, perceived as deviants from a somewhat lower socioeconomic class, seem to have less respect for the established rules and way of being in the community spaces, as defined by older members. Such tensions and perceptions reflected a larger societal issue embodied in the social construction of the community—where people who are homeless, drug using, and of lower economic status are policed and stigmatized for their behaviors.

Stigma and Syndemic Interactions

This proposed syndemic examines how HIV-related stigma contributes to damaging interactions between risky sexual behavior (resulting in increased risks for additional STIs), substance abuse, and reduced medication adherence—all of which are known to compound each other. These interactions have resulting negative health consequences for sufferers. The social factors contributing to these interactions in the proposed syndemic include the specific forms of HIV stigma perceived and experienced within groups of MSM living with HIV, often determined by the era of their diagnosis, perceived sexual practices, and assumptions about substance use. These forms of stigma allow some groups of HIV-positive MSM to be perceived by fellow MSM as differentially 'responsible' for having acquired HIV, depending on their assumed sexual or substance use behavior, or based on aspects of their background. Stigma is further reinforced based on how people within the community are perceived to be 'managing' their HIV, substance use, or other bodily or health conditions—each carrying biomedical and moral implications.

The stigma that some HIV-positive MSM perceive, both in existing literature and in this original data, may not solely affect their social place in HIV communities; stigma can contribute to a worsening of their overall disease burden. Perceived stigma related to an HIV-positive diagnosis may contribute to increased substance use and high-risk sexual behaviors, such as unprotected anal sex, which increases risks for additional STIs (Drumright et al. 2007; Mao et al. 2015; Patterson et al. 2005). Among HIV-positive MSM, unsafe injection drug use may further contribute to Hepatitis C (HCV) risk, one element in a known HIV/STI syndemic (Singer 2009; Morano, Gibson, and Altice 2013). Liver disease caused by Hepatitis C virus is the second leading cause of death in HIV-positive people (Merrill Singer 2009, 81). Central to the syndemic proposed here is the idea that an awareness of hegemonic biomedical expectations about HIV management, and resulting embodiment of biomedical moralities within HIV communities, further compound the effects of stigma, systematically marginalizing individuals whose behaviors are seen as not compliant both HIV-positive and/or biomedical "community" rules and standards.

Longtime FAB members could be heard scoffing at the people who filed into the community center for free meals and other services at the end of the month because their welfare checks had run out. Such classist judgments seemed largely due to a perceived lack of 'cultivating one's self' or engaging in the kind of bodily self-care that was valued among the more established members who are highly aware of biomedical moralities in HIV care. Grant spoke about a dichotomy that divides the HIV-positive community not only in Boston, but also in other places where he had lived:

> In New York, in Chelsea, I was told that there's the A side of the street—8th Avenue—and there's a B-side of the street. A-listers walk on one side of the street, and everybody else walks on the other. I said, "Are you kidding me?" This is just too much! But then a friend told me, "just to let you know, like within the gay community, within the HIV community there's an A-list and a B-list." (*Grant*)

Grant explained that the 'A-list' and 'B-list' separated MSM who function with HIV in "good" and "bad" ways. The A-listers are people who are "high-functioning" and have successful jobs, while B-listers are "commoners," or rather, people who represent marginalized sections of society. Though many members of FAB now represent B-listers by virtue of their income or class status, they attempt to climb the social ladder by achieving the best possible biomedical health. The notion of "A-list and B-list" or "better" and "worse" ways of living with HIV produces biomedical moralities. Such convictions echo Willen's (2012) work on health-related "deservingness" and was an underlying theme that contributed to the stigma some members of the community perceived. Through standards of social, medical, and sexual etiquette, within-group HIV stigma perpetuates expectations for a morally appropriate self that exhibits the "good" way of living with HIV.

Sexual Risk-Taking and STIs

One component of this syndemic involves the interaction between in-group stigma, sexual risk taking, and increases risk for STIs. Current literature documents increased sexual risk behavior among HIV-positive individuals and their resulting risks for other STIs that may exacerbate HIV symptoms and overall disease burden (Crepaz and Marks 2002; Dougan, Evans, and Elford 2007). High-risk behaviors among HIV-positive individuals can be related to their perception of stigma as measured by loneliness; individuals who reported more loneliness were also more likely to engage in unprotected anal intercourse (Hubach et al. 2015). These high-risk bio-behavioral factors, combined with the structural factor of social stigma toward HIV-positive MSM can worsen the overall social environment for HIV-positive MSM (Drabkin et al. 2013), and help exacerbate their overall burden of disease—the hallmark of a syndemic.

Within group settings, the combination of stigma and increased sexual risk-taking can further isolate certain individuals and contribute to loneliness. Additionally, such loneliness further increases risk-taking behaviors in a vicious and potentially dangerous cycle of risk. Moral and social judgments may then be placed on individuals who are thought to be reckless or careless with their sexual partners. Many HIV-positive MSM seek to protect partners during sexual activity, but those who do not put themselves and others at greater risk for additional sexually transmitted infections (Crepaz et al. 2009). Such behavior can also further contribute to the stigma they receive from community members. Social implications for increased stigma are embedded in the structural nature of in-group community settings, contributing to cyclic forms of stigma. Such perceived stigma contributes to risky behaviors that interact with other disease and behavioral factors leading in turn to more stigmatization, as seen in Paco's account below.

PACO'S STORY

Paco, a Puerto Rican-born citizen, was diagnosed with HIV shortly after arriving in Boston. His peppery black hair and square framed glasses mask the face of someone who suffered through years of drug use, depression, and self-isolation. While Paco's case to some extent aligns with current literature (Shoptaw and Reback 2007; Pappas and Halkitis 2011; Gideonse 2013), the details of his lived experience with HIV were also unique, as with many of participants—illustrating the value of ethnographic research on syndemics. Paco's emergence into the drug world began, according to him, as a result of internalized stigma he felt from being HIV-positive. During the interview he noted that when living with HIV, people go through different stages, or ways of being comfortable with one's self. Despite living with HIV for 20 years, Paco still considers himself in a time of transition. He says, "I think I am still going through a lot of stuff . . . I think I have some time still till I get to a more comfortable place. That's what I am feeling." Paco is referring to a comfortable place he hopes to reach with both his post-HIV-positive [diagnosis] life, and his sexual activity.

He discusses, "for some reason I thought I'm not, I can't [be sexually active] because I have HIV, you know, so I went and did meth" implying that his substance use is what allowed him to engage in sexual activity without thinking about the risks he posed to his partners. Paco maintained his substance use, in particular meth in sexual encounters, because, as he notes, he "wanted to feel":

> I didn't care about anything. I just wanted to feel. And I thought that, you know, by doing that, by taking meth and having sexual partners it was a coping mechanism because I wasn't thinking about anything else. It was just blocked. There was just one purpose. So, I didn't have to think about anything else . . . honestly, you do hear people when they say, "Oh my god, you're so beautiful." Or you're so this and you're so that, when you're doing that stuff and that stood out to me. Believe it or not, I remember and even when you are under the influence, you hear those words. They are very clear. It's very strange but that was the easiest way for me. That was the easiest way. (*Paco*)

Paco's drug use was a means of dealing with his HIV status. He knowingly engaged in sexual behavior that was risky because he was not always using condoms. His loneliness and avoidance of emotional attachment reinforced his risk-taking habits as well as the superficial social affirmation he perceived while under the influence of methamphetamine. This confirms Courtenay-Quirk et al.'s finding that, "[s]ettings that facilitate anonymous sex may be used by some men to protect themselves from emotional involvement with sex partners and expectations to share personal information such as HIV status" (2006, 65).

SEXUAL RISK-TAKING AND SUBSTANCE USE

For MSM, such increased substance use—frequently near the time of HIV (or other STI) diagnosis as an apparent coping mechanism—is associated with increased sexual risk behaviors (Campsmith, Nakashima, and Jones 2000; Parsons et al. 2003; Pathela et al. 2015). Semple, Patterson, and Grant (2002, 149) noted motivations for methamphetamine use associated with high-risk behavior including "sexual enhancement; and self-medication of negative affect associated with HIV-positive serostatus" among MSM. The use of so-called party drugs such as methamphetamine, nitrate inhalants (poppers), ketamine, and gamma-hydroxybutyrate correlates with greater sexual risk behaviors among HIV-positive men and their unknown serostatus partners (Purcell et al. 2005, S37). Campsmith, Nakashima, and Jones (2000) explored the use of crack cocaine among HIV-infected populations, noting that its use correlated with having multiple partners, transactional sex (trading sex for money), and more unprotected sex. The use of methamphetamine and other injectable substances, especially in the context of risky sex (Green and Halkitis 2006; Molitor et al. 1998; Semple et al. 2012; Wohl, Frye, and Johnson 2008; Halkitis et al. 2009), contributes to known syndemic interactions between HIV and other STIs—especially in relation to biological and social vulnerabilities (Ostrach and Singer 2012). Thus, drug use can contribute to or exacerbate biological factors that put individuals at risk for known HIV/STI syndemics, while simultaneously contributing to the stigma that affected individuals perceive (Singer 2007).

These cycles further contribute to social stigma from both outside and within MSM and HIV-positive communities. Despite the inescapability of larger structural risk factors that reinforce and exacerbate stigma, many HIV-positive individuals come to be "blamed" for their own suffering. In the following sections I further delineate specific interactions between perceived stigma from substance use within group settings and its effects with HIV medication adherence are explored.

"OH, THAT GROUP"

Jeff, an outspoken member of the center, talked about the perceived stigma associated with substance use within the community. He explains that meetings where members discuss sobriety and recovery can create unnecessary tensions, especially for people who make assumptions about the center's services.

> [A]s soon as a person reaches a certain level of whatever it be sobriety, recovery, and end homelessness, they become very judgmental about everybody who

> had not reached that level . . . I have heard people say that the morning group, when I was interviewing for the [Member Advisory Committee.] MAC here, they said:
>
> "Why do you think you'd be a good member for the[Committee] MAC?"
>
> I said, "Well, I attend Connections [a morning support group at FAB][4] every day and I think I have a good pulse of what the people in the FAB are feeling."
>
> A board member commented, "Oh, *that group*, I thought that was just for homeless drug addicts . . ." (*Jeff*)

Jeff's application to the Member Advisory Committee[5] (MAC) was stereotyped because of his association with the "morning group," which he said welcomes "homeless drug addicts" but is for everyone in the community. This iteration of stigma creates a dichotomy between FAB members who are seen as "users" and those who are not. The board member's comment about sobriety reflected certain members' attitudes about being associated with former or recovering drug users, "that group" of people. Though substance use is used as a coping mechanism for an HIV diagnosis, in many contexts, especially within FAB, it also denotes a lack of achieving a "disciplined body" in the Foucauldian sense and is therefore stigmatized within the community (Bourgois and Schonberg 2009).

In-Group HIV Stigma and Medication Adherence

As Paco's story indicates, HIV stigma can exacerbate an individual's sense of loneliness and marginalization, adding to the feeling that one needs to hide his diagnosis from family and partners or cope with it by using substances or engaging in higher-risk sexual behavior. From the interviews and participant-observation data this also appears to increase risks of depression for some. Together, these challenges can compromise an HIV-positive person's ability or willingness to adhere to anti-retroviral medication regimen to manage their HIV.

Reduced antiretroviral medication adherence is associated with HIV-related stigma (Rao et al. 2007; Rintamaki et al. 2006; Vanable et al. 2006). Such HIV-related stigma may mediate the relationship between syndemic and viral load (Friedman et al. 2015). According to Adolescent Trials Network research, depression and stigma are predictors of high-risk behavior and lack of medication adherence among youth living with HIV (Tanney et al. 2012). Perceived social stigma can affect medication adherence, contributing to feelings of marginalization, loneliness, and depression (Waite et al. 2008; Ware, Wyatt, and Tugenberg 2006; Gonzalez et al. 2004)—especially for MSM who chose to conceal their HIV status. Among HIV-positive individuals, those with high concerns about social stigma were more likely to be non-adherent to medication (Rintamaki et al. 2006)—this stigma, in turn, can affect one's behavior in other ways. For example, those who are depressed or marginalized may also be less likely to participate in community activities and receive services. Individuals with concerns about HIV stigma may be less inclined to disclose their status to sexual partners, a point of contention within HIV-positive group settings, and arguably a risk factor for HIV/STI syndemics. Despite all the reasons someone might struggle to take their medication on schedule or correctly—depression, stigma fear of disclosure, or side effects—being seen as non-adherent with HIV medication can also become a source of stigma within HIV communities like FAB.

Vinny describes a situation with an African-American friend with Kaposi's sarcoma that denotes many of the attitudes and behaviors members display in regards to medication adherence. After his friend had died of AIDS, Vinny was cleaning his apartment and found bottles of anti-retroviral medication that had been never opened.

> I was so angry after he passed away—at myself. I knew what Kaposi's sarcoma looked like on my skin tone, but I didn't know what it looked like on a Black person's skin [tone]. So, I felt horribly guilty for the longest times, like I could have did something.
>
> And then, I went through this whole anger period with him with the AIDS thing. Where [it's] like how can you not take one pill? I know, I know the psychological part of it. How? I used to have to take over 40 pills [a day]. How can you not take one?! How can you forget to take a pill? In this day in age we have so many ways to remind you. I get crazy about this! I went through such an anger period after he died. He didn't want to live, ya know? He didn't want to live. (*Vinny*)

Vinny's own inability to recognize his friend's tell-tale signs of Kaposi's sarcoma angers him, likely in a form of survivor's guilt. Additionally, being a long-term survivor, Vinny internalized managing his HIV 'well,' he prioritizes medication regimens and does not sympathize with people who do not take their medication. Going from taking 40 pills per day back in the early 90's to just one today is astronomical for him. As he mentions, "How can you not take one [pill]?" In the end, he concludes that his long-time friend died because he had given up and did not "want to live." Vinny considers his friend apathetic and careless, demonstrating a change in generational attitudes about HIV/AIDS and bodily expectations. Battling HIV/AIDS in the 80's meant multiple pill regimens and faulty medications, but more recently, the availability of multi-drug cocktails (in the United States) perpetrates biomedical moralities that make living with HIV seem "as easy as" taking a pill a day to those who can successfully do so.

Vinny asks, rhetorically, "How could you not take one pill?" This was a sentiment shared among many members at FAB. Jeff jokingly displays a common elitism about viral suppression saying, "so that's my HIV story it is so much like many of peoples, y'know? And actually I'm undetectable . . . At Mass General, we are more precise, you've become "non-detectable," but I don't share that with other people cuz I don't want to make it a status thing."

Jeff mockingly states that he's "non-detectable"—even said in jest this reaffirms a biomedical hierarchy and moral expectation. Saying, "I don't want to make it a status thing," he acknowledges a zero viral load has become a sign of status within HIV communities, hinting at the stigma that underpins the proposed syndemic. His statement demonstrates powerfully that biomedical moral 'statuses' exist within the FAB community, though Jeff claims he does not want to engage in them.

Often members discussed their viral loads and CD4+ cell counts as a way of claiming their health and well-being. Such affirmations implied the ways that biomedical moralities work within the community; being responsible implies taking one's medicine—adhering to biomedical standards—and working to rehabilitate one's self. As one staff member said, "Ya, everyone here will tell you they are 'undetectable'. . ."—everyone at FAB wants to be a "good" HIV-positive member. Such justifications are a way to avoid in-group stigma, a way to avoid being an "irresponsible," and thus "immoral," HIV patient.

BIOMEDICAL MORALITIES: REINFORCING SYNDEMIC INTERACTIONS

One particular interview illustrated how in-group stigma can drive interactions between HIV, substance use, risky sexual behavior, other STIs, and medication adherence. "Trouble,"[6] a particularly active member of FAB, showcased the hierarchies that persist in the community. Trouble stands about five foot seven inches tall, and often wears a baseball cap to cover his brown buzzcut, which was usually accompanied by a hunter green fur-lined jacket and worn jeans. He is as lean as an Olympic distance runner, and smokes a pack of cigarettes a day—a habit he picked up as a truck driver. Trouble and I had a great rapport. I inquired about HIV status within the community:

> A [author]: Do you agree or disagree that how you received your HIV status affects how you're seen at FAB?
>
> Trouble: I say, yes, because I got it from having sex with another guy. That's about it.

A: So like, if someone got it from using drugs do you think that's different? Or it's still the same?

T: Well, I'm undetectable.

A: Ya . . .

T: I think it's totally different from having sex and doing needles.

A: You think so? How so?

T: Cuz most of them still have it [a drug addiction] when they come in here. Ya know, people like me and "Joe." Well—Joe's neutered anyways. He hasn't had sex in years but he still has the virus, which will never go away. He doesn't have sex anymore. He doesn't do drugs. You know what, everybody has their own opinion, and their own stats on how they got it. [I have] HIV my way and that's it.

Trouble's remarks further demonstrate the ways that 'biomedical moralities' can be mapped onto the psyches of community members. Trouble asserts that many members of the community come in with addiction issues, which he says are "*totally different*" from having sex. He also states that he is "*undetectable*," implying he is fully compliant with his medication. Trouble meanwhile suggests his friend "Joe" demonstrates an alternate embodiment of biomedical moralities by abstaining from drug use and not having sexual intercourse. By this reading, Joe reincorporated a self that is contained and not "unruly," but one that causes Trouble to refer to him as "neutered"—no longer having sex. Trouble recognizes that Joe still has the virus, but recognizes he is trying in multiple ways to safeguard others from it. In this instance, both Trouble and Joe are group members demonstrating "good" ways to live with HIV/AIDS—complying with biomedical moralities. Others, who use substances or have risky sex, encompass "bad" ways of living with HIV, because they fail to reincorporate contained selves and adhere to moral, biomedical standards.

In FAB's case, syndemics theory helped to identify and address the larger structural factors that perpetuate and reinforce biomedical moralities, enacted through stigma, that influence pathways of bio-behavioral interaction and damage health. As many HIV-positive community members re-create and reincorporate new versions of "moral" biomedical selves, being adherent to medication, practicing "safe" sexual habits, and abstaining from substance use all become "good" ways of living with HIV and avoiding stigma from within the community. The embodiment of biomedical standards thus creates, contributes to, and perpetuates existing hierarchies that exacerbate within-group stigma for those who fail to embody "good" HIV-positive standards.

Much has been written about individual and unidirectional social and biological relationships between high-risk or 'casual' sex, substance use (especially methamphetamine), and HIV status among MSM. The bulk of this research focuses on how HIV-positive MSM manage perceived HIV stigma or homophobia from the dominant heterosexual culture around them. Yet, the existing literature does not adequately address dimensions of stigma as it affects MSM who similarly encounter HIV stigma *within* the MSM community. The community of peers can be where HIV-positive MSM seek affirming, socially protective connections and *relief* from external stigma. When or if HIV-positive MSM then encounter similarly stigmatizing and potentially syndemic-producing dynamics within a community where they expect support, the enforcement of biomedical moralities can be especially damaging to health. Building on existing research and enriched by the data I was able to gather, the in-group HIV-positive MSM syndemic presented consists of precisely these structural-biological-behavioral dynamics among HIV-positive MSM who perpetuate stigma affecting their own community.

These interactions are dynamic and fluid, existing in certain contexts, not necessarily uniformly throughout the community or equally for all members of an affected group. The syndemic model should be taken into account in certain social contexts and in light of variations within social groups and among individuals, which may not exist outside of the nexus of other structural or social conditions.

LIMITATIONS

This qualitative study was limited to a particular long-standing microcosm of Boston's HIV community (FAB), so its applicability may not be widespread. However, some existing literature supports the participants' attitudes and perceptions about HIV stigma (Haile, Padilla, and Parker 2011; Frey et al. 2000). Many of participants were older men (>50 years) and had been living with HIV for over 10 years, which may have skewed their perceptions of stigma. Certainly, added perspectives from younger voices are needed, but were not readily available during the period of data collection. It is also important to note that participants who felt most stigmatized may not have talked to me due to my status as a researcher, my affiliations with long-time members, or assumptions made about me based on his position as a younger, white male.

CONCLUSION AND RECOMMENDATIONS

Recognizing, examining, and documenting the role of stigma in HIV treatment and care is increasingly important not only for HIV-positive individuals' day-to-day lives but also for promoting supportive environments within HIV communities. As Earnshaw et al. (2013, 10) explain, "[d]ifferentiating between HIV stigma mechanisms within research may have especially significant implications for interventions to improve health and well-being among [people living with HIV] (PLWH)." Understanding the nuances of stigma and its impact on health can help advocates and policymakers plan interventions to improve outcomes. HIV stigma can create a negative feedback loop from both outside of, and within, HIV-positive communities to further isolate certain populations, adversely affect their health, interfere with the effectiveness of ART, and increase HIV and STI transmissibility. In HIV community settings where shared knowledge of diagnosis and status may contribute to stigma, HIV stigma campaigns should be designed to combat stigma both within and outside of HIV-positive community organizations.

Many existing anti-stigma campaigns target HIV-positive audiences in terms of addressing one's HIV status when dating, using appropriate language, and heightening education about HIV to the general public. However, addressing the various overlapping and intersecting stigmas that may come to be associated with aspects of being HIV-positive, such as being stigmatized for being a gay African-American man, or being an HIV-positive substance user, need to be further addressed from the structural perspective, not just in individual terms. Bowleg's (2008) work on intersectionality states "social identities and inequality are interdependent for [certain] groups" (312). Thus, stigmatization also comes layered with the social, political, and economic inequalities many HIV-positive individuals' face, which may not be mutually exclusive from aspects of their HIV-positive or MSM identities (Singer and Clair 2003). Many of the accounts presented stemmed from the social structure of the community center and how new members felt less integrated into community dynamics.

Overcoming these divides within HIV communities will be a key factor in combating HIV stigma to improve public health and quality of life. A truly intersectional prevention and treatment effort will require confronting structural, biological, behavioral, and biosocial factors, and the damaging health interactions between these. Multiple, inextricable social stigmas affect HIV-positive MSM, each of which can affect their biological and behavioral risk factors.

Working with HIV communities and their members to address and reduce each type of stigma is long overdue, and thankfully underway. But there is more to be done. Boston area HIV community centers, such as FAB, do work to combat stigma by: addressing and navigating romantic relationship communication and status disclosure for HIV-positive MSM, providing community groups to voice concerns and address issues, and creating stigma awareness blogs, Tumblr pages, and other social media websites. However, as a result of in-group HIV stigma syndemics that produce biological and behavioral interactions the effects of in-group HIV stigma can still be detrimental to the health of HIV-positive MSM and reinforce unrealistic expectations about how people should be able to 'manage' their HIV despite structural factors.

FAB's anti-stigma campaign that predated this research did address multiple aspects of stigma, but was not able to address the social and health intersections of stigma highlighted in this chapter. Although FAB created a member-centered anti-stigma campaign that addressed ways to identify and talk about perceived stigma, community members who participated in the study did not speak about stigma, explicitly. For community members, reporting stigma would imply that there was an internal problem with their community—the place they go for support. Instead, they talked about other problems, other symptoms of stigma—discrimination, othering, cliques, "better" and "worse" ways of being HIV-positive, "that group," who uses substances, and those who don't take their medications—revealing much deeper consequences of stigma.

Though FAB staff recognized and challenged the stigmas attached to marginalized communities (e.g., drug use) their attempts to challenge such notions were limited because of the biomedical values internalized and embodied by members. Additionally, while many members recognized the divide in the community, they did not elaborate on what caused such divides, or that it may be a product of stigma. The author recommends that staff and members at HIV-positive community members identify ways to identify and address *how* stigma manifests in their particular settings, to become a product of and vehicle for community values. Figuring out what the "A group" and "B group" are in a given setting could be helpful in determining how best to support each group and narrow gaps in how people are treated.

Taking a ground-up approach in defining and recognizing stigma, may be an essential part to addressing the "multiplicity of stigma." Because stigma may mean different things to different people, addressing its fluidity and how it is enacted and embodied, can help members conceptualize what defines stigma and how it manifests. Creating truly intersectional, biosocially effective campaigns to "end HIV stigma" from outside as well as inside the community will be highly beneficial within and among HIV-positive MSM and others impacted by HIV. Doing so would help address the dominant discourse around HIV management and care that produces biomedical moralities. Forums where HIV-positive members discuss the stigmas that manifest with medical providers can be a step in addressing these biomedical moralities and how they shape HIV management and health consequences.

Mendenhall echoes Good (1994), saying "just as syndromes are situated within cultural and historical contexts, so too biomedical constructions of disease are culturally and historically contingent" (2012, 22). The narratives presented come from cultural perspectives of a Boston-specific HIV community. They recount the stigma and biomedical morality present in Massachusetts, which may be exacerbated due to relatively widespread access to health care and social services. These individuals were "lucky" enough to be able to comply with medical regimens, gain a physical space to connect with similar individuals, and be referred to health-related services like needle exchanges and housing authorities. Many HIV-positive individuals—abroad and in the United States—cannot access these resources. Though specific structural factors reinforce stigma within these communities, there is still more work to be done beyond simply reducing stigma. Creating a dialogue where HIV can be talked about and treated, without enforcing biomedically hegemonic standards of conduct may be a good start. Anthropological research may not be able to remove the stigma that substance users, gay men, or HIV-positive individuals face, but it can highlight the factors that reinforce such stigma—driving HIV syndemics—and give voice to individuals and communities suffering from such inequalities.[7]

NOTES

1. To protect their privacy, the names of all people and organizations have been replaced with pseudonyms.
2. In addition to extensive literature review and analysis of extant publications from anthropology, biomedical, and social science databases on each aspect of the syndemic I propose.
3. The author collected original data to inform this chapter, including semi-structured interviews ($n = 12$) and participant-observation carried out as a volunteer intern in the site over the course of an academic year. He recruited participants—members who frequented the center—using a combination of opportunistic and convenience sampling, and conducted interviews using grounded theory techniques. Grounded theory allowed for "open-ended yet directed, shaped yet emergent, and paced yet unrestricted" interviews and help further inform my literature analysis with my participants' voices (Charmaz 2014, 85). He used a combination of discourse and narrative analysis to code the data. To supplement qualitative data from interviews, I also collected basic demographic surveys. To contextualize and triangulate data (Creswell 2013), I also collected basic demographic surveys from a larger set of community members ($n = 30$). In distributing the short anonymous surveys, I sought to better define the demographics of the sample population, including age, education, time since diagnosis, sexual orientation, drug use, and other health conditions. Though findings from the surveys are not specifically reported in this chapter, they informed the data and the development of the syndemic model in important ways. Surveys enhanced the overall findings as well as helping to identify and expand on themes that emerged in

relation to current syndemics literature. Participant-observation was a significant part of data collection, as it allowed me to develop rapport with prospective participants, and further refine the direction of the project to focus on community members' experiences with stigma. The author suspects that he achieved "successful" participant-observation in part through the liminality of his position—many members assumed he was a member or client advocate. All aspects of the study received institutional review board approval from the Boston University School of Medicine in early 2015.

4. Connections is a daily peer support open to all members, rooted in Harm Reduction concepts and holistic approaches. The group addresses stressful things that affect ability to live healthily with HIV/AIDS, including: housing, substance use, and emotional health, isolation and medication side effects. A different topic is discussed each day.

5. The MAC is a group of members who meet regularly to discuss concerns about what's going on at FAB, make recommendations to the staff on policies, and plan social events.

6. A pseudonym he chose.

7. Infinite thanks to Drs. Shir Lerman, Bayla Ostrach, and Merrill Singer for sharing their brilliance, wisdom, and guidance throughout this process. I am also indebted to the Medical Anthropology and Cross-Cultural Pracice program (Boston University School of Medicine), especially my cohort, for their research support and expertise in all writing matters. This chapter would not have been possible without all of you.

REFERENCES

Bourdieu, Pierre. "The Force of Law: Toward a Sociology of the Juridical Field." *Hastings LJ* 38 (1986): 805.

Bourdieu, Pierre, and Loïc JD Wacquant. *An Invitation to Reflexive Sociology*. University of Chicago Press, 1992.

Bourgois, Philippe I., and Jeffrey Schonberg. *Righteous Dopefiend*. University of California Press, 2009.

Bowleg, Lisa. "When Black+ Lesbian+ Woman ≠ Black Lesbian Woman: The Methodological Challenges of Qualitative and Quantitative Intersectionality Research." *Sex Roles* 59, nos. 5–6 (2008): 312–325.

———. "The Problem with the Phrase Women and Minorities: Intersectionality—an Important Theoretical Framework for Public Health." *American Journal of Public Health* 102, no. 7 (2012): 1267–1273.

Brouard, Pierre, and Caroline Wills. "A Closer Look: The Internalization of Stigma Related to HIV." 2006. http://www.popline.org/node/170983.

Campsmith, Michael L., Allyn K. Nakashima, and Jeffrey L. Jones. "Association between Crack Cocaine Use and High-Risk Sexual Behaviors After HIV Diagnosis." *JAIDS Journal of Acquired Immune Deficiency Syndromes* 25, no. 2 (2000): 192–198.

Charmaz, Kathy. *Constructing Grounded Theory*. Sage, 2014.

Courtenay-Quirk, Cari, Richard J. Wolitski, Jeffrey T. Parsons, Cynthia A. Gomez, and others. "Is HIV/AIDS Stigma Dividing the Gay Community? Perceptions of HIV-Positive Men Who Have Sex with Men." *AIDS Education and Prevention* 18, no. 1 (2006): 56.

Crenshaw, K. W. "The Structural and Political Dimensions of Intersectional Oppression." *Intersectionality: A Foundations and Frontiers Reader* (2014): 17–22.

Crenshaw, Kimberle. "Mapping the Margins: Intersectionality, Identity Politics, and Violence against Women of Color." *Stanford Law Review* (1991): 1241–1299.

Crepaz, Nicole, and Gary Marks. "Towards an Understanding of Sexual Risk Behavior in People Living with HIV: A Review of Social, Psychological, and Medical Findings." *Aids* 16, no. 2 (2002): 135–149.

Crepaz, Nicole, Gary Marks, Adrian Liau, Mary M. Mullins, Latrina W. Aupont, Khiya J. Marshall, Elizabeth D. Jacobs, Richard J. Wolitski, HIV/AIDS Prevention Research Synthesis (PRS) Team, et al. "Prevalence of Unprotected Anal Intercourse among HIV-Diagnosed MSM in the United States: A Meta-Analysis." *Aids* 23, no. 13 (2009): 1617–1629.

Creswell, John W. *Qualitative Inquiry and Research Design: Choosing Among Five Approaches*. Los Angeles, 2013.

Dougan, Sarah, Barry G. Evans, and Jonathan Elford. "Sexually Transmitted Infections in Western Europe among HIV-Positive Men Who Have Sex with Men." *Sexually Transmitted Diseases* 34, no. 10 (2007): 783–790.

Drabkin, Anya S., Kathleen J. Sikkema, Patrick A. Wilson, Christina S. Meade, Nathan B. Hansen, Allyson DeLorenzo, Arlene Kochman, et al. "Risk Patterns Preceding Diagnosis among Newly HIV-Diagnosed Men Who Have Sex with Men in New York City." *AIDS Patient Care and STDs* 27, no. 6 (2013): 333–341.

Drumright, Lydia N., Steffanie A. Strathdee, Susan J. Little, Maria Rosario G. Araneta, Donald J. Slymen, Vanessa L. Malcarne, Eric S. Daar, and Pamina M. Gorbach. "Unprotected Anal Intercourse and Substance Use Before and After HIV Diagnosis Among Recently HIV-Infected Men Who Have Sex with Men." *Sexually Transmitted Diseases* 34, no. 6 (2007): 401–407.

Dyer, Typhanye Penniman, Steve Shoptaw, Thomas E. Guadamuz, Michael Plankey, Uyen Kao, David Ostrow, Joan S. Chmiel, Amy Herrick, and Ron Stall. "Application of Syndemic Theory to Black Men Who Have Sex with Men in the Multicenter AIDS Cohort Study." *Journal of Urban Health* 89, no. 4 (2012): 697–708.

Earnshaw, Valerie A., Laramie R. Smith, Stephenie R. Chaudoir, K. Rivet Amico, and Michael M. Copenhaver. "HIV Stigma Mechanisms and Well-Being among PLWH: A Test of the HIV Stigma Framework." *AIDS and Behavior* 17, no. 5 (2013): 1785–1795.

Frey, Lawrence R., Mara B. Adelman, Lyle J. Flint, and Jim L. Query. "Weaving Meanings Together in an AIDS Residence: Communicative Practices, Perceived Health Outcomes, and the Symbolic Construction of Community." *Journal of Health Communication* 5, no. 1 (2000): 53–72.

Friedman, M. Reuel, Ron Stall, Anthony J. Silvestre, Chongyi Wei, Steve Shoptaw, Amy Herrick, Pamela J. Surkan, Linda Teplin, and Michael W. Plankey. "Effects of Syndemics on HIV Viral Load and Medication Adherence in the Multicentre AIDS Cohort Study." *AIDS* 29, no. 9 (2015): 1087–1096.

Gideonse, Theodore Karwoski. "Risky Subjectivity: The Effects of Cultural Discourses of Addiction on Methamphetamine Using HIV+ Men Who Have Sex with Men in San Diego." 2013. http://escholarship.org/uc/item/0x61w1jt.pdf.

Goffman, Erving. *Stigma: Notes on the Management of Spoiled Identity*. Englewood Cliffs, NJ, 1963.

Gonzalez, Jeffrey S., Frank J. Penedo, Michael H. Antoni, Ron E. Durán, Shvawn McPherson-Baker, Gail Ironson, Maria Isabel Fernandez, Nancy G. Klimas, Mary Ann Fletcher, and Neil Schneiderman. "Social Support, Positive States of Mind, and HIV Treatment Adherence in Men and Women Living with HIV/AIDS." *Health Psychology* 23, no. 4 (2004): 413.

Good, Byron J. *Medicine, Rationality and Experience: An Anthropological Perspective*. Cambridge University Press, 1994.

Gray, Alison J. "Stigma in Psychiatry." *Journal of the Royal Society of Medicine* 95, no. 2 (2002): 72–76.

Haile, Rahwa, Mark B. Padilla, and Edith A. Parker. "'Stuck in the Quagmire of an HIV Ghetto': The Meaning of Stigma in the Lives of Older Black Gay and Bisexual Men Living with HIV in New York City." *Culture, Health & Sexuality* 13, no. 4 (2011): 429–442.

Halkitis, Perry N., Sandra A. Kupprat, Melvin B. Hampton, Rafael Perez-Figueroa, Molly Kingdon, Jessica A. Eddy, and Danielle C. Ompad. "Evidence for a Syndemic in Aging Hiv-Positive Gay, Bisexual, and Other MSM: Implications for a Holistic Approach to Prevention and Health Care." *Annals of Anthropological Practice* 36, no. 2 (2012): 365–386.

Halkitis, Perry N., Todd M. Solomon, Robert W. Moeller, Stephanie AR Doig, Lindsay S. Espinosa, Daniel Siconolfi, and Bruce D. Homer. "Methamphetamine Use among Gay, Bisexual and Non-Identified Men-Who-Have-Sex-with-Men An Analysis of Daily Patterns." *Journal of Health Psychology* 14, no. 2 (2009): 222–231.

Hubach, Randolph D., Brian Dodge, Michael J. Li, Vanessa Schick, Debby Herbenick, William D. Ramos, Thea Cola, and Michael Reece. "Loneliness, HIV-Related Stigma, and Condom Use among a Predominantly Rural Sample of HIV-Positive Men Who Have Sex with Men (MSM)." *AIDS Education and Prevention* 27, no. 1 (2015): 72.

Isaiah Green, Adam, and Perry N. Halkitis. "Crystal Methamphetamine and Sexual Sociality in an Urban Gay Subculture: An Elective Affinity." *Culture, Health & Sexuality* 8, no. 4 (2006): 317–333.

Jeffries, William L., Ebony Symone Townsend, Deborah J. Gelaude, Elizabeth A. Torrone, Mari Gasiorowicz, and Jeanne Bertolli. "HIV Stigma Experienced by Young Men Who Have Sex with Men (MSM) Living with HIV Infection." *AIDS Education and Prevention* 27, no. 1 (2015): 58.

Lee, Rachel S., Arlene Kochman, and Kathleen J. Sikkema. "Internalized Stigma among People Living with HIV-AIDS." *AIDS and Behavior* 6, no. 4 (2002): 309–319.

Lekas, Helen-Maria, Karolynn Siegel, and Jason Leider. 2011. "Felt and Enacted Stigma among HIV/HCV-Coinfected Adults the Impact of Stigma Layering." *Qualitative Health Research* 21, no. 9 (2011): 1205–1219.

Lyons, Thomas, Amy K. Johnson, and Robert Garofalo. "'What Could Have Been Different': A Qualitative Study of Syndemic Theory and HIV Prevention Among Young Men Who Have Sex With Men." *Journal of HIV/AIDS & Social Services* 12, nos. 3–4 (2013): 368–383.

Mao, L., J. B. Wit, S. C. Kippax, G. Prestage, and M. Holt. "Younger Age, Recent HIV Diagnosis, No Welfare Support and No Annual Sexually Transmissible Infection Screening Are Associated with Nonuse of Antiretroviral Therapy among HIV-Positive Gay Men in Australia." *HIV Medicine* 16, no. 1 (2015): 32–37.

Mendenhall, Emily. 2012. *Syndemic Suffering: Social Distress, Depression, and Diabetes among Mexican Immigrant Women*. Vol. 4. Walnut Creek, CA: Left Coast Press.

Molitor, Fred, Steven R. Truax, Juan D. Ruiz, and Richard K. Sun. "Association of Methamphetamine Use During Sex with Risky Sexual Behaviors and HIV Infection Among Non-Injection Drug Users." *Western Journal of Medicine* 168, no. 2 (1998): 93.

Morano, Jamie P., Britton A. Gibson, and Frederick L. Altice. "The Burgeoning HIV/HCV Syndemic in the Urban Northeast: HCV, HIV, and HIV/HCV Coinfection in an Urban Setting." *PLoS ONE* 8, no. 5 (2013): e64321.

O'Leary, Dale. "The Syndemic of AIDS and STDS Among MSM." *The Linacre Quarterly* 81, no. 1 (2014): 12–37.

Ostrach, Bayla, and Merrill Singer. "At Special Risk: Biopolitical Vulnerability and HIV/STI Syndemics Among Women." *Health Sociology Review* 21, no. 3 (2012): 258–271.

Padilla, MARK B. "The Limits of 'Heterosexual AIDS': Ethnographic Research on Tourism and Male Sexual Labor in the Dominican Republic." *Anthropology and Public Health: Bridging Differences in Culture and Society* (2009): 142–164.

Pappas, Molly K., and Perry N. Halkitis. "Sexual Risk Taking and Club Drug Use across Three Age Cohorts of HIV-Positive Gay and Bisexual Men in New York City." *AIDS Care* 23, no. 11 (2011): 1410–1416.

Parker, Richard, and Peter Aggleton. "HIV and AIDS-Related Stigma and Discrimination: A Conceptual Framework and Implications for Action." *Social Science & Medicine* 57, no. 1 (2003): 13–24.

Parsons, Jeffrey T., Perry N. Halkitis, Richard J. Wolitski, and Cynthia A. Gómez. 2003. "Correlates of Sexual Risk Behaviors among HIV-Positive Men Who Have Sex with Men." *AIDS Education and Prevention* 15, no. 5 (2003): 383.

Pathela, Preeti, Sarah L. Braunstein, Susan Blank, Colin Shepard, and Julia A. Schillinger. "The High Risk of an HIV Diagnosis Following a Diagnosis of Syphilis: A Population-Level Analysis of New York City Men." *Clinical Infectious Diseases* 61, no. 2 (2015): 281–287.

Patterson, Thomas L., Shirley J. Semple, James K. Zians, and Steffanie A. Strathdee. "Methamphetamine-Using HIV-Positive Men Who Have Sex with Men: Correlates of Polydrug Use." *Journal of Urban Health* 82, no. 1 (2005): i120–i126.

Purcell, David W., Susan Moss, Robert H. Remien, William J. Woods, and Jeffrey T. Parsons. "Illicit Substance Use, Sexual Risk, and HIV-Positive Gay and Bisexual Men: Differences by Serostatus of Casual Partners." *Aids* 19 (2005): S37–S47.

Rao, D., T. C. Kekwaletswe, S. Hosek, J. Martinez, and F. Rodriguez. "Stigma and Social Barriers to Medication Adherence with Urban Youth Living with HIV." *AIDS Care* 19 no. 1 (2007): 28–33.

Rintamaki, Lance S., Terry C. Davis, Silvia Skripkauskas, Charles L. Bennett, and Michael S. Wolf. "Social Stigma Concerns and HIV Medication Adherence." *AIDS Patient Care & STDs* 20 no. 5 (2006): 359–368.

Ritsher, Jennifer Boyd and Jo C. Phelan. "Internalized Stigma Predicts Erosion of Morale Among Psychiatric Outpatients." *Psychiatry Research* 129, no. 3 (2004): 257–265.

Scambler, Graham. "Health-Related Stigma." *Sociology of Health & Illness* 31, no. 3 (2009): 441–455.

Semple, Shirley J., Thomas L. Patterson, and Igor Grant. "Motivations Associated with Methamphetamine Use among HIV Men Who Have Sex with Men." *Journal of Substance Abuse Treatment* 22, no. 3 (2002): 149–156.

Semple, Shirley J., Steffanie A. Strathdee, Jim Zians, and Thomas L. Patterson. "Factors Associated with Experiences of Stigma in a Sample of HIV-Positive, Methamphetamine-Using Men Who Have Sex with Men." *Drug and Alcohol Dependence* 125, no. 1 (2012): 154–159.

Shilts, Randy. *And the Band Played On: Politics, People, and the AIDS Epidemic*. St. Martin's Press, 1987.

Shoptaw, Steven and Cathy J. Reback. "Methamphetamine Use and Infectious Disease-Related Behaviors in Men Who Have Sex with Men: Implications for Interventions." *Addiction* 102, no. s1 (2007): 130–135.

Singer, Merrill and Scott Clair. "Syndemics and Public Health: Reconceptualizing Disease in Bio-Social Context." *Medical Anthropology Quarterly* 17, no. 4 (2003): 423–441.

Singer, Merrill. "A Dose of Drugs, a Touch of Violence, a Case of AIDS, Part 2: Further Conceptualizing the SAVA Syndemic." *Free Inquiry in Creative Sociology* 34, no. 1 (2006): 39–54.

———. *Drugging the Poor: Legal and Illegal Drugs and Social Inequality*. Prospect Heights, IL: Waveland Press, 2007.

———. *Introduction to Syndemics: A Critical Systems Approach to Public and Community Health*. John Wiley & Sons, 2009.

Smith, Dawn K., Lauren Toledo, Donna Jo Smith, Mary Anne Adams, and Richard Rothenberg. "Attitudes and Program Preferences of African-American Urban Young Adults about Pre-Exposure Prophylaxis (PrEP)." *AIDS Education and Prevention* 24, no. 5 (2012): 408.

Stall, Ron, Mark Friedman, and Joseph A. Catania. "Interacting Epidemics and Gay Men's Health: A Theory of Syndemic Production among Urban Gay Men." *Unequal Opportunity: Health Disparities Affecting Gay and Bisexual Men in the United States* 1 (2008): 251–274.

Stall, Ron, Thomas C. Mills, John Williamson, Trevor Hart, Greg Greenwood, Jay Paul, Lance Pollack, Diane Binson, Dennis Osmond, and Joseph A. Catania. "Association of Co-Occurring Psychosocial Health Problems and Increased Vulnerability to HIV/AIDS among Urban Men Who Have Sex with Men." *American Journal of Public Health* 93, no. 6 (2003): 939–942.

Steward, Wayne T., Gregory M. Herek, Jayashree Ramakrishna, Shalini Bharat, Sara Chandy, Judith Wrubel, and Maria L. Ekstrand. "HIV-Related Stigma: Adapting a Theoretical Framework for Use in India." *Social Science & Medicine* 67, no. 8 (2008): 1225–1235.

Tanney, Mary R., Sylvie Naar-King, Karen MacDonnel, Adolescent Trials Network for HIV/AIDS Interventions 004 Protocol Team, et al. "Depression and Stigma in High-Risk Youth Living with HIV: A Multi-Site Study." *Journal of Pediatric Health Care* 26, no. 4 (2012): 300–305.

Van Der Straten, Ariane, K. A. Vernon, K. R. Knight, C. A. Gomez, and N. S. Padian. "Managing HIV among Serodiscordant Heterosexual Couples: Serostatus, Stigma and Sex." *Aids Care* 10, no. 5 (1998): 533–548.

Vanable, Peter A., Michael P. Carey, Donald C. Blair, and Rae A. Littlewood. "Impact of HIV-Related Stigma on Health Behaviors and Psychological Adjustment among HIV-Positive Men and Women." *AIDS and Behavior* 10, no. 5 (2006): 473–482.

Waite, Katherine R., Michael Paasche-Orlow, Lance S. Rintamaki, Terry C. Davis, and Michael S. Wolf. "Literacy, Social Stigma, and HIV Medication Adherence." *Journal of General Internal Medicine* 23, no. 9 (2008): 1367–1372.

Ware, Norma C., Monique A. Wyatt, and Toni Tugenberg. "Social Relationships, Stigma and Adherence to Antiretroviral Therapy for HIV/AIDS." *AIDS Care* 18, no. 8 (2006): 904–910.

Wohl, Amy Rock, Douglas M. Frye, and Denise F. Johnson. "Demographic Characteristics and Sexual Behaviors Associated with Methamphetamine Use among MSM and Non-MSM Diagnosed with AIDS in Los Angeles County." *AIDS and Behavior* 12, no. 5 (2008): 705–712.

Chapter Eight

Methamphetamine Addiction, HIV Infection, and Gay Men

Stigma and Suffering

Theodore K. Gideonse

Sam[1] smoked meth for the first time when he was 13, not long after being molested by a neighbor; he started turning tricks at 17, tested positive for HIV at 23, received an AIDS diagnosis at 30, and at 43 had been mostly homeless in San Diego for 25 years. Jorge left home in Guadalajara at 18 because of his parents' violent reaction to him coming out as gay; he tested positive and received an AIDS diagnosis in San Diego ten years later, started using meth at 42, and was in a halfway house at 47. Jonathan came out in his teens in Los Angeles and did meth for the first time at 25 and tested positive five years later; at 50 he was couch surfing in San Diego and living off checks from his aged father who did not know why Jonathan needed the money. Max's first long-term partner persuaded him to smoke meth during sex when Max was 33; Max left his partner when he discovered that his partner had graduated to injecting the drug. Max started living on streets, and when he tested positive for HIV and received an AIDS diagnosis, a case manager persuaded him to go into substance abuse treatment.

These stories were typical of the 14 men who participated in an ethnographic study of methamphetamine-using HIV-positive men who have sex with men in San Diego that I conducted from 2009 to 2012.[2] They each were subjects of person-centered ethnographies, sitting for five or more in-depth interviews regarding their life histories and illness trajectories, as seen in table 8.1.

They were all participants in what has been called a "double epidemic" for American gay men, the intertwining of infection with the human immunodeficiency virus (HIV), which causes acquired immunodeficiency syndrome (AIDS), and the abuse of the powerful synthetic stimulant methamphetamine (Halkitis, Parsons, and Stirratt 2001). It is a syndemic, "the concentration

Table 8.1. Participants in the Study with Demographic Descriptors

Name (Pseudonym)	*Place of Birth*	*Race/Ethnicity*	*Age at First Interview*	*Age Tested HIV+*	*Age of First Meth Use*	*Ever Homeless*	*Ever Incarcerated*
Adam	Michigan	White	31	31	22	Yes	Yes
Brandon	California	White	22	20	12	No	Yes
Charles	California	Native American	41	17	15	Yes	Yes
Darrell	California	African-American	36	34	17	No	No
Eric*	Tennessee	White	46	22	25	No	No
Glenn	California	White	42	31	34	No	No
Jonathan	California	White	50	30	25	No	No
Jorge	Jalisco, Mexico	Hispanic	47	28	42	Yes	No
Matthew	California	White	32	26	12	No	Yes
Max	The Philippines	Pacific Islander	38	37	34	Yes	Yes
Richard	California	Hispanic	49	34	42	No	Yes
Sam	California	White	43	23	13	Yes	Yes
Walter	California	African-American	49	36	49	No	Yes
William	California	African-American	43	23	17	Yes	Yes

* Eric sat for two one-hour interviews in 2010 and did not return. He died the next summer in an altercation with police.

Source: Compiled by the author.

and deleterious interaction of two or more diseases or other health conditions in a population, especially as a consequence of social inequity and the unjust exercise of power" (Singer 2009). Not only is there strong evidence that methamphetamine augments the replication of HIV by enhancing HIV infection in microphages (Liang et al. 2008), but with an increased libido and decreased inhibitions methamphetamine users are much more likely to practice sexual behaviors that increase the risk of HIV infection (Volkow et al. 2007). The emotional reaction to an HIV diagnosis has been described as one reason some men seek out the drug (Reback 1997; Semple, Patterson, and Grant 2002). HIV infection and meth abuse are often only the dominant problems in the syndemic, with other sexually transmitted diseases, depression, poverty, and violence also linked and interacting with meth addiction and health complications from HIV.

Central to this syndemic are multiple, competing, and interrelated stigmas targeting HIV/AIDS, meth addiction, homosexuality, mental illness, poverty, and homelessness. Individually, these diseases and problems are difficult to manage on a quotidian basis, and the interaction of the stigmas compounds these difficulties. The stigmas create internal shame and mandate external management, both of which are made more problematic by the psychological and cognitive difficulties that HIV and meth create. That said, the men who took part in this study managed all of these problems—because they had to. Some were more or less successful than others, but all had to do it at a historical moment when the HIV-positive gay meth addict had become a folk devil of a moral panic, a pariah in the gay community. Their stigma was more than the sum its parts; it was worse because of its combination.

In this chapter, I describe how the men I worked with entered into this syndemic and how they responded to their illnesses, stigmas, and struggles, focusing on three exemplary cases. First, I describe the stigmas of AIDS and of methamphetamine addiction, and how the combination of the two, with meth leading the way, produced something worse. Then, I explain the epidemiological and sociostructural associations between HIV and meth among gay men. Finally, I illustrate these interactions and their health consequences through the stories of Charles, Andrew, and Glenn, three men who have different experiences but whose struggles create archetypes of social suffering. This ethnographic description of the syndemic of HIV disease and stigmatized meth addiction among gay men exemplifies the profoundly painful interactions between psychosocial behaviors, neurobiological experiences, and psychoculturally embedded stigmas. Disentangling the syndemic's causes and their combined effects may be able to help us ease the pain it brings.

HIV/AIDS STIGMA

"In its fullest sense," Philip Setel wrote, "the paradox of AIDS is that this *new* disease is enmeshed in *historically shaped* social environments" (2000, 4). When AIDS appeared in the early 1980s, those who initially suffered from it belonged to already oppressed or stigmatized groups (Shilts 1987; Treichler 1999; Farmer 1992): gay men, long considered dangerous sexual deviants; injection drug users, the worst of the victim-perpetrators of the then-new Drug War; and people from Haiti, the "basket case" of the Western Hemisphere. A fourth group, hemophiliacs, were considered by many to be innocent victims; it was not a coincidence that the 1990 Ryan White Comprehensive AIDS Resources Emergency Act, which provides medical care for under- and uninsured people with HIV, is named after a "compelling and nonthreatening" teenaged hemophiliac (Keeler 2007, 616). While White and other seemingly innocent people with AIDS helped turn scorn into pity, the remaining fears of people with AIDS, of their bodily fluids, their breath, and their simple proximity made treating AIDS, raising money for research, and preventing new infections extremely difficult.

Because of the severe stigma in the early years of the epidemic, people with HIV or AIDS quickly determined how they would communicate, or *not* communicate, their status to others, focusing on what Goffman called "information control" (Goffman 1963). Green and Sobo explain that, in general, "Chronic illness requires strategic management to minimize the impact of illness on social interaction. Social risk, which everyone must manage, is compounded in the chronically ill by the stigmas associated with various chronic illnesses and the indeterminacy of their definition of self and of events" (2000, 71). Because many people with HIV/AIDS internalize the stigma, many of them put great energy in hiding their status and, if necessary, their symptoms. Then and now, they try to preserve normalcy for as long as possible by simply not telling anyone and by hiding any symptom or developing cover stories, like a diabetes or cancer diagnosis, to explain doctor or hospital visit (Sandstrom 1990; Adam and Sears 1996; Cowles and Rodgers 1997; Green and Sobo 2000). Others will carefully decide who can and will be trusted with the information, weighing the possibility of rejection or discrimination with the ethical duty to tell, particularly, a family member or partner (Siegel and Krauss 1991).

HIV can become a "master status," dwarfing all other identities and markers. For some, embracing the stigma—through advocacy, activism, or art—is a way of disrupting the stigma's power (Gould 2009; Chambers 2004). It is often, however, a source of shame, and not just because of the stigmatized routes of infection, like homosexual sex or drug use. Loss of memory, continence, looks, and other "personal competences, taken for granted by almost any adult, challenges the sense of control over one's life and even personal worth (Adam and Sears 1996, 36). Managing and hiding such symptoms become a major concern, and it can lead to isolation and depression, denial of possible support, and delaying treatment (Alonzo and Reynolds 1995).

In the mid-1990s, after years of massive public health campaigns, unprecedented activism by people with AIDS and their communities, and enormous support from the entertainment industry, incredibly effective anti-retroviral treatments arrived, lessening symptoms, likelihood of death, and for many, fear. But the stigma persists, even if its power has waned. The stigma surrounding HIV/AIDS is still an "impediment to public health" (Valdiserri 2002). Fear of HIV and AIDS makes people less likely to be tested for the disease, and fear that others will find out about the infection makes many HIV-positive people avoid seeing doctors for treatment. The stigma of HIV/AIDS makes even discussing it difficult many people, leading to behaviors that put them at risk for infection.

METH STIGMA

In *Methland*, Nick Reding described the impetus for using meth in terms of American culture and political economy. Not only was meth not a surprising drug for people to take, it was also a sensible reaction to American labor conditions—as a reaction to the American dream.

> until the early 1980s, meth was a highly acceptable drug in America, one of the reasons being that it helped . . ."the salt of the earth"—soldiers, truck drivers, slaughterhouse employees, farmers, auto and construction works, and day laborers—work harder, longer, and more efficiently. It's one thing for a drug to be associated with sloth, like heroin. But it's wholly another when a formerly legal and accepted narcotic exists in a one-to-one ratio with defining ideal of American culture. . . . [The] ability to make something in your basement that promised work, success, wealth, thinness, and happiness was not necessarily too good to be true. (Reding 2009, 54)

But as Reding details, it *was* too good to be true. Addiction and the criminal, medical, and social results of the spreading addiction led to a social suffering in especially rural America that compounded the economic conditions that Reding claims encouraged its use.

Meth became an "epidemic" in the late 1990s and early 2000s as its use spread from Hawaii and California's coastal cities, across the entire West Coast, and then into eastern gay enclaves and particularly into the rural Plains

States and the Midwest, from the Dakotas to Tennessee. Once sleepy communities were amazed by the increased crime, the swelling population of addicts, and the misery that followed. To many observers, meth was doing to white, rural Middle America what crack had done to some black inner cities in the 1980s, and the construction of the meth addict resembled that of the crack addict. "Skinny, crazed urban blacks" were simply replaced by "prematurely aged, toothless, pockmarked rural whites" in media reports and shared fears. "[By] 2005," Reding writes, "thousands of stories across the country blaming meth for delusional violence, moral depravity, extreme sexual perversion, and an almost otherworldly, hallucinogenic dimension of evil" (2009, 43).

The media, not surprisingly, focused greatly on the worst case scenarios of meth use, from the horrible burns caused by meth lab accidents to abandoned children of meth addicts. Famous public health campaigns focused on the infamous "meth mouth," in which meth addicts lose their teeth because of incessant grinding. Others focused the potential for irrational violence, such as the ad from the Montana Meth Project that depicted a bloodied woman on the floor of a kitchen with the slogan, "My mom knows I'd never hurt her. Then she got in the way" ("Mother" 2011). Meanwhile, gay men were said to be in denial as they practiced "sexual roulette" (Cheshes 1999) and possibly starting a "rebound epidemic" of HIV (Torassa 2001). The *Village Voice* expressed its moral outrage about the hedonism of gay men: "Amid flashing lights and pounding music, untutored freelance pharmacologists conduct experiments on their own bodies to determine what happens when one consumes a bewildering array of pills and powders in the confined and humid setting of a nightclub. The results are not always pretty" (Owen 1999). The caricature of gay men as pathological narcissists who care only about pleasure, the men blamed for being the incubators of AIDS in the 1970s, was back.

Moral panic theory calls these enemies of society "folk devils" (Cohen 2011), not only a "them" that stands in opposition to an "us" but a repository of blame, fear, and immorality. Drug users are common folk devils, from the Mexican marijuana users in the 1930s to black crack addicts in the 1980s. Singer and Page argue that these drug users serve a social function, if a nefarious one, as they are Othered. "Despite the routine and redundant depiction of drug users as wasted and worthless, closer examination reveals that they regularly are put to good social use in multiple ways," they say. Drug users can "exist as negative role models who help define the boundaries of approved behavior [and] as evidence of the unassailability of dominant understandings and values, and as conveniently scapegoated objects of blame for an array of social ills" (Singer and Page 2013, 22). It must be stated, however, that not all moral panics, not all folk devils, and not all Others are conjured out of nothing simply to further the goals of the dominant group (Cohen 2011, xliii). For every satanic cult that never existed, there are tangibly, empirically important problems, like AIDS and the meth epidemic. How extreme and imbalanced the response is the critical issue. But the general public, however defined, was not wrong to be alarmed the increase in the numbers of meth addicts and meth's role in HIV infection.

Public health researchers were alarmed, too. In one early and influential article, meth was described as a "substantial threat to HIV/AIDS prevention," because meth encourages risky sexual behavior. The authors point to the use of the drug in the creation of the "instant bottom" (implying the drug's influence on MSM's willingness to engage in sexual activities thought to carry greater risks for contracting HIV, such as receptive anal penetration) and in facilitating sexual marathons, group sex, fisting, and "a greater likelihood of having 50 or more sexual partners . . . as compared to their heterosexual counterparts" (Halkitis, Parsons, and Stirratt 2001, 25). The authors conclude that meth is at the center of behaviors that will exacerbate the AIDS epidemic, possibly by helping to create resistant versions of HIV:

> With the development of new treatment regimens for HIV infection, such as protease inhibitors, methamphetamine-related risky sexual behavior among HIV-positive gay and bisexual men presents the likelihood that newer seroconversions will occur with antiretroviral-treated and potentially mutated HIV virus (Halkitis 1998). The spread of drug-resistant strains of HIV will further complicate and prolong the HIV/AIDS epidemic. (Halkitis, Parsons, and Stirratt 2001, 28)

When a resistant strain seemed to arrive in the winter of 2005, the hysteria of the AIDS reportage from the 1980s was reproduced. The event easily fit into the narrative being created by the moralistic and angry anti-meth public health campaigns and the alarming academic research implicating meth use in new HIV infections. In turn, the media helped create a short, but intense moral panic that winter and spring. A man recently infected with HIV developed full-blown AIDS in few months, and he was resistant to three of the four classes of anti-retroviral drugs used to treat HIV. On February 11, 2005, health officials in New York City put out a press release announcing the case, with a quote from city's health commissioner: "This is a wakeup call to men who have sex with men" (New York City Health Commissioner). *The New York Daily News,* in a language typical of the press coverage around the country, railed, "Such reckless foolishness is the most extreme manifestation of a complacency toward AIDS" (*New York Daily News* 2005). While the panic that the super-strain garnered may have increased vigilance about HIV and meth and certainly was a factor in increased spending on anti-meth public health campaigns, interventions, and studies, it was not, in hindsight, something worth panicking over. The media response, however, was not surprising: as in the original AIDS panic of the early 1980s (Patton 1985), the discourse focused on the irresponsibility of gay men, on out of control sexual behavior, on the danger that what gay men have wrought will lead to an second epidemic, and implicitly, this would be yet another epidemic that threatens the "general" and "innocent" population.

The meth-HIV panic was different from the original AIDS panic in that it was created and supported by gay men in positions of power in academia and the media. Gay men had made enormous progress in the 25 years since the beginning of the AIDS epidemic, not only structurally within institutions like large media conglomerates and research universities, but also in winning unprecedented healthcare for people with HIV and in the shockingly swift social acceptance of same-sex marriage. The disproportionately high numbers of meth users in the gay community, and the publicizing of this, threatened the hard-fought image of gay men as respected and responsible members of society. In turn, gay men crafted messaging that differentiated good gays from bad gays. For example, several gay AIDS activists were quoted in a front-page article in *The New York Times* advocating hunting HIV-positive gay meth users and incarcerating them (Jacobs 2005), and the noted gay sex advice columnist and political commentator/memoirist Dan Savage spoke out in favor of this (Conan 2005). Controversial posters created by New York City's Crystal Meth Working Group depicted a demented, bug-eyed man holding a giant meth pipe with the slogan "Crystal Meth Makes Me Sexy" and smiling, healthy looking man holding a sign saying "Crystal Free" (Halkitis 2009, 75). Memoirs like Patrick Moore's Tweaked (2006) depict meth addiction as a cautionary tale, with sobriety an idealized state, while Larry Kramer's the 2004 speech "The Tragedy of Today's Gays," lambasting gay men for not honoring those who fell before them by participating in a hedonistic culture of sex and drugs, was published as a book and reviewed in numerous publications, many quoting: "we are murdering each other" (Towle 2004; Kramer 2005). The stigmatization of meth use and condomless sex succeeded in making "No PNP" (No Party and Play) a fixture in online profiles for gay men seeking sexual and romantic partners, which in turn succeeded in shoving men who wanted to PNP and have condomless sex into both actual (underground sex clubs) and virtual (websites like BarebackRealTime) venues that would cater to them without stigma.

As the moral panic about meth and HIV in the gay community died down, the stigma set in. The general public and most gay men stopped paying attention; the anti-meth ads and messages became rote, omnipresent, like wall paper. The largest and most expensive anti-meth campaign in the country, 2008's California's $17.5 million "Me Not Meth" campaign, barely registered in the mainstream media and the gay media was only slightly concerned (for example, *The Gay and Lesbian Times* 2008). Visitors on gay discussion sites like DataLounge typically mocked gay meth addicts without criticism from other site users, while a storyline on *Law & Order: Special Victims Unit* depicting meth-using gay men infected with the super strain as sociopaths (Makris 2005) was not challenged by the activists who had fought against AIDS stigma so valiantly. This particular panic dissipated, but the ideology that fed the panic remained, as did the scorned folk devil the panic created.

Meth Use and HIV-Positive MSM

HIV and meth abuse among MSM is one of several AIDS-related syndemics. Singer identified the Substance Abuse, Violence, and AIDS (SAVA) syndemic in studying the inner city Puerto Rican community of Hartford, CT (Singer 1994, 1996), and Stall described the syndemic of mental illness and HIV (Stall et al. 2003) in addition to joining Halkitis and others identifying HIV and meth abuse among MSM as a syndemic (Stall and Purcell 2000; Halkitis, Parsons, and Stirratt 2001). Halkitis has also described a broader syndemic of substance abuse, STIs, and mental health disorders among young MSM (Halkitis et al. 2015; Halkitis et al. 2013). In Africa, the syndemics of hookworm, malaria, and HIV (Hotez 2008) have been identified along with diabetes, depression, and HIV (Mendenhall et al. 2015) as well as HIV, tuberculosis, and poverty (Kwan and Ernst 2011) and HIV and food insecurity (Himmelgreen et al. 2009).

Stigma is involved in all of these syndemics, though in different ways and at varying intensities. In the meth and HIV syndemic, the intertwining stigmas combine cultural prohibitions on promiscuity, fear of infection, and distrust of seemingly irrational behavior. They also help create situations that perpetuate the syndemic in parts and as a whole. The stigma around HIV/AIDS helps to promote HIV infections and complications, while stigma around meth use encourages meth users to hide (Halkitis, Parsons, and Stirratt 2001; Link et al. 1997; Ahern, Stuber, and Galea 2007; Katz et al. 2013; *The Lancet* 2014). The stigma around homosexuality has been repeatedly linked to depression and anxiety, which can lead to sexual behaviors that can cause both HIV infection and substance abuse (Herek 2009; Hatzenbuehler, Nolen-Hoeksema, and Erickson 2008; Cabaj 2000). The stigmas are markers of social attitudes that create social situations that in turn create biological events, and these in turn create behaviors, appearances, and more social situations which can double back to the beginning of the cycle.

The various parts of the syndemic—the diverse stigmas, the interacting biologies and psychologies of infection and addiction—are not equal players and do not function the same across the population. For example, meth was often the accelerant for problems the men I worked with had; HIV management tended not to be difficult, while meth addiction was an exceptional struggle. The reasons for using meth are varied, but most MSM seem to use meth to self-medicate for emotional problems, to enhance sexual experiences, and to improve and facilitate socialization (Halkitis 2009, 85; Reback 1997; Reback, Larkins, and Shoptaw 2004; Semple, Patterson, and Grant 2002; Semple et al. 2006a; Shoptaw, Reback, and Freese 2001). These are not mutually exclusive, of course, as most men are likely to have multiple and overlapping reasons.

Depression, self-esteem problems, anxiety, and stress are all indicated as precursors to meth use, with robust findings of co-morbidity of meth use and depression (Ross 2004; Looby and Earleywine 2007; El-Bassel et al. 2001). As Halkitis writes, "Not only may methamphetamine directly impact depression by alleviating the mood disturbances engendered by this condition, but it may also mask feelings of fatigue as well as lack of concentration, both characteristic of a depressive state" (2009, 92). Since people with HIV are more likely to experience depression—for numerous reasons—meth is often used as a coping tool, particularly after seroconversion (Halkitis, Fischgrund, and Parsons 2005; Reback 1997). Unfortunately, meth exacerbates these symptoms; depression is both a cause and an effect of meth use (Rabkin 2006).

All of my informants all used meth to cope with depression. While not all of them described themselves as depressed prior to using meth, either using the term "depressed" or by describing emotional states that sounded to be depressive, during periods of abstinence from use or recovery from meth addiction, those who returned to meth did so to treat, alleviate, or mask their depression. Many seemed to have been prone to depression since childhood, indicating a possible genetic or biological basis. For others, their daily lives are extremely difficult, and like many who suffer under structural inequalities, they used drugs to temper the experience (Singer 2007). Some described the depression as a reaction of upsetting or traumatic events, like an HIV diagnosis or the death of a loved one. Adam, whose experience is described below, discovered as an adolescent that alcohol and drugs were the most effective tools for helping him survive his severe depression and anxiety, sometimes manifested in boredom. Meth was even better. "When I'm not high, actually," he said, "I feel really uncomfortable. I hate it because I'm bored, nothing to do. There's many people that don't do drugs that live everyday like that. . . . But I don't want to do that because it's boring. It's a messed up world. Too much hurt and too much sadness." Jonathan was enormously depressed and distressed by recovery and relapsed repeatedly. Sam was probably the most negative about his chances for recovery and the most depressive in his statements, saying during one interview, "I often think I should kill myself. But whenever I have enough heroin to do it, I forget."

Suffering from attention-deficit/hyperactivity disorder (ADHD) is considered a major risk factor for meth dependence. Methamphetamine was once used as a treatment for ADHD, which may lead some people with untreated ADHD to be drawn to it (Khantzian 1985). In addition, ADHD is associated with defective or lower levels of dopamine receptors, reducing the capacity to feel pleasure. Taking meth floods the brain with dopamine and prevents its reuptake, boosting pleasure (Volkow et al. 2001). Several of my informants described being much clearer and focused on meth and recalled diagnoses, formal and informal, of ADD or ADHD. Sam was given Ritalin as a child for hyperactivity and Andrew was diagnosed with ADHD, while Glenn, Charles, and Eric were never given actual diagnoses as children, but in interviews, all claimed to have ADHD and to find that meth helped focus them. Both Charles and Andrew say that they only feel "normal" when they are on meth. Sam explains, "You know, I used to be down, and you put me on speed, I usually get calm. I mean, it depends on the deal, but . . . really, it's pharmaceutical."

Studies also indicate that some gay men use meth and other drugs as a means for coping with the stress of homophobia, loneliness, HIV disease, and social situations (Reback 1997; Semple, Patterson, and Grant 2002; Halkitis, Fischgrund, and Parsons 2005). Post-traumatic stress disorder is also associated with drug abuse and addiction; long-term sufferers of HIV who have many AIDS related losses show signs of trauma, PTSD, and existential crises (Nord 1998; Machado 2012). Cathy Reback argues, in her ethnography of meth use among gay and bisexual men in Los Angeles, that some tried to manage the physical, psychological, and social effects of having HIV/AIDS with meth. For men who had AIDS and lowered energy, meth gave them vigor. Meth helped others forget that they were grieving the loss of friends and lovers. In their study of HIV-positive men who used meth, Semple et al. found similar motivations. They quote one informant who used meth to escape HIV: "Everywhere you go, you're reminded of HIV. Can I have one day when I'm not reminded that I'm HIV-positive? Meth gives me that" (2002, 153).

I conducted my ethnographic research 13 years after Reback's ethnography was published, and none of them talked about HIV being the main stressor in their lives, at least not in 2010 and 2011.[3] I often found it hard to untangle stress from anxiety and depression in the informants' narratives, but several of them described the joys of using meth after a stressful week, as a way to take away their worries, or to disassociate from the "real world." Richard, who worked as an administrative assistant, constantly described his weekend meth binges as antidotes to the stress of his job. When I interviewed him, he was in recovery, not working, and living in a sober living facility. He was calm and happy and was planning for the future. When he went back to work within a month, the stress of the job, he said, led him to relapse. Adam, who had begun using meth partly because of its successful masking of depression, also used meth to cope with the stress and anxiety of his life, which ranged from not knowing where he will sleep or how he will eat to dealing with an emotionally abusive boyfriend or his needy sex work clients.

These reasons people offer for their meth use are individualistic, and many of the researchers who have described them underplay the role that interpersonal influences, particularly within the family, have in encouraging meth use. Halkitis (2009, 102) argues that the composition and processes of the family can influence meth abuse, citing the work by Hawkins et al. (1992) that connects to meth use by children to meth use by family members, poor family management practices, heightened family conflict, and weak family bonds. These patterns, in their individualistic detail, certainly can be seen among the participants. Both Brandon and Matthew had family members who used meth. Dylan's mother was a dealer and his father had spent time in jail for possession. After his mother abandoned him, Glenn grew up in numerous foster homes, several of which were either or both physically and emotional abusive. Charles, Richard, William, Jonathan, and Jorge had missing parents, either dead, estranged, or far away. Max and Eric had enormous levels of conflict within their respective families. Max ran away from home as a child, and Eric was beaten. However, it bears mentioning that Sam and Adam, two of the most troubled of my informants, had intact nuclear families with parents who were not drug users not abusive, suggesting the importance of other factors.

Of course, peer influence is incredibly important, particularly among gay men, whose feelings of difference as a child often lead to social insecurity as an adult. Brandon, who always worried about being abandoned, used his drug connections to make and keep friends as a teenager and used with friends as an adult. Darrell's gay friends in high school encouraged him to take meth to lose weight. Richard was introduced to meth by men he met in West Hollywood. Eric first used meth when men he met online raved about the sex they had on it. He went to a hotel room to meet one of them and the man had a syringe full of meth ready for him.

Sexual experiences that seem impossible while not high are commonplace on meth. Since meth is such a powerful stimulant that intensifies the senses and dramatically increases dopamine levels, the physical experience of sex is enormously powerful. One of Reback's informants described the sex: "All your senses are ascending, suddenly awakened and not dormant. Like being born; really cool, warm, everything is new and exciting, like the first time." Another echoes, "It's just every nerve in your body is standing at attention" (Reback 1997, 25). In addition, meth enables many men to have anal sex more easily, to experiment sexually, or to have sex for longer durations of time. Semple et al. quote one man for whom meth was "about pushing my limits. It's about seeing how far I can take it. The nastier sex, the better. Nastier being multiple partners, a lot of exchange of body fluids. I have to have multiple partners, one right after the other for hours and hours, and sexual marathons up to 20 hours of rough sex" (Semple, Patterson, and Grant 2002, 152). The informants echo these kinds of comments. Jonathan said, giggling, "I would do the craziest things on meth." Jorge said, "Oh, yes, all I wanted to do was bottom. And I would do it forever."

In the introduction to Reback's ethnography, the Los Angeles AIDS Coordinator Ferd Eggan, who commissioned the study, suggests that the "outlawry" inherent in the mythos of gay sex is partly to blame for this destructive behavior. He argues, "[My] readings of the narratives provided by the men in this study is that the lives they have constructed and had constructed for them involve internalization of stigma, a sexualized definition of self, and mechanisms to resist the internalized negative feelings" (Reback 1997, ii). Meth use may not simply increase risk-taking in otherwise risk-averse men. Rather, research suggests that "methamphetamine attracts a hypersexual risk-taking group of men who engage in unprotected sexual behaviors regardless of their methamphetamine use" (Halkitis, Shrem, and Martin 2005, 703). This possibility is supported by another study that shows a correlation between meth use and both impulsivity and sexual compulsion (Semple et al. 2006a; Semple et al. 2006b; Semple et al. 2008). It is not surprising that since self-control is so valued in American culture many gay meth users feel shame about their drug use and sexual behavior, and those who quit rarely have anything but extremely negative memories of their meth use (Reback 1997; Mimiaga et al. 2008; Menza et al. 2007). Several gay cultural critics (Halperin 2007; Warner 1999) have argued that this shame, which comes from pathologizing both gay sexual adventure and the use of illegal psychoactive drugs, is precisely what many men are resisting, probably more unconsciously than consciously, by using meth and having sex that is called "risky." Many of the men in this study described themselves as rebellious as children and cited their drug use as evidence of that rebelliousness, but it was unclear whether rebelliousness was an external description of their abnormal behavior by parents and teachers or a self-aware, agentive state of being in opposition to control or oppression.

The effects of meth abuse often perpetuate the social, psychological, and biological bases that encouraged the initial meth use, creating a cycle that is difficult to escape. Prolonged use can change the dopamine system; it can take many months, even years, for the dopamine system to recover following cessation (De Vito and Wagner 1989). By reducing the dopamine transporters, more meth is needed to feel pleasure, furthering addiction to the drug. The decrease in dopamine transporters also can hurt motor functioning, memory, and verbal learning. Cognitive impairment is also common among meth abusers, from increasing distractibility to decreasing the ability to think abstractly (Simon et al. 2000). Dental problems, caused by decreased saliva and increased grinding (among other issues), are famously common among chronic meth users (Klasser and Epstein 2005), as are skin problems, often the result of obsessively picking the skin because of the common hallucination that bugs are crawling all of the body (Rusyniak 2013). Prolonged use can also impair social skills, making it difficult to "read" another's emotions and encourage awkward social interactions (though ADHD may also influence or intersect with/exacerbate these problems) (Homer et al. 2008). Withdrawal from meth leads to a depletion of catecholamines (Meredith et al. 2005), which can cause to a number of psychiatric problems—depression, anxiety, social impairment, psychosis, hallucinations, and both homicidal and suicidal ideation—that can lead directly to conflict with other people, especially the police. And the addiction to meth compounds problems associated with HIV. Studies have shown that meth users are much more likely to fail to adhere to treatment regimens, further compromising their immune systems (Carrico et al. 2007). Thus the increased likelihood of contracting STDs, because of sexual compulsivity associated with the drug, is much more problematic (Shoptaw and Reback 2007), as are the potential problems associated with toxic substances, like lead, found in impure meth (Halkitis 2009, 65). Meth is also associated directly with an increased replication of HIV and the replication of two of the 23 opportunistic infections that define AIDS: candida albicans, or thrush, and a fungus that causes meningitis, cryptococcus neoformans (Tallóczy et al. 2008). As health problems, illness, pain, and depression are drivers for meth use, these complications from HIV associated with long-term meth use can further encourage the use of meth or other drugs.

These affective, behavioral, and physical changes signal to many observers, especially in communities with large meth problems, who is a meth addict. While some react to the stigma with empathy, others become afraid and work to distance themselves. Shunning and incarcerating meth addicts out of fear or disgust is both a result of and driver for stigma, and the consequence is isolating the meth addicts from their larger communities, making them less likely to seek help or treatment and more likely to socialize with other meth users, which will only further the addiction.

Three Pathways of Interaction

In the three narratives that follow, I demonstrate how Charles, Andrew, and Glenn deal with social, psychological, and biological interactions between methamphetamine addiction, HIV, depression, and stigma, to illustrate the syndemic proposed in this chapter. Their stories depict the individualized and idiosyncratic nature of this syndemic, but these individuals also have a good deal in common: stigma, shame, and an uneasy, sometimes hostile, relationship with the potential for recovery from addiction. These commonalities need to be understood not only through their different iterations but also through the ways they are structured by cultural, political and economic forces that drive the syndemic.

Charles

Of the informants discussed in this chapter, Charles had the most extensive psychotherapy, and through it he developed a great deal of insight. During the study, Charles was the only informant who saw a psychiatrist every week. The others saw drug counselors, had medical doctors prescribing anti-depressants, or were members of at least one support group. Charles did all of these, as well as psychotherapy. Charles seemed to have the most self-awareness of anyone in my study, but at no point did he stop using meth for longer than a few months. Still, he was rather high-functioning; had his own apartment, picked up monthly federal disability checks, and always kept his appointments. But despite having analyzed his past and his emotions so thoroughly, and despite being on numerous psychotropic medications, Charles had an almost exclusively negative, if not depressive, analysis of his psychodynamic narrative.

Charles grew up in the northern part of California's Central Valley. When asked about his earliest memories, he discussed being left at his grandparents' house often: "I would sit and stare out the window," he said, "waiting for my parents to come pick me up. They would never show up." He explained to me that is why he was always early for interviews. "Now I have to be early, or they won't wait." "They" referred to anyone he might rely on. Charles links this fear of being left behind with his fear of his family discovering that he was gay; they suspected it early on because of his effeminate mannerisms: "To my dad's parents, who were dumb rednecks, I was devil spawn." Instead of disappearing into himself and hiding, he became an extrovert. "I was afraid of being found out and afraid of being forgotten, so I would be as obnoxious as I possibly could." In his self-analysis, he sees this extroversion, much of which was a clown-like performance, as a defense mechanism. "They could never know how depressed I was," he said. "It takes so much effort to put on that happy face. I have a hard time attaching myself to people. That's why I had to be outlandish." But that didn't always work. Charles was always acting out as a child, and was not treated well because of it. "When I was 12, I went on a crazy rant—ADHD stuff—and one of the teachers slapped me." On meth, his mind is quieted. "Meth calms me down; I can focus."

What he refers to as a pathological fear of abandonment is his explanation for two key moments in the narrative of his illness. He found out he was HIV-positive in his early 20s and he told no one after he got the results. He was too afraid and too ashamed. "I never talked about it until I was 35," he said, not even to his partner of many years, Greg. "I never told him. I knew for sure he would leave me." The cruel irony was that Greg was actually dying of Hepatitis C, which he did not tell Charles about until it was killing him, at which time Greg revealed he also had HIV. When Greg died, Charles' fear was realized: "Greg told me he loved me no matter what. He told me he would never leave. And then he died." In response, Charles says, he focused on a combination of denial and self-destruction: He spent all of his money and all of the money Greg left him on drugs, eventually becoming homeless and finding himself in jail.

As he explained his behavior, he repeated the various analyses offered him by his therapists and counselors. His current therapist told him, "You're not crazy, you just do crazy things." In one support group, which used an intervention curriculum designed at UCLA, he said, "We were trying to figure out why a lot of us have underlying reasons for using. You're supposed to be responsible to yourself." This responsibility meant that, as Charles came to believe, "I made my life this way." In analyzing himself, both through years of psychotherapy and in various interventions, from groups to one-on-one sessions of motivation interviews, he has learned to narrate his life. But he is not the good guy in his own story. He feels shame for letting these events and situations make him—and others—suffer. He said: "I have to stop using my past as an excuse for being bad."

But an argument can be made for Charles' past experiences being partly to blame for some of his problems, a past (and present) with stigmas, depression, and HIV biologically and socially interacting and influencing each other. Untreated childhood ADHD coupled with depression resulting from his family and community's homophobia may have led not just to meth use but also to risky sexual behavior and HIV infection. The stigma around HIV encouraged Charles not to tell anyone about his status, and that internalized shame, fear, and sadness only made it more likely that he would seek solace in meth. Charles completely internalized the stigmas of the syndemic he suffered. He hated himself for being depressed, for being addicted to drugs, for having HIV, for lying, for failing. Considering how well-managed his HIV and his meth addiction was, it was actually the depression and the multiple stigmas that brought Charles the most suffering. It made sense why he periodically went back to the drug. When I asked Charles to describe the feeling of meth, he focused on its ability to take away his worries. "Oh, it's like every care in the world is just gone," Charles said. "You're not worried about anything. For that moment, it's just perfect."

Adam

The author met Adam at the syringe exchange where I volunteered. He was a tall, lanky man in his late 20s, wearing a tank top and shorts and eyeing me suspiciously while smoking a cigarette. Adam told me during their first meeting that he was living with friends, was working for a landscaper, and was looking into going back to school. These were not exactly false statements. In a way, the men he lived with were his friends, but they were friendships forged in drug use and had numerous strings attached. Adam was thinking about working: one of his other friends had said he could help him get a job assisting a landscaper. As for school, this was a goal, or rather an idea of a goal, that he had been told over and over again to have, by drug counselors, case workers, and probation officers. Because of who I resembled—a researcher, a therapist, a drug counselor—he seemed like the kind of person who wanted to hear that Adam was thinking about going back to school. Otherwise, Adam did not contemplate the future very much. He was more concerned with where his meth would come from, where he was going to sleep the next time he decided to sleep, where he was going to be able to find money, who was going to give it to him, and what he would have to exchange for it. Adam had been doing meth for more than a decade.

As a child, Adam had felt disconnected from his family. "I'm not their blood, you know?" he said. "I'm not their biological son. I'm adopted. So, that kind of threw me off. It made me feel like, you know, I don't have parents. Ever since I was little, I've felt that way. So, that kind of made me feel like I was less than. . . . It screwed me up." He thinks it led him to look outside for social kinship. He grew up upper middle class, the son of a lawyer and a doctor in suburban Michigan. His parents, he said, were obsessed with being good at being parents. But when he was 12, he became fascinated with the other side of the tracks—literally. The kids from that side of town smoked cigarettes before school, they drank a lot, and they did whatever they wanted to. By 14, Adam was getting arrested, and he was using all kinds of drugs and copious amounts of alcohol to self-medicate for severe depression, anxiety, and ADHD. His parents paid for psychiatry, rehabilitation, and lawyers, and they pulled strings to keep him out of jail multiple times. But no treatment, no prescription psychopharmacological substance worked to soothe him the way that the drugs and alcohol did. Finally, his parents put their feet down: If he would not cooperate, they would not take care of him anymore. He left Michigan when a warrant was issued for his arrest for writing bad checks.

Adam and his then-girlfriend decided to come to San Diego. They spent days on buses and arrived at her father's door expecting a bed to sleep on. But her father did not want to see her or help her, and they spent the next couple of weeks sleeping on sidewalks downtown before cobbling together enough money to rent a unit at an SRO. It was in the lobby that he met his first boyfriend, who introduced him to meth.

> We start smoking meth and then we had sex. So on that night I had sex, anal sex for the first time. And smoked meth. He was a drug dealer and he liked me, and shortly after that I moved in. And I had a really bizarre fun time for . . . a couple years. So that was my introduction. Selling meth, unprotected sex. I got warned of like HIV or something like that. I don't even know if that was true or not. I just didn't care, that is really sick. That is how I was thinking. (*Adam*)

After that relationship ended, Adam discovered that his good looks and mostly mellow demeanor gave him an advantage; he could easily trade sex for drugs, for a bed, for cash. Some of the men were nice, many were not. Some would get him involved in the drug trade. He found himself carrying drugs for dealers, selling some on the side, and one day, at a Wal-Mart, he was arrested with a duffle bag full of meth, ecstasy, marijuana, and cash. He had been high when he went into the store, and paranoid and agitated, and he easily piqued the suspicions of the security staff. This was not the first time he ended up in jail, but it did lead to his longest stay.

As with the vast majority of people who are incarcerated for drug offenses in California, Adam received no drug counseling while he was in jail. When he was released, he was sent to an in-patient rehabilitation program. Understaffed by under-educated and under-paid drug counselors, the program was useless for Adam. After learning the vocabulary of recovery, after learning that only he has the power to end his addiction using drugs, he walked out, violating his parole; the prescription drugs meant to quell the agony of his emotional state were no comparison to the illegal, "recreational" ones he knew from the street. This pattern repeated itself more than a dozen times: He would wander the city, couch hopping and scrounging for drugs and money, before eventually doing something—shoplifting, loitering, or just looking weird and out of place—that caught the attention of the police. After an arrest or a conviction, he would be funneled to treatment that failed to stick, and Adam would leave, violating probation or his parole.

During the months that Adam met with me, he would discuss his depression frequently. This was the depression that even the meth couldn't mask. He often said he didn't see any point in trying, that he expected failure, that he didn't see anyone interested or willing or able to help. One day Adam came to the my office covered in bruises and dried blood; he was incredibly agitated and terrified. His boyfriend, who he called Psycho, had crossed a gang in a check-kiting scheme, and the gang had held them and Psycho's brother hostage for two days. They were beaten and tortured before, for no seeming reason, and then they were released. Adam seemed to have a concussion; he needed medical attention. But he was terrified to go to the hospital because the last time he went—for bronchitis—he ended up with $50,000 in bills. He repeatedly stopped himself from crying, which was most difficult for him when I said I wanted to help him.

He said, "I can't go on like this. I really feel bad. I don't know what to do." I spent the rest of the interview convincing Adam to let me help him find emergency crisis housing. Adam agreed to meet me in an hour. But he never showed up. For a week, I agonized that Adam might be dead. I dreamed about him and couldn't stop talking about him. Then Adam showed up for his next appointment as if nothing had happened. He told me he had gone to get some meth to calm himself down before meeting me. One thing led to another and he was back sleeping at Psycho's apartment. After that week, I tried repeatedly to convince him to try to get into crisis housing, to get him to go see his doctor's appointments, to get him to find some method of excising himself from Psycho's home and grasp. And he simply could not.

During this period, as I contemplated why Adam would refuse help I was reminded not only of Reback's conclusion, that meth made sense in the lives of meth users, but also of the stack of studies (referenced above) about meth users using the drug to self-medicate their clinical depression, other mental health disorders, and their existential dread, as well as to cope with the knowledge that meth was not actually helping relieve the depression (Looby and Earleywine 2007). Adam was addicted to meth, and that physical need was the most powerful drive for his continued use of the drug, but when he was sober, he didn't utilize the resources, however weak and ineffective, that might have helped him. Those resources came from institutions that told him he was a failure, a criminal, that his struggle was deserved and necessary; the people that were charged with helping Adam recover were also the ones that most powerfully reinforced the stigma of being a meth-addicted, HIV-positive gay man. Being sober did not make sense to Adam. Sobriety meant feeling all of the stigmas, hating himself, having panic attacks, and having to make Herculean efforts to do things as mundane as grocery shopping. Even though staying on meth would have other, negative consequences, from self-loathing to physical pain, it made sense to Adam to continue to use.

Glenn

Glenn grew up in and around San Diego, bouncing from foster parents to an uncle who touched him inappropriately, then to more foster parents. His father was gone and his mother had been incapable of taking care of him; his temporary families were only slightly better. Some were violent. Many he cannot remember. One family stuck the longest, and he refers to the other boy his age who lived there as his brother, still, more than 30 years after he left the system. When he was younger, he was always getting into trouble, either because of his anger or sometimes, because he made passes at father figures. "I thought that that's how you loved a father figure," he explained. "I was a kid. I just wanted to be loved." Glenn experienced a great deal of chaos and emotional violence as a child. He said that when he is high on meth he is most sexually turned on by degradation and humiliation (as explained below). When asked if there was a connection, he said, "I don't see that as a reflection on my childhood."

In his late teens, Glenn found himself in Kansas, engaged to a woman, even though he had long before realized he was gay. He got married anyway, had two children in quick succession—a boy and a girl—but was divorced by age 22. Constantly looking for stability and for family, he found a boyfriend and, long before it was both politically possible and socially acceptable, had a commitment ceremony at a branch of the Metropolitan Community Church in Wichita. They were together for two years, and it was his addiction to crack cocaine that split them apart. He moved to Texas, where he was drugged in a club and raped, and he believes this is when he was infected with HIV. He'd always had trouble with drugs, using them, he said with hindsight honed by 12-step programs, to masque his anxiety and loneliness, to fill the hole ripped into him when his mother abandoned him. This is not a completely logical explanation, of course, and jumping over that disconnect, he also said he took drugs, "to get higher and higher. I don't ever think I've been high enough. I'm hooked on the idea of not looking at reality."

When his kids graduated from high school, he saw his responsibility to them lessened, and he and his brother decided to get a fresh start back in San Diego. They packed everything up, and without jobs or a plan, just an imagined belief that San Diego really was American's Finest City, they drove west. But like the wannabe starlet who arrives on a bus in Hollywood and is promptly introduced to sex, drugs, and rock and roll, Glenn's return to San Diego was also his arrival to meth. The night they arrived, Glenn went to Montage, a gay club not far from San Diego's airport, and he drank and danced, thrilling by his new old home. He met two men on the dance floor, roommates who invited him back to their apartment for an after party of more booze and sex. When they got to the men's home, the roommates disappeared into one of their bedrooms, where unbeknownst to him they injected meth, while Glenn waited in the living room. Then, they opened the door, revealing themselves to Glenn both naked and in ecstasy. Glenn looked at them and saw freedom from care and constraint, from sadness and anxiety, and he thought, "I want to feel like that."

So, he did. And he did it over and over again, though he would never feel like he did that night. Shortly after Glenn became addicted to meth, his brother returned to Kansas. Left completely to his own devices, Glenn devoted his time to meth and to sex, to finding money to pay for meth, and to finding people who might give it to him. He spent time in motels and hotels and flop houses with other men who were also doing meth. He asked men to act out rape scenes with him, to rape him. "That's what I was pursuing in all of my addiction, pursuing hurtful sex. The idea of being held down and injected, it turns me on. In my addiction, I wanted hands around my neck, to be spit on, spanked. I wanted to be hurt and to be loved."

Glenn had sex with men who he'd never have looked twice at while sober, he crashed on couches, he spent his savings, and he started finding and reselling junk to make ends meet. After four years of this, after a couple fits and starts attempting recovery, he says he hit bottom in an SRO, crying all night long because he knew he was killing himself, destroying his children, ruining his life. When he came to our first interview, Glenn was crashing on a friend's couch and applying to sober living housing, for social security, and making plans for the future. He went to meetings every day, volunteered at a community health center, and said he wanted to become an addiction counselor. He was positive, focused, full of goals. He was also dishonest, both with me and with himself and with the sober living programs. He outlined one life story over three interviews, and then during the fourth, he read the addiction narrative he had written for San Diego's Crystal Meth Anonymous Book, and the tale was different. In the addiction narrative, he had been a crack addict in Kansas and to me, he'd said that he'd tried cocaine once. I asked about the discrepancy and he mentioned, off-handedly, that he probably had wanted me to like him.

Glenn had seemed so excited about his future and his recovery, had thrown himself so fully into the recovery community, repeating their mantras in our interviews, volunteering at meetings, and declaring his desire to make a career as a former addict. He acted like a veteran of 12-step programs, but he was barely two months into his sobriety when he started sitting for interviews with me. He would also beat himself up after every set back, blaming himself for his failure to recover more quickly. After six interviews, Glenn and I took a break from interviews; I had planned on doing two or three follow-up interviews after six months. But a couple of weeks after the sixth interview, another interview subject, who was living in the same recovery housing for people with HIV, told me that Glenn had left the complex. He had relapsed; he left one night, shot up meth, and returned a few days later to pick up his stuff. Within a week, he was back in Kansas, out of contact with his friends at the complex. Brandon, a 22-year-old who Glenn had suggested for this study and who was in love with him, was livid: "He just gave up. He couldn't handle it. He couldn't be sober."

Aside from never having been arrested and never spending time incarcerated, Glenn's story was typical of my other subjects, who were in turn typical of HIV-positive MSM who use meth, at least in epidemiological terms. Before using meth, he had a long history of emotional trauma, depression, instability, and substance abuse. He was drawn to meth not only for purpose of pleasure, but also because of the freedom from earthly worries, from anxiety and sadness and unease. It also allowed him to feel things he'd never allow himself to feel while sober. The ecstasy of sex and meth provided just that freedom. For a while. When he had tried to stop using, he had received minimal counseling and treatment by either experienced psychotherapists or addiction specialists. He relapsed not because of lack of willpower, morality, or ethics, but because he had neither the cognitive nor practical skills to manage the depression, anxiety, rootlessness, and insecurity of being an indigent addict.

"If I had never had consequences, I'd do meth again. But it will kill me." Glenn said a few weeks before the relapse that led him, first, to leave the recovery program where he lived, and second, to leave San Diego and return to Kansas, where he lives as of this writing. It did not kill him. We are friends on Facebook, and in the last two years since we last spoke, he has posted numerous mantras from recovery programs, photos of him and his children and grandchildren, a series of updates about a visit with his estranged mother, and a number of updates about his first weeks as a freshman at the University of Kansas.

> Today is "New Student Orientation Day" at the University of Kansas. I'm up, showered and ready to go. There is a "little" voice in my head telling me that I'm too old to go back to school, people are going to laugh at me, I can't do this and so on. It's the same "little" voice that said I wasn't good enough and so I spent years of my life running from that belief with drugs and alcohol. So, today I'm not going to listen to that voice. Today I'm going to hear the voices of all those who are supportive and encouraging to me (and let me just say that there are several of you that believe I can do this). I will let you know how it goes. :) Have a great day everyone. (*Glenn*)

Glenn's path to recovery was a long one. He mentioned during one interview that he'd introduced himself as a new member of Alcoholics Anonymous eight times; he'd relapsed seven times so far. This time, it seems, the program, both as a series of meetings and exercises and a series of cognitive scripts and behavior modifications, has worked. He has stopped using. For now. Perhaps for good.

CONCLUSION

Like Charles and Andrew, and the other men in this study, Glenn's addiction has been powerfully individualistic experience. As they describe it, the desire for the drugs is theirs alone, the triggers are theirs to avoid, the use of drugs is theirs to end; they deserve their stigmas. The discourse of addiction promoted by the 12-step programs, popular culture, and anti-drug campaigns expresses drug use as an individual choice; you choose to follow the path of recovery or you choose to follow the path of addiction. The informants who were not able to follow the path of substance use recovery often described experiencing disastrous consequences for which they blamed themselves despite larger structural circumstances, from Adam's assault and torture to Charles' constant sadness and anxiety, from Glenn's internalized stigma manifested as self-loathing to others' incarceration, homelessness, or even death. With few exceptions, the informants describe walking their paths to addiction under their own moral power.

Neither biological nor structural reasons were addressed, likely because the informants were never told about them or because they were told to minimize them. I never heard that untreated childhood ADHD was a major risk fact for methamphetamine abuse; that it was methamphetamine that increased libido and decreased inhibitions, not one's moral failing or lack of self-control; that methamphetamine itself made HIV more likely to replicate, that the harm to cognition made it harder to remember to take medications. Rarely did anyone discuss the structural poverty that contributed to many of their difficult childhoods, and rarely did they talk about the structural violence of the governmentalities of the Drug War. Glenn did not see the state's failure to provide him with a safe foster family or to treat his mental health problems as a child as having anything to do with the trauma he is still dealing with. He did not see how state-sponsored recovery programs push 12-step ideologies on him not because they are the most effective, but because they are the cheapest.[4] He does not see how the shame, guilt, sadness and despair that he felt during his recovery is partially determined by these programs, not because one needs to feel these things in order to overcome an addiction but rather because the

Drug War, and the cultural, political, and economic processes that started and perpetuate it, need the shame, guilt, sadness and despair in order to justify itself (Singer 2007; Singer and Page 2013). As Glenn said, in describing his rapes at the hands of men who drugged him, "I didn't deserve it. But it happened because I put myself in that situation."

Glenn, like other participants, was indoctrinated structurally and culturally to individualize his life experience rather than to consider genetic predispositions, structural factors, and hierarchical social influences; he was taught to blame himself for "poor choices" and life failures, for creating his own life situation. What this individuation of causation cannot explain, however, are the structural patterns across the lives of the men in this study. It is the study of these patterns that leads us to a useful assessment of the role of structural factors in interactions between meth use, HIV, their individual and compounded stiamas, and other biological and behavioral aspects of illness, addiction, and suffering.

The stigmas against HIV, meth addiction, and homosexuality stem from and are embedded in entrenched cultural ideologies, which in turn influence state and non-government structures and systems that further reproduce the stigmas. These stigmas serve a function, as Singer and Page argue: "Othering is purposeful; it has practical benefits. Specifically, it serves interests and rewards its perpetrators. Othering, in short, has its advocates, its operators, its benefactors" (2013, 208) The institutionalized legal and cultural heterosexism of Western culture (despite recent marriage equality) *needs* homophobia, either overt or covert, to define itself (Foucault 1976). The hostility to substance users, whether of marijuana or meth, helps to define what is normal, rational, and acceptable. And HIV—which seemed to come from already racially, sexually, and behaviorally problematic peoples—worked as the danger that defined the purity of the ideal American family (Patton 1985). The forces that promote these ideologies and produce the stigmas have interacted with the biological, psychological, and social manifestations of meth addiction and HIV to create a syndemic that behaves almost like a perpetual motion machine. Stigma toward HIV, however lessened since the mid-1990s, continues to make prevention, care, and treatment difficult. The stigma of methamphetamine addiction, based not only on the imagined monster of the meth addict but also on the embarrassment that addiction brings to the gay community, is fresher but also currently more resistant to critique. It drives meth addicts underground; they are less likely to talk about it, harder to reach because of it, and more likely to get sicker, progress faster, and die from it. Perhaps only by reducing these stigmas, fighting the cultural logic that structures them, and reforming structures that support them, we might be able to address the syndemic they help to fuel.

NOTES

1. The names of the study participants have been changed to protect their anonymity.

2. This chapter includes sections that appear in different forms in other publications (Gideonse 2015a, 2015b, 2016).

3. Eric and Jorge, both of whom contracted HIV in the 1980s and identified greatly with being gay and with the gay community, would have been the most likely to provide me with data that would match Reback's, but they did not describe their meth use as having such meaning. William was old enough and has had HIV long enough, but he did not identify himself as part of a gay community.

4. As Carr explains, "by prescribing talk that can only reference the inner states of speakers, addiction counselors effectively, if not intentionally, enervate clients' institutional critiques and discourage social commentary" (2010, 5).

REFERENCES

Adam, Barry D., and Alan Sears. *Experiencing HIV*. New York: Columbia University Press, 1996.

Ahern, Jennifer, Jennifer Stuber, and Sandro Galea. "Stigma, Discrimination and the Health of Illicit Drug Users." *Drug and Alcohol Dependence* 88, nos. 2–3 (2007): 188–96. DOI:10.1016/j.drugalcdep.2006.10.014.

Alonzo, Angelo A., and Nancy R. Reynolds. "Stigma, HIV and AIDS: An Exploration and Elaboration of a Stigma Trajectory." *Social Science & Medicine* 41, no. 3 (1995) 303–15. DOI:10.1016/0277-9536(94)00384-6.

Cabaj, Robert Paul. 2000. "Substance Abuse, Internalized Homophobia, and Gay Men and Lesbians." *Journal of Gay & Lesbian Psychotherapy* 3, nos. 3–4 (2000): 5–24. DOI:10.1300/J236v03n03_02.

Carr, E. Summerson. *Scripting Addiction: The Politics of Therapeutic Talk and American Sobriety*. Princeton, NJ: Princeton University Press, 2010.

Carrico, Adam W., Mallory O. Johnson, Judith T. Moskowitz, Torsten B. Neilands, Stephen F. Morin, Edwin D. Charlebois, Wayne T. Steward, et al. 2007. "Affect Regulation, Stimulant Use, and Viral Load Among HIV-Positive Persons on Anti-Retroviral Therapy." *Psychosomatic Medicine* 69, no. 8 (2007): 785–92.

Chambers, Ross. *Untimely Interventions: AIDS Writing, Testimonial, and the Rhetoric of Haunting*. Ann Arbor, MI: University of Michigan Press, 2004.

Cheshes, Jay. "Sexual Roulette; Despite the Risk, HIV-Positive Gay Men Are Engaging in Unsafe Sex in the Wake of Improved AIDS Medications. Don't Believe Us? Check Out South Florida's Backroom Bars." *New Times Broward-Palm Beach (Florida)*, 1999.

Cohen, Stanley. *Folk Devils and Moral Panics*. New York: Routledge, 2011.

Conan, Neal. 2005. "AIDS and Personal Responsibility." *National Public Radio (NPR)*, March 10, 2005. Accessed August 31, 2016. http://www.npr.org/templates/story/story.php?storyId=4529981.

Cowles, Kathleen V., and Beth L. Rodgers. "Struggling to Keep on Top: Meeting the Everyday Challenges of AIDS." *Qualitative Health Research* 7, no. 1 (1997): 98–120.

De Vito, Michael J., and G. C. Wagner. "Methamphetamine-Induced Neuronal Damage: A Possible Role for Free Radicals." *Neuropharmacology* 28, no. 10 (1989): 1145–50.

El-Bassel, Nabila, Susan S. Witte, Takeshi Wada, Louisa Gilbert, and Joyce Wallace. "Correlates of Partner Violence Among Female Street-Based Sex Workers: Substance Abuse, History of Childhood Abuse, and HIV Risks." *AIDS Patient Care and STDs* 15, no. 1 (2001): 41–51.

Farmer, Paul. *AIDS and Accusation: Haiti and the Geography of Blame*. Comparative Studies of Health Systems and Medical Care. Berkeley, CA: University of California Press, 1992.

Foucault, Michel. *The History of Sexuality, Vol. 1*. Translated by R. Hurley. New York: Pantheon, 1976.

Gideonse, Theodore K. "Survival Tactics and Strategies of Meth-Using HIV+ Men Who Have Sex with Men in San Diego." *PLoS ONE* 10, no. 9 (2015a): e0139239.

———. "Pride, Shame, and the Trouble with Trying to Be Normal." *Ethos* 43, no. 4 (2015b): 332–52.

———. "Framing Samuel See: The Discursive Detritus of the Moral Panic Over the 'Double Epidemic' of Methamphetamines and HIV Among Gay Men." *International Journal of Drug Policy*, 28 (February 2016): 98–105. DOI:10.1016/j.drugpo.2015.10.010.

Goffman, Erving. *Stigma: Notes on the Management of Spoiled Identity*. New York: Prentice-Hall, 1963.

Gould, Deborah B. *Moving Politics: Emotion and ACT-UP's Fight Against AIDS*. Chicago: University of Chicago Press, 2009.

Green, Gill, and E. J. Sobo. *The Endangered Self: Managing the Social Risks of HIV*. Health, Risk and Society. London: Routledge, 2000.

Halkitis, Perry N. "Advances in the Treatment of HIV Disease: Complexities of Adherence and Complications for Prevention." *The Health Psychologist* 20, no. 1 (1998): 6–14.

———. *Methamphetamine Addiction: Biological Foundations, Psychological Factors, and Social Consequences*. Washington, DC: American Psychological Association, 2009.

Halkitis, Perry N., Beth N. Fischgrund, and Jeffrey T. Parsons. "Explanations for Methamphetamine Use Among Gay and Bisexual Men in New York City." *Substance Use & Misuse* 40, nos. 9–10 (2005): 1331–45. DOI:10.1081/JA-200066900.

Halkitis, Perry N., Farzana Kapadia, Kristen L. Bub, Staci Barton, Alvaro D. Moreira, and Christopher B. Stults. "A Longitudinal Investigation of Syndemic Conditions Among Young Gay, Bisexual, and Other Msm: The P18 Cohort Study." *AIDS and Behavior* 19, no. 6 (2015): 970–80. DOI:10.1007/s10461-014-0892-y.

Halkitis, Perry N., Robert W. Moeller, Daniel E. Siconolfi, Erik D. Storholm, Todd M. Solomon, and Kristen L. Bub. "Measurement Model Exploring a Syndemic in

Emerging Adult Gay and Bisexual Men." *AIDS and Behavior* 17, no. 2 (2013): 662–73. DOI:10.1007/s10461-012-0273-3.

Halkitis, Perry N., Jeffrey T. Parsons, and Michael J. Stirratt. "A Double Epidemic: Crystal Methamphetamine Drug Use in Relation to HIV Transmission Among Gay Men." *Journal of Homosexuality* 41, no. 2 (2001): 17–35.

Halkitis, Perry N., Michael T. Shrem, and Frederick W. Martin. "Sexual Behavior Patterns of Methamphetamine-Using Gay and Bisexual Men." *Substance Use & Misuse* 40, no. 5 (2005): 703–19.

Halperin, David M. *What Do Gay Men Want? An Essay on Sex, Risk, and Subjectivity*. Ann Arbor, MI: University of Michigan Press, 2007.

Hatzenbuehler, Mark L., Susan Nolen-Hoeksema, and Sarah J. Erickson. "Minority Stress Predictors of HIV Risk Behavior, Substance Use, and Depressive Symptoms: Results from a Prospective Study of Bereaved Gay Men." *Health Psychology* 27, no. 4 (2008): 455–62. DOI:10.1037/0278-6133.27.4.455.

Hawkins, J. David, Richard F. Catalano, and Janet Y. Miller. "Risk and Protective Factors for Alcohol and Other Drug Problems in Adolescence and Early Adulthood: Implications for Substance Abuse Prevention." *Psychological Bulletin* 112, no. 1 (1992): 64–105. DOI: http://dx.doi.org/10.1037/0033-2909.112.1.64.

Herek, Gregory M. "Sexual Stigma and Sexual Prejudice in the United States: A Conceptual Framework." In *Contemporary Perspectives on Lesbian, Gay, and Bisexual Identities*, edited by Debra Hope, 65–111. Vol. 54. New York, NY: Springer, 2009.

Himmelgreen, David A., Nancy Romero-Daza, David Turkon, Sharon Watson, Ipolto Okello-Uma, and Daniel Sellen. "Addressing the HIV/AIDS—Food Insecurity Syndemic in Sub-Saharan Africa." *African Journal of AIDS Research* 8, no. 4 (2009): 401–12. DOI:10.2989/AJAR.2009.8.4.4.1041.

Homer, Bruce D., Todd M. Solomon, Robert W. Moeller, Amy Mascia, Lauren DeRaleau, and Perry N. Halkitis. "Methamphetamine Abuse and Impairment of Social Functioning: A Review of the Underlying Neurophysiological Causes and Behavioral Implications." *Psychological Bulletin* 134, no. 2 (2008): 301–10. DOI:10.1037/0033-2909.134.2.301.

Hotez, Peter. "Hookworm and Poverty." *Annals of the New York Academy of Sciences* 1136, no. 1 (2008): 38–44. DOI:10.1196/annals.1425.000.

Jacobs, Andrew. 2005. "Gays Debate Radical Steps to Curb Unsafe Sex." *The New York Times*, February 15, 2005. Accessed September 1, 2016. http://www.nytimes.com/2005/02/15/health/gays-debate-radical-steps-to-curb-unsafe-sex.html?_r=0.

Katz, Ingrid T., Annemarie E. Ryu, Afiachukwu G. Onuegbu, Christina Psaros, Sheri D. Weiser, David R. Bangsberg, and Alexander C. Tsai. "Impact of HIV-Related Stigma on Treatment Adherence: Systematic Review and Meta-Synthesis." *Journal of the International AIDS Society* 16, no. 3 (2013). DOI:10.7448/ias.16.3.18640.

Keeler, Rebecca L. "Analysis of Logic Categories of People in U.S. HIV/AIDS Policy." *Administration & Society* 39, no. 5 (2007): 612–30. DOI:10.1177/0095399707303637.

Khantzian, E. J. "The Self-Medication Hypothesis of Addictive Disorders: Focus on Heroin and Cocaine Dependence." *American Journal Psychiatry* 142, no. 11 (1985): 1259–1264.

Klasser, Gary D., and Joel Epstein. "Methamphetamine and Its Impact on Dental Care." *Journal of Canadian Dental Association* 71, no. 10 (2005): 759–62.

Kramer, Larry. *The Tragedy of Today's Gays*. New York: Jeremy P. Tarcher/Penguin, 2005.

Kwan, Candice K., and Joel D. Ernst. "HIV and Tuberculosis: A Deadly Human Syndemic." *Clinical Microbiology Reviews* 24, no. 2 (2011): 351–76. DOI:10.1128/CMR.00042-10.

Liang, Hao, Xu Wang, Hui Chen, Li Song, Li Ye, Shi-Hong Wang, Yan-Jian Wang, Lin Zhou, and Wen-Zhe Ho. "Methamphetamine Enhances HIV Infection of Macrophages." *The American Journal of Pathology* 172, no. 6 (2008): 1617–24. DOI:10.2353/ajpath.2008.070971.

Link, B. G., E. L. Struening, M. Rahav, J. C. Phelan, and L. Nuttbrock. "On Stigma and Its Consequences: Evidence from a Longitudinal Study of Men with Dual Diagnoses of Mental Illness and Substance Abuse." *Journal of Health and Social Behavior* 38, no. 2 (1997): 177–90.

Looby, Alison, and Mitch Earleywine. "The Impact of Methamphetamine Use on Subjective Well-Being in an Internet Survey: Preliminary Findings." *Human Psychopharmacology: Clinical and Experimental* 22, no. 3 (2007): 167–72. DOI:10.1002/hup.831.

Machado, Silvio. "Existential Dimensions of Surviving HIV The Experience of Gay Long-Term Survivors." *Journal of Humanistic Psychology* 52, no. 1 (2012): 6–29. DOI:10.1177/0022167810389049.

Makris, Constantine. "Strain." *Law & Order: Special Victims Unit*. NBC, 2005.

Mendenhall, Emily, Gregory Barnabas Omondi, Edna Bosire, Gitonga Isaiah, Abednego Musau, David Ndetei, and Victoria Mutiso. "Stress, Diabetes, and Infection: Syndemic Suffering at an Urban Kenyan Hospital." *Social Science & Medicine* 146 (December 2015): 11–20. DOI:10.1016/j.socscimed.2015.10.015.

Menza, Timothy W., Grant Colfax, Steven Shoptaw, Mark Fleming, Robert Guzman, Jeffrey D. Klausner, Pamina Gorbach, and Matthew R. Golden. "Interest in a Methamphetamine Intervention Among Men Who Have Sex with Men." *Sexually Transmitted Diseases* 34, no. 4 (2007): 209–14. DOI:10.1097/01.olq.0000233643.66138.b9.

Meredith, Charles W., Craig Jaffe, Kathleen Ang-Lee, and Andrew J. Saxon. "Implications of Chronic Methamphetamine Use: A Literature Review." *Harvard Review of Psychiatry* 13, no. 3 (2005): 141–54. DOI:10.1080/10673220591003605.

Mimiaga, Matthew J., Andrew D. Fair, Kenneth H. Mayer, Karestan Koenen, Steven Gortmaker, Ashley M. Tetu, Jeremy Hobson, and Steven A. Safren. "Experiences and Sexual Behaviors of HIV-Infected Msm Who Acquired HIV in the Context of Crystal Methamphetamine Use." *AIDS Education and Prevention: Official Publication of the International Society for AIDS Education* 20, no. 1 (2008): 30–41. DOI:10.1521/aeap.2008.20.1.30.

Moore, Patrick. *Tweaked: A Crystal Memoir*. New York: Kensington Press, 2006.

"Mother." 2011. *MethProject.org*. http://www.methproject.org/ads/print/mother.html.

New York Daily News. 2005. "Deadly Disease, Deadly Behavior."

Nord, David. "Traumatization in Survivors of Multiple Aids-Related Loss." *OMEGA—Journal of Death and Dying* 37, no. 3 (1998): 215–40. DOI:10.2190/BLCP-VY5K-FV01-2AVY.

Owen, Frank. "Higher and Higher." *Village Voice (New York, NY)*, July 20, 1999. Accessed August 31, 2016. http://www.villagevoice.com/news/higher-and-higher-6421355.

Patton, Cindy. *Sex and Germs*. Boston: South End Press, 1985.

Rabkin, Judith. "HIV and Mood Disorders." *ACRIA Update* 15, no. 3 (2006): 1, 3–5.

Reback, Cathy J. *The Social Construction of a Gay Drug: Methamphetamine Use Among Gay and Bisexual Males in Los Angeles*. Los Angeles: City of Los Angeles, Office of the AIDS Coordinator. 1997.

Reback, Cathy J., Sherry Larkins, and Steven Shoptaw. "Changes in the Meaning of Sexual Risk Behaviors Among Gay and Bisexual Male Methamphetamine Abusers Before and After Drug Treatment." *AIDS and Behavior* 8, no. 1 (2004): 87–98. DOI:10.1023/B:AIBE.0000017528.39338.75.

Reding, Nick. *Methland: The Death and Life of an American Small Town*. New York: Bloomsbury USA, 2009.

Ross, Luana. "Native Women, Mean-Spirited Drugs, and Punishing Policies." *Social Justice*. 32, no. 3 (2005): 54–62.

Rusyniak, Daniel E. "Neurologic Manifestations of Chronic Methamphetamine Abuse." *Psychiatric Clinics of North America* 36, no. 2 (2013): 261–75.

Sandstrom, Kent L. "Confronting Deadly Disease: The Drama of Identity Construction Among Gay Men with AIDS." *Journal of Contemporary Ethnography* 19, no. 3 (1990): 271–94.

Semple, Shirley J., Thomas L. Patterson, and Igor Grant. "Motivations Associated with Methamphetamine Use Among HIV Men Who Have Sex with Men." *Journal of Substance Abuse Treatment* 22, no. 3 (2002): 149–56. DOI:10.1016/S0740-5472(02)00223-4.

Semple, Shirley J., Jim Zians, Igor Grant, and Thomas L. Patterson. "Methamphetamine Use, Impulsivity, and Sexual Risk Behavior among HIV-Positive Men Who Have Sex with Men." *Journal of Addictive Diseases* 25, no. 4 (2006a): 105–14.

———. Sexual Compulsivity in a Sample of HIV-Positive Methamphetamine-Using Gay and Bisexual Men." *AIDS and Behavior* 10, no. 5 (2006b): 587–98. DOI:10.1007/s10461-006-9127-1.

Semple, Shirley J., Jim Zians, Steffanie Strathdee, and Thomas L. Patterson. "Sexual Marathons and Methamphetamine Use Among HIV-Positive Men Who Have Sex with Men." *Archives of Sexual Behavior*, January 2008. DOI:10.1007/s10508-007-9292-y.

Setel, Philip W. *A Plague of Paradoxes: AIDS, Culture, and Demography in Northern Tanzania*. Chicago: University of Chicago Press, 2000.

Shilts, Randy. *And the Band Played On*. New York: Penguin, 1987.

Shoptaw, Steven, and Cathy J. Reback. "Methamphetamine Use and Infectious Disease-Related Behaviors in Men Who Have Sex with Men: Implications for Interventions." *Addiction* 102, no. s1 (2007): 130–35.

Shoptaw, Steven, Cathy J. Reback, and Thomas E. Freese. "Patient Characteristics, HIV Serostatus, and Risk Behaviors Among Gay and Bisexual Males Seeking Treatment for Methamphetamine Abuse and Dependence in Los Angeles." *Journal of Addictive Diseases* 21, no. 1 (2001): 91–105.

Siegel, Karolynn, and Beatrice J. Krauss. "Living with HIV Infection: Adaptive Tasks of Seropositive Gay Men." *Journal of Health and Social Behavior* 32, no. 1 (1991): 17–32.

Simon, Sara L., Catherine Domier, Jennifer Carnell, Paul Brethen, Richard Rawson, and Walter Ling. "Cognitive Impairment in Individuals Currently Using Methamphetamine." *The American Journal on Addictions* 9, no. 3 (2000): 222–31. DOI:10.1080/10550490050148053.

Singer, Merrill. "AIDS and the Health Crisis of the U.S. Urban Poor; the Perspective of Critical Medical Anthropology." *Social Science & Medicine* 39, no. 7 (1994): 931–48. DOI:10.1016/0277-9536(94)90205-4.

———. A Dose of Drugs, a Touch of Violence, a Case of AIDS: Conceptualizing the Sava Syndemic." *Free Inquiry in Creative Sociology* 24, no. 2 (1996): 99–110.

———. *Drugging the Poor: Legal and Illegal Drugs and Social Inequality*. Waveland Press, 2007.

———. *Introduction to Syndemics: A Critical Systems Approach to Public and Community Health*. San Francisco, CA: Jossey-Bass, 2009.

Singer, Merrill, and J. Bryan Page. *Social Value of Drug Addicts: Uses of the Useless*. Left Coast Press, 2013.

Stall, Ron, Thomas C. Mills, John Williamson, Trevor Hart, Greg Greenwood, Jay Paul, Lance Pollack, Diane Binson, Dennis Osmond, and Joseph A. Catania. "Association of Co-Occurring Psychosocial Health Problems and Increased Vulnerability to HIV/AIDS Among Urban Men Who Have Sex with Men." *American Journal of Public Health* 93, no. 6 (2003): 939–42.

Stall, Ron, and David W. Purcell. "Intertwining Epidemics: A Review of Research on Substance Use Among Men Who Have Sex with Men and Its Connection the AIDS Epidemic." *AIDS and Behavior* 4, no. 2 (2000): 181–92.

Tallóczy, Zsolt, Jose Martinez, Danielle Joset, Yonaton Ray, Attila Gácser, Sima Toussi, Noboru Mizushima, et al. "Methamphetamine Inhibits Antigen Processing, Presentation, and Phagocytosis." *PLoS Pathog* 4, no. 2 (2008): e28.

The Gay and Lesbian Times. 2008. "Meth Doesn't Discriminate," March 27.

The Lancet. "HIV: Science and Stigma." *The Lancet* 384, no. 9939 (2014): 207. DOI:10.1016/S0140-6736(14)61193-4.

Torassa, Ulysses. "'Rebound Epidemic' Feared as HIV Rate Jumps in S.F." *The San Francisco Chronicle*, January 24, 2001. Accessed September 1, 2016. http://www.sfgate.com/health/article/Rebound-Epidemic-Feared-As-HIV-Rate-Jumps-in-3195220.php.

Towle, Andy. "Larry Kramer Speech at Cooper Union." *Towleroad*. November 10, 2004. Accessed August 30, 2016. http://www.towleroad.com/2004/11/larry_kramer_sp/

Treichler, Paula A. *How to Have Theory in an Epidemic: Cultural Chronicles of AIDS*. Durham, NC: Duke University Press, 1999.

Valdiserri, Ronald O. "HIV/AIDS Stigma: An Impediment to Public Health." *American Journal of Public Health* 92, no. 3 (2002): 341–42.

Volkow, Nora D., Linda Chang, Gene-Jack Wang, Joanna S. Fowler, Yu-Sin Ding, Mark Sedler, Jean Logan, et al. "Low Level of Brain Dopamine D2 Receptors in Methamphetamine Abusers: Association with Metabolism in the Orbitofrontal Cortex." *American Journal of Psychiatry* 158, no. 12 (2001): 2015–21. DOI:10.1176/appi.ajp.158.12.2015.

Volkow, Nora D., Gene-Jack Wang, Joanna S. Fowler, Frank Telang, Millard Jayne, and Christopher Wong. "Stimulant-Induced Enhanced Sexual Desire as a Potential Contributing Factor in HIV Transmission." *American Journal of Psychiatry,* 164, no. 1 (2007). http://ajp.psychiatryonline.org/doi/pdf/10.1176/ajp.2007.164.1.157.

Warner, Michael. *The Trouble with Normal: Sex, Politics, and the Ethics of Queer Life*. New York, NY: The Free Press, 1999.

Conclusion

Shir Lerman, Merrill Singer, and Bayla Ostrach

In this volume, the contributors provided a detailed examination of the foundations, mechanisms, and varieties of stigma syndemics. They demonstrated both the frequency with which stigma promotes syndemic interaction, and the array of diseases ensnared in these critical biosocial threats to health. Specifically, the chapters in this volume highlighted the complex structural, social, and biological interactions that form stigma-related, syndemics and trace the myriad ways in which vulnerable populations are stigmatized by the very social organizations that produce syndemic environments, producing those vulnerable populations. Each chapter analyzed a different set of stigma-driven disease and structural interactions and illuminates the unfortunately numerous manifestations of syndemic oppression. All of the contributors in this volume trace the multiple ways in which stigma is embedded in everyday life and interacts with structural and biologized inequalities to promulgate syndemics.

Through these chapters the contributors reiterate the need for researchers, policy makers, and healthcare practitioners to take a critical look at the social conditions that underlie syndemic disease clusters, and particularly at the role of stigma, which is socially constructed (Kleinman and Hall-Clifford, 2009) and plays fundamental roles in the syndemics discussed in this volume. Many of the examples discussed here expand on the theoretical contributions of classic, long-recognized syndemics by mirroring and expanding on the role of stigma in relation to some aspect of the first-identified syndemic of *Substance Abuse, Violence, and AIDS (SAVA)* (Singer, 1996). These chapters highlight the increasing opportunities for exposure through which the physical and emotional sequelae of adverse social conditions are biologized, illuminating the conditions in a fully delineated syndemic that interact to deleteriously affect health.

The chapters in this volume provided a detailed guide to the myriad ways in which complex socio-political-economic environments to produce stigma-syndemics interactions. Until now, stigma has not constituted a significant element in syndemics research; this volume exemplifies the urgent need to acknowledge stigma in both the identification of additional syndemics and when creating policies and treatments to combat the underlying factors of syndemics. This volume, in providing a discussion of "classic" syndemics, showcases the imperative for a closer look at the role of stigma in the structural and biological foundations of syndemics, and overall illness and health. The authors build on the original syndemic example—substance abuse, violence, and AIDS—and delve deeply into the social, biological, structural, political, and environmental factors that form both the original syndemic example and the ensuing early syndemic examples, such as diabetes and depression (e.g., Everett 2009; Mendenhall 2012). The authors in this volume stress the importance of both situating syndemics in historical contexts and drawing on current-day contexts to understand how and why stigmatized syndemics continue to emerge and afflict. The compelling presence of stigma in syndemics research requires a closer personal look at how policy makers, healthcare providers, and researchers interact with stigmatized populations and the laws and environments which should protect these populations.

REFERENCES

Everett, Margaret. "Diabetes Among Oaxaca's Transnational Indigenous Population: An Emerging Syndemic." *Annals of Anthropological Practice* 36, no. 2 (2009): 295–311.

Herrick, A., S. Lim, M. Plankey, J. Chmiel, T. Guadamuz, U. Kao, et al. "Adversity, and Syndemic Production Among Men Participating in the Multicenter AIDS Cohort Study: A Life-Course Approach." *American Journal of Public Health* 103, no. 1 (2010): 79–85.

Kleinman, Arthur, and Rachel Hall-Clifford. "Stigma: A Social, Cultural and Moral Process." *Journal of Epidemiology & Community Health* 63, no. 6 (2009): 418–19.

Mendenhall, Emily. *Syndemic Suffering: Social Distress, Depression, and Diabetes among Mexican Immigrant Women* Walnut Creek, CA: Left Coast Press, 2012.

Singer, Merrill. 1996 "A Dose of Drugs, A Touch of Violence, A Case of AIDS: Conceptualizing the SAVA Syndemic." *Free Inquiry in Creative Sociology* 24 (2): 99–110.

Stall, R., M. Friedman, and J. A. Catania. 2008. "Interacting Epidemics and Gay Men's Health: A Theory of Syndemic Production Among Urban Gay Men." *Unequal Opportunity: Health Disparities Affecting Gay and Bisexual Men in the United States* 1(2008): 251–274.

Index

About the Contributors

Alexandra Brewis is the President's Professor in the School of Human Evolution and Social Change at Arizona State University, as well as Co-Director of the MC-ASU Obesity Solutions initiative. Trained as a medical and biological anthropologist (PhD 1992, Arizona), she has lead major field-based projects in the Pacific islands, Mexico, and the United States. Currently she is conducting a global study of weight-related stigma, examining why its health impacts are spreading and deepening.

Nicholas Emard received his Master's of Science in Medical Anthropology and Cross Cultural Practice from Boston University School of Medicine. He has worked with HIV-specific community organizations as well as with Boston's National HIV Behavioral Surveillance system (NHBS) interviewing individuals at risk from HIV-infection. He is currently working at Brown University's School of Public Health on a study examining how social media may be used to reach African Americans and Latinos to help improve Treatment as Prevention and Pre-Exposure Prophylaxis uptake.

A medical and psychological anthropologist, **Theodore K. Gideonse** is interested in how political structures and moral ideologies impact both mental and physical health, particularly among addicts, the homeless, and people with chronic illnesses like HIV. Dr. Gideonse was awarded funding by UCLA's Center for HIV Identification, Prevention, and Treatment Services (CHIPTS) for a pilot study on the risk behaviors of drug offending HIV+ men who have sex with men who were inmates in Los Angeles County Jail. He also studies cultural barriers to the use of Pre-Exposure Prophylaxis (PrEP) among high-risk MSM and the role physical and virtual gay venues have in substance abuse among MSM.

Seung Yong Han is an Assistant Research Scientist in the MC-ASU Obesity Solutions initiative. Seung Yong is a social demographer with more than eight years' experience researching population and environment, livelihood, migration and inequality. He also has extensive experience in data analysis and project management in diverse contexts in both developed and developing countries. He graduated from Arizona State University with a PhD in sociology and a certificate in statistics.

Shir Lerman, PhD, MPH is a PRACCTIS postdoctoral fellow in implementation science at the University of Massachusetts Medical School. Trained as a medical anthropologist, her research centers on chronic illness syndemics in Puerto Rico, particularly framed within Puerto Rico's political and economic crises. More broadly, her research focuses on mental health, syndemics, and structural inequalities in ethnic minorities. She also conducts research on mindfulness in underserved communities and on the Zika Virus in Puerto Rico.

Harrison M. K. Maithya holds PhD in Anthropology specializing in Medical Anthropology from the University of London at University College London. He is currently an Associate Professor in the Department of Sociology and Anthropology and Dean, School of Humanities and Social Sciences of the South Eastern Kenya University. Before joining South Eastern Kenya University, Maithya taught at Moi University where he was Associate Professor and head of the Department of Anthropology and Human Ecology.

Ruthanne Marcus, PhD, MPH, is an epidemiologist and medical anthropologist with over 30 years of experience conducting quantitative and qualitative research on infectious diseases. She worked at the Centers for Disease Control and Prevention in Atlanta coordinating research activities on occupational transmission of HIV/AIDS. More recently she was a lecturer and epidemiologist at the Yale School of Public Health with the Connecticut Emerging Infections Program as Director of the Connecticut Foodborne Diseases Active Surveillance Network (FoodNet). She is currently the Associate Director of Clinical and Community Research with the Yale School of Medicine, Infectious Diseases Section, AIDS Program, conducting domestic and international behavioral research on HIV, substance use disorders, and mental health. Her primary interest is in using a syndemic approach to conduct implementation science research that addresses health inequality and health disparities affecting people who are homeless, with substance use disorders, mental illness, and infectious diseases.

Gerald McKinley is a medical anthropologist who specializes in the social determinants of mental health and Indigenous youth suicide prevention in Ontario, Canada. Dr. McKinley conducts research as part of the Canadian Biomarker Integration Network on Depression's Indigenous Outreach project. This community-based project is building a sustainable suicide prevention program in partnership with Mnaamodzawin Health Services on Manitoulin Island. Dr. McKinley is also a member of the Walpole Island First Nation/Western University Ecosystem Health Research Team which is studying the long-term health effects of environmental stress on the community.

Bayla Ostrach, MA, PhD, is an Assistant Professor of Medical Anthropology and Cross-Culture Practice in the Family Medicine Department at Boston University School of Medicine, and Affiliated Faculty at Boston University's Department of Anthropology. A Full Fellow of the Society of Family Planning, her research explores reproductive justice, publicly funded health systems, syndemics, and the role of social and mutual support in people's ability to overcome obstacles. She began working directly in the field of reproductive health and abortion care in 1999, and has since worked with and volunteered at multiple clinics in Oregon, Connecticut, and Catalunya. Dr. Ostrach's ongoing fieldwork primarily occurs in Catalunya, focused on publicly funded reproductive health care and community-based solidarity movements focused on inclusivity. She is the author of *Health Policy in a Time of Crisis: Abortion, Austerity, and Access*.

Elizabeth J. Pfeiffer is a socio-cultural anthropologist with specializations in medical anthropology and African Studies. She recently completed a National Institutes of Health postdoctoral fellowship in HIV/AIDS research at the Indiana University School of Medicine, and is currently an Instructor of Anthropology in the Department of History and Anthropology at Butler University in Indianapolis, IN.

Mary A. Ott is an Associate Professor of Pediatrics at the Indiana University School of Medicine. She is board certified in Pediatrics and Adolescent Medicine, and provides both general adolescent medical care and specialty adolescent reproductive health care at Riley Hospital for Children, the HealthNet Pediatric and Adolescent Care Center, and the Eskenazi Health—Pecar Health Center Teen Clinic. Dr. Ott consults on adolescent health policies and programs at IU Health, locally in central Indiana, and nationally. She has a Master's degree in Philosophy and Bioethics.

Merrill Singer, PhD, Professor in the Department of Anthropology at the University of Connecticut and Senior Research Scientist at the UConn Center for Health, Intervention and Prevention, University of Connecticut, is an applied medical anthropologist and co-founder of Critical Medical Anthropology. Dr. Singer developed the concept of syndemics and was the first to publish the term in 1996. His research focuses on structural and biosocial factors in health, syndemics, health effects of substance use and HIV/AIDS, anthropogenic climate change and ecosyndemics, and health inequality. He is the author of more than 20 books and more than 200 articles.

Sarah Trainer is a Post-Doctoral Researcher in the MC-ASU Obesity Solutions initiative. Sarah Trainer completed a PhD in medical and biocultural anthropology at the University of Arizona in 2013. Her research interests the interplay between the personal, the local, and the global, by using the specific lenses of stigma, food, health, and related body changes. She has worked in locations as diverse as the United Arab Emirates, Egypt, the American Southwest, and the American Pacific Northwest.

Kara Wools-Kaloustian is the Director of the Division of Infectious Diseases at Indiana University School of Medicine the Co-Director Emerita of Field Research in Infectious Diseases within the Academic Model Providing Access to Healthcare (AMPATH) Partnership in western Kenya and the Co-PI of the International Epidemiologic Databases to Evaluate AIDS (IeDEA) East Africa Consortium.

Amber Wutich is an Associate Professor in Arizona State University's Anthropology and Global Health programs. She has been awarded the Carnegie CASE U.S. Professor of the Year Award for Arizona and ASU's Award for Excellence in Classroom Performance. Her research examines the nexus of injustice, resource insecurity, and adaptability, with a focus on water and food in Bolivia, Paraguay, and the US. She is Associate Editor of the journal, Field Methods, and is on the faculty of the National Science Foundation's research methods programs in cultural anthropology.

James Ziegler is a cultural anthropologist in the PhD program at the University of Connecticut. His research involves concepts of addiction, drug use, and drug use treatment in coastal China and the American Southwest. His prior work involved medicinal cannabis and experience of hidden violence among Denver methadone maintenance clients.

CPSIA information can be obtained
at www.ICGtesting.com
Printed in the USA
BVOW09*0723280417
482302BV00002B/6/P

9 781498 552110